CLINICAL NEUROLOGY
FOR PSYCHIATRISTS

CLINICAL NEUROLOGY FOR PSYCHIATRISTS

Second Edition

David Myland Kaufman, M.D.

Department of Neurology
Montefiore Medical Center
Albert Einstein College of Medicine
Bronx, New York

Grune & Stratton, Inc.
Harcourt Brace Jovanovich, Publishers
Orlando   New York   San Diego   London
San Francisco   Tokyo   Sydney   Toronto

Library of Congress Cataloging-in-Publication Data
Kaufman, David Myland.
    Clinical neurology for psychiatrists.

    Includes bibliographies and index.
    1. Nervous system—Diseases.   2. Neurology.
3. Psychiatrists.   I. Title.   [DNLM: 1. Nervous
System Diseases.   2. Psychiatry. WL 100 K205c]
RC346.K38   1985   616.8   85-17753
ISBN   0-8089-1733-1

Grune & Stratton, Inc.
Orlando, FL 32887

Distributed in the United Kingdom by
Grune & Stratton, Ltd.
24/28 Oval Road, London NW 1

Library of Congress Catalog Number 85-17753
International Standard Book Number 0-8089-1733-1
Printed in the United States of America

86   87   88   10   9   8   7   6   5   4   3   2

To my wife, Rita Gail Kaufman. She has been the love of my life, and also first suggested and continually helped with the book.

Contents

Acknowledgments

Mr. Michael Lipton and Dr. Marc Singer provided editorial assistance that was both critical and creative. Mr. Barry Morden and Ms. Anne Mannato were the artists who provided the wonderful illustrations. Ms. Louise Wolkis and her staff typed the manuscript diligently and thoughtfully.

Valuable suggestions and reviews have been made by my students and colleagues at Montefiore Medical Center, the Albert Einstein College of Medicine, and the course on which this book is based, "Clinical Neurology for Psychiatrists."

Preface

The text of this second edition of *Clinical Neurology for Psychiatrists* is completely rewritten and adds material on recent developments in dementia, pain control, seizure management, computed tomography, and neurologic conditions that affect the elderly. It also offers expanded reviews of several classic neurologic conditions with prominent psychologic symptoms, such as headaches, nondominant hemisphere injuries, and sleep disorders. Despite the additions, my aim remains to provide an *explicit, pragmatic,* and *concise* presentation of clinical neurology in a format combining traditional neuroanatomic correlations with clinically useful symptom-oriented discussions.

Since neurology is so much a visual specialty (whereas psychiatry may be the quintessential verbal specialty), I have again provided a large number of illustrations of anatomic relationships, lifelike clinical examples, and examinations that elicit particular findings. These illustrations, which reinforce the text and graphically portray numerous illnesses, may offer to many readers their first sight of several uncommon but important neurologic disorders.

This book will first describe how a physician might approach the patient who possibly has a neurologic disorder. It will explain how to decide if there is disease in either the central or peripheral nervous system, and in what way certain neurologic illnesses may be associated with mental impairments.

The book's second half will offer discussions of the most commonly encountered neurologically based symptoms. For each symptom, e.g., headaches, a chapter describes the relevant history and neurologic findings, and then discusses the usefulness and costs of the pertinent laboratory tests. After considering the differential diagnoses, each chapter will suggest specific and easily implemented plans for initial management. Sample histories, short lists of common differential diagnoses, names of self-help groups, and references to recent reviews and landmark articles are included in virtually every chapter. Finally, for those readers who wish to test their knowledge, an expanded series of questions is included at the conclusion of each chapter and at the end of the book.

DAVID MYLAND KAUFMAN, M.D.

Note About the References

Specific references are provided at the conclusion of most chapters, but some neurologic textbooks are standard references works that might be consulted for detailed information about many topics:

Adams RD, Victor M: *Principles of Neurology* (ed 3). New York, McGraw-Hill Book Co., 1985.

Baker AB, Baker LH (eds): *Clinical Neurology.* Philadelphia, Harper & Row, 1985.

Jefferson JW, Marshal JR: *Neuropsychiatric Features of Medical Disorders.* New York, Plenum Medical Book Co., 1981.

Rowland L: *Merritt's Textbook of Neurology.* Philadelphia, Lea and Febiger, 1984.

Swaiman KF, Wright FS: *The Practice of Pediatric Neurology.* St. Louis, The C. V. Mosby Co., 1982.

CLINICAL NEUROLOGY
FOR PSYCHIATRISTS

SECTION 1

Classical Anatomic Neurology

1

First Encounter with a Patient: Examination and Formulation

Patients with an apparent or possible disease of the nervous system should be examined in the same systematic manner as is employed in other branches of medicine. A history is taken in the customary methodical fashion. The physical examination is performed so that areas of interest may be tested in detail, while the major components of the nervous system are examined sequentially.

Undeviating adherence to routine is vital if omission, duplication, and confusion are to be avoided. Despite obvious disease in one part of the nervous system, all areas must be evaluated. An initial or screening neurologic examination can be completed in 20 minutes, after which detailed testing of areas of concern may be performed. The examiner, for example, might return to perform full mental status testing or to review inconsistent results. After a preliminary evaluation, a formulation of the case should be prepared.

EXAMINATION

The examiner should obtain the patient's age, sex, and handedness. He or she should then review the chief complaint, present illness, past medical history, and family and social history. Some patients cannot relate the necessary information, but further evaluation of these patients may reveal that intellectual, language, or memory impairments were the reason that they could not comply. With the majority of patients who are able to relate a history, detailed questioning should follow the line of the chief complaint, which is likely to be one of several common symptoms, e.g., headaches, seizures, or weakness. A brief series of specific standard questions is asked about the primary symptom, associated symptoms, and possible etiologic factors. Section 2 of this book, which deals with these common symptoms, contains outlines for obtaining pertinent history and making a general evaluation.

While obtaining the history, the examiner should consider the possible types of neurologic deficits the patient may display during the subsequent physical examination. The examiner should be prepared, for instance, to look for disease primarily of

3

the central nervous system (CNS) or of the peripheral nervous system (PNS). In other words, without yielding to rigid preconceptions, some feeling for the problem at hand should be acquired after eliciting the patient's history.

The routine physical examination is outlined in Table 1-1. Its basis is a sequential evaluation of the functional anatomy of the nervous system: mental status, cranial nerves, motor system, reflexes, sensation, and cerebellar system. This format should be followed during every examination. Until this outline can be memorized, a copy should be taken to the patient's bedside, where it will serve both as a reminder and a place to record neurologic findings.

In the first part of the examination, during testing of the mental status, the examiner should assess the patient's general intellectual function and exclude specific intellectual deficits, such as language impairment. These examinations are detailed in Chapters 7 and 8. Tests of cranial nerves may reveal malfunctions of either single nerves or groups of nerves. These nerves are tested for particular abnormalities, some of which are virtually diagnostic of lesions in certain areas of the nervous system. The intricate tests and implication of abnormal findings are discussed in Chapter 4.

Table 1-1
Neurologic Examination

Mental Status
  Cooperation
  Orientation
  Language
  Memory for immediate, recent, and past events
  Higher intellectual functions, e.g., arithmetic, similarities/differences

Cranial nerves
  I   Smell
  II   Visual acuity, visual fields, optic fundi
  III, IV, VI   Pupils' size and reactivity, extraocular motion
  V   Corneal reflex and facial sensation
  VII   Strength of upper and lower facial muscles, taste
  VIII   Hearing
  IX–XI   Articulation, palate movement, gag reflex
  XII   Tongue movement

Motor System
  Limb strength
  Spasticity, flaccidity, or fasciculations
  Abnormal movements, e.g., tremor, chorea

Reflexes
  Deep tendon reflexes (DTRs): biceps, triceps, brachioradialis, quadriceps, Achilles
  Pathologic reflexes: extensor plantar response (Babinski sign); frontal lobe release
    signs

Sensation
  Position, vibration, stereognosis
  Pain (pin)

Cerebellar system
  Finger–nose, heel–shin, and rapid alternating movements
  Gait

Examination of the motor system is usually performed to detect general patterns of weakness, that is, paresis. The distribution of paresis has major implications in the assessment of neurologic problems. For example, if the lower face, arm, and leg on one side are weak, it is hemiparesis. If both legs are weak, it is paraparesis. Severe weakness is plegia, e.g., hemiplegia or paraplegia.

Two categories of reflexes are usually tested. Deep tendon reflexes (DTRs) are normally present with uniform reactivity in all limbs. In neurologic disorders, their activity, symmetry, or both will be altered. Moreover, paresis is almost always associated with change in the DTRs. In general, with CNS injury (with corticospinal tract damage) DTRs are hyperactive, whereas with PNS injury they are hypoactive.

In contrast to DTRs, "pathologic" reflexes are not normally found in persons older than 1 year. If present, they are signs of damage to the CNS (see Fig. 2-2). The most generally accepted indication of CNS injury is the Babinski sign. A clear understanding of terminology is important. With plantar stimulation, the great toe normally moves downward, i.e., a flexor response. With disease of the CNS, plantar stimulation might cause the great toe to move upward, i.e., an extensor response. The abnormal extensor response is a Babinski sign. This sign and others may be "present" or "elicited," but they are never "positive" or "negative." For example, a traffic stop sign is either present or not, but it is never positive or negative.

Other pathologic reflexes indicate impairment of the frontal lobes. As will be discussed later (Chapter 7), the presence of such signs is helpful in indicating "organic" causes of changes in personality and intellect.

The examination of the sensory system is long and tedious. In addition, unlike abnormal DTRs and Babinski signs, which are reproducible, objective, and virtually impossible to mimic, the sensory examination relies almost entirely on the patient's report. The best approach under most circumstances is to perform tests of major modalities of sensation in a clear anatomic order.

Sensation of position, vibration, and stereognosis (appreciation of form by touch), all of which are carried in the posterior columns of the spinal cord, are each routinely tested. Pain (pin prick) sensation, which is carried in the lateral columns, is usually tested with a pin.

The examiner should be able to recognize when a sensory deficit stems from a disorder of the CNS or PNS. When it does stem from CNS damage, the examiner should know the characteristic patterns of loss associated with lesions of the cerebral cortex, brainstem, and spinal cord.

Cerebellar function is evaluated by observing the patient for intention tremor and incoordination during several standard maneuvers that include the finger–nose test and rapid repetition of alternating movement test (Chapter 2). Finally, the patient's walk (gait) is observed for signs not only of incoordination, i.e., ataxia, but also for indications of paresis, involuntary movement disorders, and hydrocephalus (see Table 2-4).

FORMULATION

The *formulation* is an appraisal of four problematic areas: the symptoms, signs, site of involvement (*localization*), and probable cause (*differential diagnosis*). A succinct and cogent formulation is the basis upon which neurologic problems are solved and cases are meaningfully presented to fellow physicians. While somewhat ritualistic, this format encourages careful and critical review.

The clinician must support his or her impression that neurologic disease is present or, sometimes more important, absent. For this first step, psychologically induced (psychogenic) symptoms and signs must be separated, if only tentatively, from neurologic ones. Evidence must be demonstrable for either impression. Neither etiology is a diagnosis of exclusion, and patients can have psychogenic signs (Chapter 3) superimposed on neurologic ones. In practice, despite neurologists' inclinations, a diagnosis of a psychogenic disturbance is usually made only after exhaustive tests have excluded obscure as well as common neurologic illnesses. During such an evaluation, psychiatric evaluation should be performed concomitantly.

Localization of neurologic lesions requires the clinician to determine if the illness affects the CNS or PNS (Chapters 2–6). Precise localization of lesions within these systems is possible and generally expected. The physician must also establish if the nervous system is affected diffusely or only in a limited, discrete area. The site and extent of neurologic damage will indicate certain diseases. For example, cerebrovascular accidents and tumors generally involve only a single area of the brain, whereas degenerative conditions, e.g., Alzheimer's disease, have a widespread and symmetric effect.

Finally, the differential diagnosis is offered as the most probable disease or diseases with which the symptoms, signs, and localization are consistent. When specific diseases cannot be determined, major categories of illnesses, such as "structural lesions," should be suggested.

A typical formulation might be: "Mr. Jones, a 56-year-old man, has had left-sided headaches for 2 months and a generalized seizure on the day before admission. He is lethargic and has papilledema, a right hemiparesis with hyperactive DTRs, and a Babinski sign. The lesion seems to be in the left cerebral hemisphere. Most likely he has a tumor, but a cerebrovascular accident (stroke) is a less likely possibility." In this formulation, the first sentence recounts the symptoms and an abbreviated relevant medical history and the second sentence details the salient physical findings. The formulation tacitly assumes that neurologic disease is present because of the obvious, objective physical findings. The localization is based on the history of seizures and the right-sided hemiparesis and reflex abnormalities. The differential diagnosis is based on the probability that the patient has a lesion of the cerebral hemisphere.

To conclude, the physician should present a formulation that answers the *Four Questions of Neurology:*

- What are the *symptoms* of *neurologic* disease?
- What are the *signs* of *neurologic* disease?
- *Where* is the lesion?
- *What* is the lesion?

2

Central Nervous System Disorders

This chapter will discuss important physical and intellectual signs accompanying frequently occurring lesions of the two components of the central nervous system (CNS): the brain and the spinal cord (Table 2-1). It will describe signs of lesions in the major areas of the brain: the cerebral hemispheres, the basal ganglia, the brainstem (midbrain, pons, and medulla), and the cerebellum. Similarly, it will discuss signs of spinal cord lesions. Chapter 3 will contrast signs of CNS lesions with those of psychogenic disturbances.

SIGNS OF CEREBRAL HEMISPHERE LESIONS

Signs indicating that a cerebral hemisphere is the site of injury may be physical, intellectual, or, in the opinion of some, emotional (Table 2-2). Usually, the most prominent sign is *contralateral hemiparesis,* paresis of the opposite face, trunk, arm, and leg, because of damage to the *corticospinal tract.* Motor function originates in each cerebral cortex in the corticospinal tract, which eventually supplies the contralateral trunk and limbs (Fig. 2-1). Within the cerebral hemisphere, the corticospinal tract passes through the internal capsule. It then descends through the brainstem, but in the medulla almost entirely crosses within the *pyramids* and then descends contralaterally in the spinal cord as the *lateral corticospinal tract.* Finally, it terminates by synapsing onto the *anterior horn cells* of the spinal cord.

During its course from the cerebral cortex to the anterior horn cells, the corticospinal tract is considered the upper motor neuron (UMN) (Fig. 2-2). The anterior horn cell of the spinal cord, the origin of the peripheral nerve, is considered the beginning of the lower motor neuron (LMN). Thus, CNS lesions that damage the corticospinal tract are associated with various signs of UMN injuries: hyperactive deep tendon reflexes (DTRs), muscle spasticity, and Babinski signs. In contrast, peripheral nerve lesions, including anterior horn cell, or "motor neuron," diseases, are associated with signs of LMN injuries: hypoactive DTRs, muscle flaccidity, and no Babinski signs (Figs. 2-3, 2-4, 2-5).

7

Table 2-1

Signs of CNS Lesions

Cerebral hemisphere*
  Hemiparesis with hyperactive DTRs and Babinski sign
  Hemisensory loss
  Homonymous hemianopsia
  Aphasias, hemi-inattention, and dementia
  Pseudobulbar palsy
Basal ganglia*
  Movement disorders: parkinsonism, athetosis, chorea, and
    hemiballismus
Brainstem
  Cranial nerve palsy with contralateral hemiparesis, hemisensory
    loss, or both, or ipsilateral or contralateral ataxia
  Internuclear ophthalmoplegia (MLF syndrome)
  Nystagmus
  Bulbar palsy
Cerebellum
  Tremor on intention
  Impaired rapid alternating movements (dysdiadochokinesia)
  Ataxic gait
  Scanning speech
Spinal cord
  Paraparesis or quadriparesis
  Sensory loss up to a "level"
  Bladder, bowel, sexual dysfunction

---

*Signs are contralateral to lesions.

Because the corticospinal tract has such a long course, the hemiparesis and other signs of damage may originate not only from lesions in the cerebral hemispheres, but also from those in the brainstem or spinal cord. Localizing them depends on other features discovered in the examination. For example, the presence of signs of cerebral injury, such as aphasia, dementia, or homonymous hemianopsia, indicate that any hemiparesis is probably of cerebral origin.

Sensory loss to certain modalities over one half of the body, i.e., a *hemisensory* loss, is usually another indication of a contralateral cerebral lesion. Characteristically,

Table 2-2

Signs of Cerebral Lesions

Either hemisphere*
  Hemiparesis with hyperactive DTRs and Babinski sign
  Hemisensory loss
  Homonymous hemianopsia
Nondominant hemisphere
  Hemi-inattention
  Anosognosia
  Constructional apraxia
Dominant hemisphere
  Aphasias
Both hemispheres
  Dementia
  Pseudobulbar palsy

---

*Signs are contralateral to lesions.

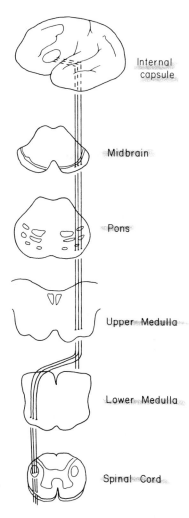

Internal
capsule

Midbrain

Pons

Upper Medulla

Lower Medulla

Spinal Cord

Fig. 2-1. The path of the corticospinal (pyramidal)
tract.

a patient with a cerebral lesion loses position sensation, two-point discrimination, and
the ability to identify objects by touch (stereognosis); however, pain sensation, which
is "perceived" in the thalamus, is largely retained in almost all instances (Fig. 2-6).

The pain-sensing role of the thalamus is clinically important. For example, a
patient with a lesion of the cerebral cortex, although possibly unable to locate the
body area that is painful, will still feel the intensity and discomfort of the pain. In
particular, patients with common cerebral infarctions are still quite able to feel pain.
Also, patients who suffer from intractable pain do not obtain relief when they undergo
surgical resection of the cerebral cortex.

Loss of vision involving the same half of the visual field in each eye, *homonymous hemianopsia* (Fig. 2-7), is another reliable sign of a contralateral cerebral
lesion. There are also characteristic patterns of visual loss associated with lesions
involving the eye, the optic nerve, or the optic tract (Chapters 4 and 12). Of course,
no visual loss accompanies brainstem, cerebellar, or spinal cord lesions.

While hemiparesis, hemisensory loss, and homonymous hemianopsia are found
with lesions of either cerebral hemisphere, several neurologic deficits are specifically

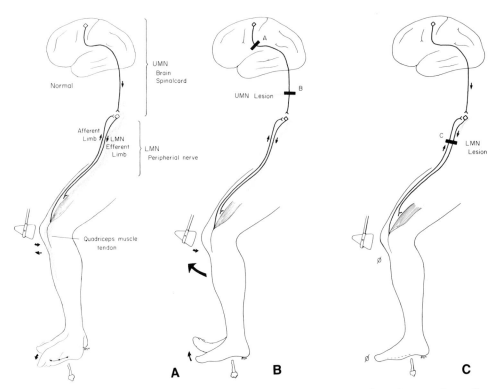

Fig. 2-2. (A) Normally, when the quadriceps tendon is percussed, a deep tendon reflex (DTR) is elicited. Also, when the sole of the foot is scratched in a certain manner to elicit a plantar reflex, the big toe bends downward (flexes). (B) When brain (A) or spinal cord (B) lesions that involve the corticospinal tract cause UMN damage, the DTR is hyperactive and the plantar reflex is extensor, i.e., a Babinski sign is present. (C) When peripheral nerve injury causes LMN damage, the DTR is hypoactive and the plantar reflex is absent.

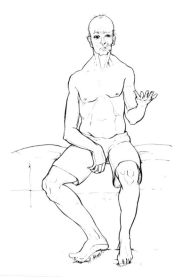

Fig. 2-3. With severe right hemiparesis, the patient typically has weakness of the right lower face, the arm, and the leg. In the face, there is right-sided widening of the palpebral fissure and flattening of the nasolabial fold, but the forehead muscles appear normal. The right arm remains limply held; the elbow, wrist, and fingers are flexed. The right leg is externally rotated, and the hip and knee are also flexed.

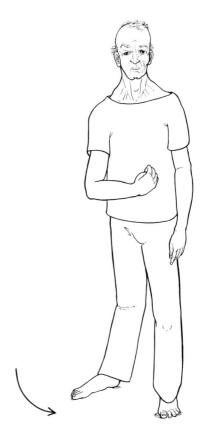

Fig. 2-4. When the patient arises, his or her weakened arm retains its flexed position. His or her leg remains externally rotated. The patient can walk by swinging the right leg in a circular path, resulting in a *circumduction* or *hemiparetic* gait.

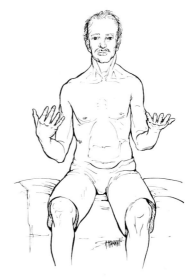

Fig. 2-5. Mild hemiparesis may not be obvious. To exaggerate a subtle hemiparesis, the examiner should ask the patient to close his or her eyes and extend both arms with the palms held upright, as though the patient were holding glasses of water on the outstretched hands. After 1 minute, the weakened arm will drift downward and the palm will turn inward (pronate). The imaginary water glass would spill from the right hand. This arm's drift and pronation is a *forme fruste* of the posture that is seen with more severe paresis (see Fig. 2-3).

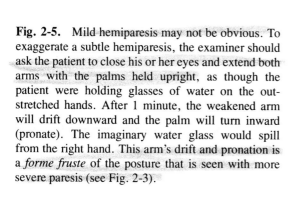

11

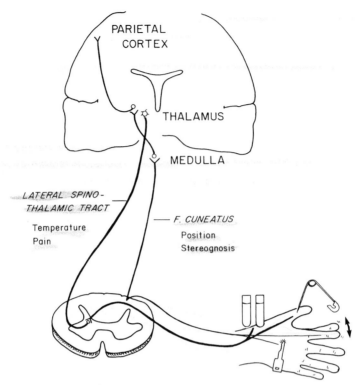

PARIETAL
CORTEX

THALAMUS

MEDULLA

LATERAL SPINO-
THALAMIC TRACT

Temperature
Pain

F. CUNEATUS

Position
Stereognosis

Fig. 2-6. Pain perception (tested by pinprick) and temperature sensation (tested by warm and cold test tubes) are carried to the spinal cord where, after a synapse, these sensations ascend in the *contralateral* lateral spinothalamic tract. For practical purposes, they terminate in the thalamus. Position sense (tested by movement of the distal finger joint) and stereognosis (tested by tactile identification of common objects) are carried in the *ipsilateral* fasciculus cuneatus and f. gracilis, which together constitute the *posterior columns*. These tracts terminate in the cortex of the contralateral parietal lobe.

referable either to the dominant or nondominant hemisphere. In almost all people, the left hemisphere is dominant because it governs the use of fine motor movements and language. Unless the physician knows otherwise, he or she should assume that a patient is left hemisphere dominant, i.e., right-handed.

Disorders of the dominant hemisphere usually cause impairment of verbal and written language, that is, *aphasia* (Chapter 8). Because language centers are so near the corticospinal tract (see Fig. 8-1), lesions in the dominant hemisphere characteristically cause a combination of aphasia and right hemiparesis.

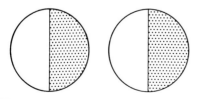

Fig. 2-7. Homonymous hemianopsia. The same half of the visual field is lost in each eye. In this case, a right homonymous hemianopsia is attributable to damage of the left cerebral hemisphere.

Disorders of the nondominant hemisphere usually cause more subtle and transient deficits. When the nondominant parietal lobe is injured, patients might have *hemi-inattention,* which is a constellation of psychologic abnormalities in which they neglect left-sided visual perceptions, touch stimulation, and hemiparesis (Chapter 8). They may not even acknowledge their (left) hemiparesis, a condition known as *anosognosia.* These patients characteristically cannot copy simple forms, which is known as *constructional apraxia* (Fig. 2-8).

All signs discussed so far are referable to one cerebral hemisphere or the other. An important sign of bilateral cerebral hemisphere damage is *pseudobulbar palsy,* in which emotional lability and other mental aberrations are accompanied by dysarthria (speech impairment) and reflex abnormalities. Pseudobulbar palsy must be distinguished from *bulbar palsy,* which does not result from cerebral damage (Chapter 4).

Dementia also clearly indicates that both cerebral hemispheres are damaged. It is

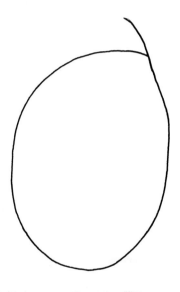

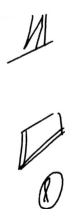

Fig. 2-8. Constructional apraxia. The patient who drew these figures was a 68-year-old woman who had just developed a right parietal lobe infarction. On request, she was able to complete a circle (top figure). She could not draw a square on request (second highest figure) or even copy one (third highest figure). She spontaneously tried to draw a circle and attempted to retrace it (bottom figure). Note the characteristic rotation of the forms, perseveration of certain lines, and the incompleteness of the second and lowest figures. Also note that the figures tend to move to the right-hand side of the page, suggesting that she is ignoring the left-hand side of the page.

usually caused by Alzheimer's disease, multiple infarctions, alcohol-related damage, or other *diffuse* structural or metabolic injury (Chapter 7).

Extensive bilateral cerebral damage usually is also associated with bilateral hyperactive DTRs and often Babinski and frontal lobe release signs, although not necessarily with hemiparesis or other lateralized findings. Whenever possible, a diagnosis of dementia or "organic mental syndrome" should be buttressed by a description of physical abnormalities.

The four conditions most likely to cause *discrete* unilateral or bilateral cerebral lesions are cerebral infarctions and other cerebrovascular accidents ("strokes"), primary or metastatic brain tumors, trauma, and multiple sclerosis. (A broader listing is offered in Table 2-3, and detailed discussions of strokes, tumors, and multiple sclerosis are presented in Section 2.)

SIGNS OF BASAL GANGLIA LESIONS

Since the corticospinal tract crosses in the pyramids, it is often called the *pyramidal* tract. The involuntary motor system that originates in the basal ganglia, in contrast, is called the *extrapyramidal* tract or extrapyramidal system. The extrapyramidal tract modulates motor tone and involuntary activity. Its major components and associated structures are the caudate nucleus, the globus pallidus, the putamen, the substantia nigra, and the subthalamic nucleus (corpus of Luysii).

Basal ganglia injury often causes the dramatic involuntary movement disorders. Pending later details (Chapter 18), the following are general descriptions:

Parkinsonism is the combination of resting tremor, rigidity, and bradykinesia (slowness of movement). Minor features including festinating gait (Table 2-4) and micrographia. Parkinsonism is associated with damage to the substantia nigra from degeneration (Parkinson's disease) or antipsychotic medications.

Athetosis is the slow continuous writhing movement of the fingers, hands, face, and throat. It is usually caused by kernicterus or other perinatal brain injury.

Chorea is intermittent jerking of limbs and trunk. The most important variety, *Huntington's* chorea, is associated with hereditary atrophy of the caudate nucleus.

Hemiballismus is the intermittent flinging of the arm and leg on one side of the body. It is associated with small infarctions of the contralateral subthalamic nucleus.

When damage is restricted to the extrapyramidal tract, as in many cases of hemiballismus and athetosis, patients have no paresis, DTR abnormalities, or Babinski signs—signs of corticospinal (pyramidal) tract damage. More important, in such cases patients will have no intellectual abnormality.

On the other hand, several illnesses in which there is injury to the cerebral cortex as well as to the basal ganglia are characterized by a notorious association of mental abnormalities with involuntary movement disorders. The most noteworthy are Huntington's chorea and Wilson's disease (see Table 7-6).

Several features common to the movement disorders should be appreciated. Involuntary movements disappear during sleep. They are exacerbated by anxiety, fatigue, and stimulants. Finally, they may be suppressed for short periods of time by voluntary action. Unfortunately, these characteristics occasionally prompt physicians to accuse patients with movement disorders of having hysteria (Chapter 3).

Unlike those that affect the cerebral hemispheres, most illnesses that affect the basal ganglia are slowly progressive and cause bilateral damage. Their cause is

Table 2-3

The Most Commonly Occurring Conditions that
Damage the CNS

Genetic
  Down's syndrome
  Wilson's disease
  Huntington's chorea
Congenital ("cerebral palsy" or mental retardation or both)
  Cerebral anoxia, kernicterus (jaundice), prematurity
Toxic
  Hepatic or renal failure
  Medications
  Illicit drugs
  Alcohol (and malnutrition)
Infectious
  Bacterial: Abscess* or meningitis
  Viral: Encephalitis or meningitis
  Tuberculous: Tuberculoma* or meningitis
Inflammatory*
  Multiple sclerosis
  Systemic lupus erythematosus (SLE)
Traumatic*
Neoplastic (tumors)*
  Primary: Glioblastoma, astrocytoma, meningioma
  Metastatic: Lung, breast, others
Vascular ("strokes")
  Infarction*
  Embolus*
  Hemorrhage*
  Anoxia from cardiopulmonary arrest
Degenerative (etiology unknown)
  Alzheimer's disease
  Creutzfeldt-Jakob disease
  Amyotrophic lateral sclerosis (ALS)

*Discrete cerebral damage.

usually a biochemical abnormality. Discrete structural lesions, such as infarctions, tumors, or multiple sclerosis lesions ("plaques"), rarely injure the basal ganglia.

When there is unilateral basal ganglia damage, the signs are found contralateral to the lesion. One example is hemiballismus, which results from infarction of the contralateral subthalamic nucleus. Another is unilateral parkinsonism ("hemiparkinsonism") from degeneration of the contralateral substantia nigra.

Table 2-4

Gait Abnormalities

Gait	Associated Illness	Figure
Apraxia	Normal pressure hydrocephalus	7-7
Astasia-Abasia	Hysteria	3-2
Ataxia	Cerebellar damage	2-13
Festinating (marche à petits pas)	Parkinson's disease	18-9
Hemiparetic	Cerebrovascular accidents	
(circumduction)		2-4
(spastic hemiparesis)		13-2

SIGNS OF BRAINSTEM LESION

The brainstem contains the nuclei of the cranial nerves, which are the "long tracts" that carry motor and sensory impulses between the cerebral hemispheres and the extremities, and also several systems contained entirely within the brainstem itself (Fig. 2-9). Massive brainstem injuries, such as those resulting from extensive infarctions or barbiturate overdoses, cause coma. The commonly encountered small brainstem injuries, however, usually do not cause intellectual or personality impairment. Again, all forms of mentation seem to be the exclusive role of the cerebral cortex.

Although brainstem injuries can cause *diplopia* (double-vision) because of cranial nerve impairment, visual acuity in each eye remains normal. This is because the visual pathways, which pass from the chiasm to the cerebral hemispheres, do not travel within the brainstem (see Fig. 4-1).

Several syndromes are important because each illustrates critical anatomic relationships, such as the location of the different cranial nerve nuclei or the course of the corticospinal tract. While each syndrome has an eponym, for practical purposes it is only necessary to identify them as the result of a lesion in the brainstem or, possibly,

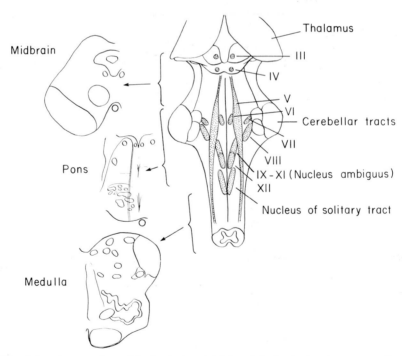

Fig. 2-9. An overview of the brainstem (right) and the brainstem in cross-section (left). The midbrain contains the nuclei of cranial nerves III and IV. The pons contains nuclei V through VIII. The medulla contains nuclei IX through XII. In addition to cranial nerve nuclei, the brainstem also contains important tracts that pass from the cerebellum and cerebral hemispheres to the brainstem and spinal cord. Many other tracts, such as the medial longitudinal fasciculus, the cerebellar tracts, and the reticular activating system, are contained within and act solely within the brainstem.

in a particular division of the brainstem—midbrain, pons, or medulla. Virtually all cases are caused by infarctions in branches of the basilar or vertebral arteries.

In the midbrain, where the oculomotor (third cranial) nerve passes through the descending corticospinal tract, both pathways can be damaged by the same small infarction. Patients with oculomotor nerve paralysis and contralateral hemiparesis typically have a midbrain lesion ipsilateral to the paretic eye (see Fig. 4-8).

Likewise, patients with abducens (sixth cranial) nerve paralysis and contralateral hemiparesis typically have a pons lesion that is also ipsilateral to the paretic eye (see Fig. 4-10).

Lateral medullary infarctions create a classic but complex picture. Patients have paralysis of the ipsilateral palate because of damage to cranial nerves IX through XII; ipsilateral facial hypalgesia because of damage to cranial nerve V with contralateral anesthesia of the body (*alternating hypalgesia*) because of ascending spinothalamic tract damage; and ipsilateral ataxia because of ipsilateral cerebellar dysfunction.

It is not necessary to recall all the features of this syndrome, just to realize that those cranial nerve palsies and the alternating hypalgesia are characteristic of lower brainstem lesions (Fig. 2-10 A and B).

While all brainstem syndromes are virtually pathognomonic of infarctions, clinically the most frequently observed sign of brainstem dysfunction is *nystagmus* (jerk-like eye movements). Resulting from any injury of the brainstem's large vestibular nuclei, nystagmus usually is a manifestation of one of the following disorders: multiple sclerosis; intoxications with alcohol, phenytoin (Dilantin), or barbiturates; Wernicke-Korsakoff syndrome; ischemia of the vertebrobasilar artery system; or merely viral labyrinthitis. Nystagmus may also be associated with *internuclear ophthalmoplegia,* a disorder of ocular motility in which the brainstem's medial longitudinal fasciculus (MLF) is damaged by multiple sclerosis or infarction (Chapters 4 and 15).

SIGNS OF CEREBELLAR LESIONS

The cerebellum is composed of two hemispheres and a central portion, the *vermis.* Each hemisphere controls motor coordination of the ipsilateral limbs and, in essence, the vermis controls coordination of the head, neck, and trunk, especially during walking.

The control of coordination of the limbs on the *same side of the body* gives the cerebellum a somewhat unique quality, which is captured by the aphorism, "Everything in the brain, except for the cerebellum, is backwards." Another unique feature of the cerebellum is that if one of its hemispheres is damaged, the other will eventually be able to perform almost all the functions for both.

Cerebellar lesions cause impaired ipsilateral coordination but not paresis or reflex abnormality. Since the cerebellum is nowhere near the cerebral hemispheres, even its total destruction does not cause intellectual abnormalities.

The primary sign of a cerebellar lesion is *intention tremor.* This characteristic tremor is elicited during the finger–nose test (Fig. 2-11) and heel–shin test (Fig. 2-12). It is present when the patient moves willfully and absent when the patient is resting. In contrast, parkinsonism causes a *resting tremor* that is typically present when the patient is sitting quietly at rest and reduced when the patient makes willful movements (Chapter 18).

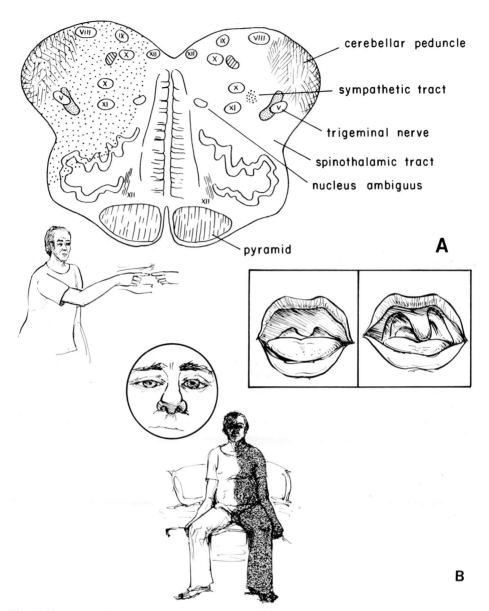

Fig. 2-10. (A) Whenever the posterior inferior cerebellar artery (PICA) is occluded, the lateral portion of the medulla suffers infarction, which damages important structures: the cerebellar peduncle, the nucleus of the trigeminal nerve, the spinothalamic tract, the nucleus ambiguus (motor nuclei of cranial nerves IX–XI), and the poorly delineated sympathetic fibers. Structures that escape damage are the corticospinal tract, the hypoglossal nerve, and the medial longitudinal fasciculus. The stippled area represents the region that would be infarcted when the right PICA or its parent artery, the vertebral artery, is occluded. (B) This patient, who suffered an infarction of the right lateral medulla, has a right-sided Wallenberg's syndrome. He has a right-sided Horner's syndrome (ptosis and miosis) because of damage to the sympathetic fibers. He has right-sided ataxia because of damage to the ipsilateral cerebellar tracts. He has an alternating hypalgesia: diminished pain sensation on the *right* side of his face accompanied by loss of pain sensation on the *left* trunk and extremities. Finally, he has hoarseness and paresis of the right soft palate because of damage to the right nucleus ambiguus: on voluntary phonation or in response to the gag reflex, the palate deviates upward toward his left because the right side of the palate is weak.

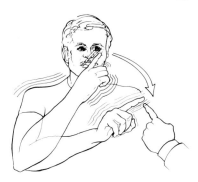

Fig. 2-11. This young man, who has a multiple sclerosis plaque (lesion) in the right cerebellar hemisphere, has a coarse, irregular *intention tremor* as his finger approaches his own nose and then the examiner's finger during the *finger–nose test.*

Another sign of a cerebellar lesion is impairment of the ability to perform rapid alternating movements, *dysdiadochokinesia.* When asked to slap the palm and then the back of the hand rapidly and alternately on his or her own knee, for example, a patient with dysdiadochokinesia will have uneven force, irregular rhythm, and breakdown of the alternating pattern.

When either the entire cerebellum or the vermis alone is damaged, incoordination of the trunk, i.e., *truncal ataxia,* will develop. This impairment will force the patient to place his or her feet widely apart when standing. A lurching, unsteady, and wide-based pattern of walking, known as *ataxic gait,* will develop (Table 2-4; Fig. 2-13). This gait abnormality is dramatically apparent in the staggering and reeling of people who are drunk.

With extensive cerebellar damage, voice production will also be impaired because of poor modulation, irregular cadence, and inability to separate adjacent sounds. This speech impairment, *scanning speech,* can be distinguished by trained personnel from the dysarthria found in bulbar and pseudobulbar palsy, other CNS conditions, and laryngeal disorders. All these forms of dysarthria must be distinguished from aphasia (Chapter 8). Finally, with cerebellar disease, DTRs have been described as being hypotonic or pendular; however, this is a subtle finding that is rarely discussed in clinical practice today.

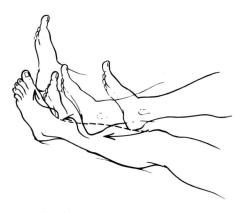

Fig. 2-12. In the *heel–shin test,* the patient with the right-sided cerebellar lesion in Fig. 2-11 displays limb *ataxia* or *tremor on intention* as his right heel wobbles when he moves it along the crest of his left shin.

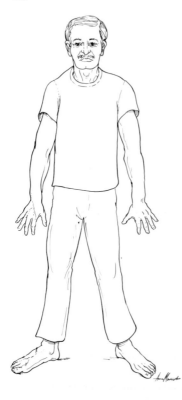

Fig. 2-13. This man, who has been a chronic alcoholic, suffers from diffuse cerebellar degeneration. His stance and his gait are broad-based and unsteady, i.e., he has an *ataxic gait*.

Three disorders—infarctions, multiple sclerosis, and tumors—which are also responsible for cerebral lesions, cause almost all discrete cerebellar lesions. The different clinical settings, associated signs, and computed tomography found in these disorders, all discussed later, make distinction among them relatively easy.

Cerebellar dysfunction probably results more frequently from excessive alcohol or certain medications, such as phenytoin (Dilantin®), than from any discrete lesion. The single most important situation is the Wernicke-Korsakoff's syndrome, in which excessive alcohol and poor nutrition lead to ataxia, nystagmus, peripheral neuropathy, and mental impairment characterized by memory loss. Any patient even suspected of having Wernicke-Korsakoff's syndrome should receive thiamine 50 mg IV to prevent serious brain injury.

SIGNS OF SPINAL CORD LESIONS

At the spinal cord's center is an H-shaped, gray matter structure composed largely of neurons that transmit nerve impulses in a horizontal plane. Surrounding it is white matter, composed of myelinated tracts conveying information in a vertical direction (Fig. 2-14). Curiously, this arrangement, gray matter on the inside, white outside, is the opposite of that found in the cerebral hemispheres.

The white matter's main contents are descending motor, *lateral corticospinal*, and ascending sensory tracts; the *posterior columns*, which carry position and vibration sensation; the *lateral spinothalamic tracts*, temperature and pain; and the *anterior spinothalamic tracts*, light touch.

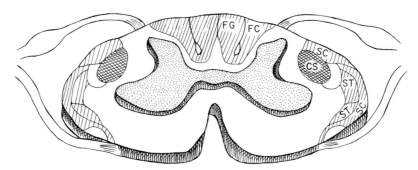

Fig. 2-14. In this drawing of the spinal cord, the centrally located gray matter is stippled. The surrounding white matter contains myelin-coated tracts that ascend and descend within the spinal cord. Clinically important ascending tracts are the spinocerebellar tracts (SC), the lateral spinothalamic tract (ST), and the posterior columns [fasciculus cuneatus (FC) and fasciculus gracilis (FG)]. The most important descending tract is the lateral corticospinal tract (CS).

A spinal cord lesion will interrupt descending motor and ascending sensory tracts. With a cervical spinal cord injury, for example, all motor function and sensation may be lost below the neck. The arms and legs, of course, will be paralyzed (*quadriparesis*). After a time, spasticity, hyperactive DTRs, and Babinski signs will develop. Also, there will be interruption of sensations, including those of bladder fullness and genital stimulation, from the trunk or limbs. With a midthoracic spinal cord injury, similarly, there will be leg paralysis (*paraparesis*), reflex changes, and sensory loss below the nipples (Fig. 2-15).

A classic, although rarely found disturbance, the *Brown-Sequard syndrome*, occurs when an injury transects the lateral half of the spinal cord (Fig. 2-16). In this condition, unilateral corticospinal tract damage causes paralysis of the ipsilateral limb(s) and lateral spinothalamic tract damage causes pain loss (*hypalgesia*) in the contralateral limb(s).

The position of the pain-carrying lateral spinothalamic tract offers an opportunity to alleviate unilateral pain. With a relatively simple neurosurgical procedure, *cordotomy*, surgeons selectively sever the lateral spinothalamic tract contralateral to the painful side to produce considerable analgesia.

With any spinal cord lesion, of course, cerebral, brainstem, and cerebellar function is preserved. For example, patients with even a complete transection of the cervical spinal cord, although quadriplegic, will still have full intellectual, visual, and verbal facilities.

Bullet wounds are a well-known cause of spinal cord injury; however, most injuries to the spinal cord now result from automobile, diving, and other civilian accidents. In these, the spinal cord is usually crushed by dislocation of the cervical vertebrae.

Two illnesses, multiple sclerosis and metastatic cancer, account for the vast majority of spinal cord diseases. Multiple sclerosis typically causes spinal cord damage alone or in combination with cerebellar, optic nerve, or brainstem damage. Metastatic lung or breast tumors, which often develop and grow in the vertebral bodies, compress the spinal cord.

With several illnesses, only certain tracts of the spinal cord may be affected (Fig.

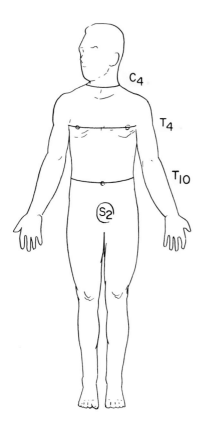

Fig. 2-15. In a patient with a spinal cord injury, the "level" of hypalgesia will indicate the site of the damage: C-4 injuries cause hypalgesia below the neck; T-4, hypalgesia below the nipples; T-10, hypalgesia below the umbilicus.

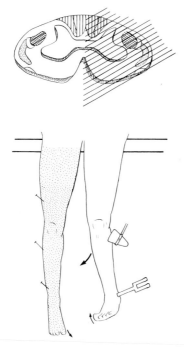

Fig. 2-16. Hemitransection of the spinal cord (Brown-Sequard syndrome). In this case, the left side of the thoracic spinal cord has been transected, as by a knife wound. Injury to the left lateral corticospinal tract results in the combination of left-sided leg paresis, hyperactive DTRs, and a Babinski sign; injury to the left posterior column results in left leg vibration and position sense impairment; and, most striking, injury to the left spinothalamic tract causes loss of temperature and pain (pinprick) sensation in the right leg. The loss of pain sensation contralateral to the paresis is the hallmark of the Brown-Sequard syndrome.

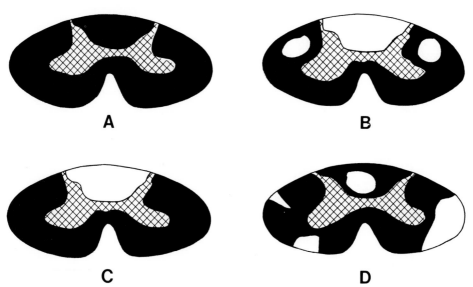

Fig. 2-17. (A) A standard spinal cord histologic preparation stains normal myelin ("white matter") black and leaves the central H-shaped column gray. (B) In combined system disease (vitamin B_{12} deficiency), damage to the posterior column and corticospinal tract causes their demyelination and loss of stain. (C) In tabes dorsalis (syphilis), damage to the posterior column causes loss of stain in that region. (D) Multiple sclerosis, however, leads to many scattered demyelination plaques.

2-17). Tabes dorsalis (syphilis) and combined system disease (B_{12} deficiency) are two good examples because both illnesses are characterized by spinal cord tract and cerebral injury. Moreover, a dementia in both conditions may be reversible to a certain extent. Freidrich's ataxia and the other rarely occurring, familial spinocerebellar degenerations are also characterized by degeneration of specific tracts. In contrast, patients with multiple sclerosis have variable, irregular patches of spinal cord involvement and, unless the disease is advanced, usually no mental impairment.

SUMMARY

Physical abnormalities, sometimes in combination with intellectual ones, indicate the presence, location, and etiology of CNS injury. The most frequent signs of cerebral injury are dementia, aphasia, pseudobulbar palsy, and homonymous hemianopsia.

CNS lesions are most often caused by stroke, tumors, trauma, or multiple sclerosis. Among disorders that cause extensive cerebral damage are Alzheimer's disease, multiple infarctions, and alcoholism. Those disorders that affect the basal ganglia as well as the cerebral hemispheres are Huntington's chorea and Wilson's disease. Those that affect the spinal cord and cerebral hemispheres are tabes dorsalis (syphilis) and combined system disease (B_{12} deficiency).

3

Psychogenic Disorders

Classic studies of hysteria, conversion reactions, and related conditions included patients who had only cursory physical examinations and minimal, if any, laboratory evaluation. Depending on the study, as many as 30 percent of patients eventually were found to have specific neurologic diseases; of these, many seem to have had dementia or mental retardation at the time of the study. Others were found to be suffering from anemia, congestive heart failure, and other medical illnesses. Another group had major psychiatric disturbances, such as psychotic depression or schizophrenia. Finally, all had a high rate of death from known neurologic or medical illnesses, suicide, or unexplainable causes.

Today, such diagnostic mistakes would not be made as readily because of better education of physicians, hesitancy in diagnosing hysteria and conversion reactions, and a general tendency to rely on laboratory tests, including computed tomography (CT) (Chapter 20). Also, many conditions thought nonneurologic in the early studies are now considered neurologic. Tourette's syndrome, torsion dystonia (dystonia musculorum deformans), writer's cramp, migraine headache, and trigeminal neuralgia, for example, are now acknowledged to be symptoms of disordered brain physiology rather than manifestations of psychologic aberrations.

The *Diagnostic and Statistical Manual of Mental Disorders,* Third Edition (DSM III) definition of "conversion disorder" carefully limits the issues and, with proscriptive criteria, sidesteps many pitfalls. It requires loss or alteration of physical function. It prohibits the diagnosis if the only symptom is pain or sexual dysfunction and excludes deficits due to a somatization disorder or schizophrenia.

This approach to diagnosis, however, still involves problems. As in the initial studies, the criteria have been based on experience with patients from psychiatric rather than from general medical or neurologic services. Thus, an unfair burden might fall on the neurologist or internist who is asked to prove that neurologic disease *is not* present. Likewise, the psychiatrist, at least during the initial evaluation, might not be able to exclude an underlying somatization disorder or schizophrenia. Overall, DSM III diagnostic criteria may be so restrictive as not to be useful to the entire medical community.

In this text, therefore, physical manifestations of mental aberrations are designated "psychogenic." This term has become accepted by neurologists, who use it to include all disturbances that have previously been called hysteric, subconscious, conversion, malingering, factitious, nonorganic, functional, or various other terms, some clearly pejorative.

For many patients whose condition is the result of combinations of underlying psychologic and neurologic factors, the relative contribution of each type is often, admittedly, indeterminate. Nevertheless, if appropriate, the diagnosis of psychogenic illness should be made. Such a designation will limit acceptable manifestations of illness and injury. It will permit appropriate diagnostic tests and therapy, eliminating those that are expensive or potentially harmful. Actually, as long as serious, progressive physical illness has been excluded, many symptoms can be treated as though they were chronic illnesses. For example, chronic low back or surgical incision pain can be treated as "pain syndromes" by using empiric combinations of antidepressants, analgesics, and psychotherapy, without expecting either to cure or determine an underlying cause.

The primary guideline neurologists use to determine whether a deficit is psychogenic is that it appears to violate neuroanatomic laws. For example, if temperature sensation is preserved while there is loss of pain sensation, the deficit is considered to be nonanatomic and therefore psychogenic. Likewise, tunnel or tubular vision is considered to be a classic psychogenic disturbance (see Fig. 12-8).

Another indication of a disturbance being psychogenic is when the deficit is not constant. For example, a patient with psychogenic paralysis might walk when unaware of being observed. Likewise, deficits are thought to be psychogenic when they disappear under the influence of hypnosis or sodium amytal.

Two practices, but ones with questionable reliability, are often followed. Disorders are considered psychogenic when they are unique or bizarre. This determination, however, may simply reflect an individual neurologist's lack of experience. Neurologists also diagnose disturbances as psychogenic if the patient has no accompanying objective physical abnormalities, such as a Babinski sign. Such a determination should likewise be accepted with some hesitancy. Many illnesses, such as migraine headaches and tic douloureux (trigeminal neuralgia), do not ordinarily have accompanying physical abnormalities. More important, there are many physical disturbances, such as multiple sclerosis, where objective signs are subtle and sometimes overshadowed by psychic distress.

PSYCHOGENIC ("HYSTERIC") SIGNS

Several motor and sensory disturbances are rightfully considered psychogenic. Classic studies indicated that psychogenic hemiparesis developed in the left limbs much more often than in the right. Psychogenic paresis on either side is often characterized by a "give-away" effort in which the patient has normal exertion for a brief (several second) period before returning to a paretic position.

Psychogenic paresis is sometimes demonstrable using the *face–hand test*. In this test, the patient's arms are raised and then released directly above his or her face. If the patient were indeed weak, the weakened hand would strike the patient's face unless caught by the examiner; however, with hysteric weakness, the patient momentarily exerts sufficient strength to deflect the hand from striking the face (Fig. 3-1).

Another indication of psychogenic weakness is marked right hemiparesis unaccompanied by aphasia or right homonymous hemianopsia. Exceptions are common. One would be, of course, if the patient were left-handed; another, if the lesion were in the deep cerebrum or upper brainstem.

Finally, patients who have difficulty walking often seem to stagger, balance momentarily, and be in great danger of falling. Instead, they grab hold of railings, chairs, and even the examiner, never seeming to fall (Fig. 3-2). This is a display of acrobatics and is a characteristic gait disturbance called *astasia-abasia* that is virtually diagnostic of a psychogenic etiology.

Several sensory abnormalities are signs of psychogenic disturbances. Loss of sensation to pinprick that stops abruptly at the middle of the face and body is called "splitting the midline." It is indicative of a psychogenic abnormality because sensory nerve fibers of the skin normally spread across the midline (Fig. 3-3). Likewise, loss of vibration sensation of half the forehead, jaw, sternum, or spine is also indicative of a psychogenic loss because vibrations always spread across these bony structures.

Another indication of psychogenic sensory loss is a discrepancy between pain and temperature sensation. This is because both sensations are normally carried together by the lateral spinothalamic tracts. (Discrepancy between pain and *position* sensation in the fingers, however, is indicative of syringomyelia, because in this condition the central fibers of the spinal cord are stretched by the expanding central canal.)

Intermittent blindness, tunnel vision, and inconsistent diplopia are also often

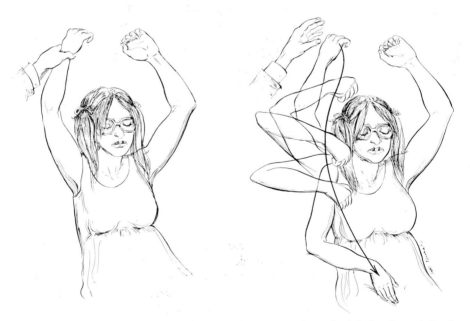

Fig. 3-1. In the face–hand test, a young woman with psychogenic right hemiparesis inadvertently demonstrates her preserved strength by deflecting her falling "paretic" arm from striking her face as it is dropped by the examiner.

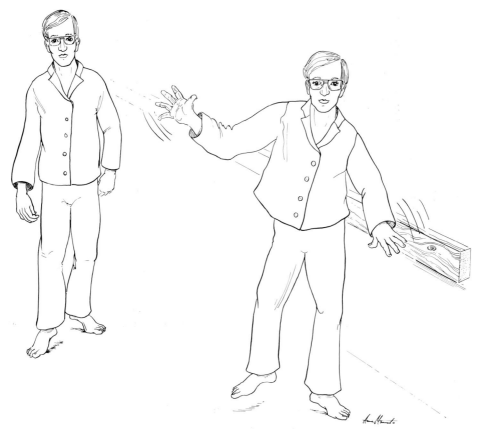

Fig. 3-2. A young man with psychogenic weakness demonstrates astasia-abasia by seeming to fall when walking, but catching himself by carefully balancing or grasping on to the railing.

signs of psychogenic disturbances. (They are contrasted to other visual system disorders in Chapter 12.) Finally, hearing loss in the ear ipsilateral to a psychogenic hemiparesis is highly suggestive of a psychogenic hearing disturbance because auditory tract synapsing is so extensive in the CNS auditory pathways (see Fig. 4-15) that some auditory tracts are almost always preserved in CNS lesions.

PROBLEM CONDITIONS

Neurologists have tended to misdiagnose several types of disturbances as psychogenic. In general, they tend to make the determination of psychogenic illness whenever there is a potential secondary gain and in patients with a known psychiatric disorder.

In particular, neurologists have misdiagnosed early cases of multiple sclerosis. The error occurs because early signs are sometimes evanescent, disparate, or exclusively sensory. The diagnosis of multiple sclerosis can now be made earlier and more

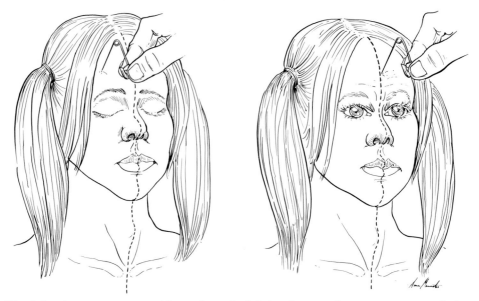

Fig. 3-3. A young woman with psychogenic left hemisensory loss appears not to feel a pinprick until the pin reaches the midline of her forehead, face, neck, or sternum, i.e., she splits the midline.

reliably with use of visual-evoked responses and cerebrospinal fluid analysis for gamma globulin concentration and "oligoclonal bands" (Chapter 15).

Another area in which neurologists are prone to err is that of involuntary movement disorders. As noted previously (Chapter 2), movement disorders are often bizarre, associated with mental abnormalities, exacerbated by anxiety, reduced by intention, and disappear during sleep. Aside from determining the ceruloplasmin level in cases of suspected Wilson's disease, there are no readily available laboratory tests. The diagnosis almost always rests on the clinical evaluation. As a general rule, however, movement disorders should always be considered neurologic.

Seizures are often diagnosed as psychogenic. Many patients with psychogenic seizures actually have an underlying seizure disorder (epilepsy) upon which they elaborate. Many cases of "intractable" seizures are a mixture of psychogenic and neurologic seizures. Of course, metabolic aberrations, cardiac arrhythmias, and other systemic disturbances must be considered in the differential diagnosis of seizures.

When seizures are psychogenic, they are usually only clonic and not accompanied by incontinence, tongue biting, or loss of body tone. More telling, after a psychogenic seizure there is usually an immediate resumption of awareness and no retrograde amnesia. Although an EEG cannot usually be obtained during the actual psychogenic episode, one done afterwards would not show typical postictal electrical slowing or depression (Chapter 10).

Emotional and thought disorders that have been diagnosed as being psychogenic have sometimes turned out to be the result of frontal lobe meningiomas and other tumors. The error has arisen because patients with such tumors often have had no overt intellectual or physical abnormalities. With the ready availability of the CT, physicians now rarely overlook any structural lesion.

CURRENT SITUATION

The patient population is now much more sophisticated than that described in the classic studies. People are better informed about psychologic mechanisms and are even willing to attribute neurologic deficits as well as emotional disturbances to psychologic factors.

Today, people rarely act in the bizarre manner of the grand hysterics. Most often the medical problems are unexplainable severe and prolonged pain and disability following apparently trivial injuries, such as "rear-end" automobile accidents, head trauma at work, and low back pain from minor injuries. Dizziness, weakness, and headaches are other common complaints requiring exhaustive, expensive evaluation for which no physical explanation is found. While these patients' disturbances are nondramatic and nonspecific, their complaints still lead to just as much disability.

SUMMARY

Since both patients and physicians can be trapped by words, physicians might simply consider psychologically based deficits as "psychogenic disturbances" until a specific psychiatric diagnosis can be determined. By simultaneously trying to exclude neurologic causes and establish a psychiatric diagnosis, physicians should not fall into the trap of overlooking important illnesses. They should readily accept the frequent combination of psychologic and neurologic etiologies and the psychic embellishment of a neurologic deficit. After appropriate evaluation, physicians should feel free to treat pain and similar disabilities as discrete entities.

Although patients may have signs indicative of psychogenic disturbances, the physician should be wary of that diagnosis in patients with movement disorders, seizures, signs consistent with multiple sclerosis, or change in both emotion and thought.

REFERENCES

Caplan LR, Nadelson T: Multiple sclerosis and hysteria: lessons learned from their association. JAMA 243:2418, 1980

Gulick RA, Spinks IP, King DW: Pseudoseizures: Ictal phenomena. Neurology 32:24, 1982

King DW, Gallagher BB, Marvin AJ, et al: Pseudoseizures: diagnostic evaluation. Neurology 32:18, 1982

Lazare A: Conversion symptoms. N Engl J Med 305:745, 1981

Mai FM, Nerskey H: Briquet's concept of hysteria: An historical perspective. Can J Psychiatry 26:57, 1981

Maloney MJ: Diagnosing hysterical conversion reactions in children. J Pediatr 97:1016, 1980

Roy A. (ed): Hysteria. New York, John Wiley & Sons, 1982

Weintraub MI: Hysterical Conversion Reactions. New York, SP Medical and Scientific Books, 1983

4

Cranial Nerve Disorders

The cranial nerves, individually, in pairs, or in groups, may be impaired by various conditions. When a cranial nerve disorder seems to be present, however, the problem might not be damage to the cranial nerve itself but rather underlying cerebral or brainstem injury or psychogenic disturbances. Determining the presence and origin of any particular cranial nerve disorder depends upon knowing the function of these nerves and signs of damage.

This chapter reviews the functional neuroanatomy of the cranial nerves, discusses appropriate examinations, and describes deficits found in commonly occurring illnesses and psychogenic disturbances. It concludes with a review of paresis resulting from injury of the lower cranial nerves, i.e., *bulbar palsy,* which is contrasted to the commonly encountered condition *pseudobulbar palsy.*

This chapter follows the customary practice of giving the twelve cranial nerves Roman numeral designations and presenting them in numerical order:

I	Olfactory	VII	Facial
II	Optic	VIII	Acoustic
III	Oculomotor	IX	Glossopharyngeal
IV	Trochlear	X	Vagus
V	Trigeminal	XI	Accessory
VI	Abducens	XII	Hypoglossal

An old mnemonic that is useful in recalling this list is "On old Olympus's towering top, a Finn and German viewed some (spinal accessory) hops."

THE OLFACTORY NERVE (FIRST CRANIAL NERVE)

The function of the olfactory nerves is to carry the sensation of smell to the brain. From sensory receptors within each nasal cavity, branches of the two olfactory nerves pass through the multiple holes of the cribriform plate of the skull to several areas of the brain. They terminate partially in the frontal cortex, where olfactory sensory areas are located, and in the hypothalamus and amygdaloid complex, which are the cornerstones of the limbic system. This input of olfactory sensation into the limbic system accounts for the influence of smell on psychosexual behavior.

When both olfactory nerves are totally impaired, complete loss of smell, *anosmia,* occurs. Usually, any person with anosmia will also find that food is largely tasteless because aroma is lost. If only one nerve is damaged, the patient will be unaware of it, since some sense of smell, and therefore taste, will be preserved.

The examiner asks the patient to smell substances through one nostril while the other is compressed. Testing must be done with substances such as tobacco and coffee, which are readily identifiable and not noxious. Irritative or volatile substances, such as ammonia and alcohol, are not suitable because they will stimulate the sensory endings of the trigeminal nerve, which are also within the nose, and elicit a reaction, thereby bypassing a (possibly damaged) olfactory nerve.

An impaired ability to smell is usually caused by trivial problems. It is found in many normal older people and in anyone with nasal congestion. Also, since the olfactory nerve can be sheared off as it passes through the cribriform plate, even minor head trauma can result in anosmia.

Unilateral anosmia, which is rare, may be the result of tumors adjacent to the olfactory nerve, such as olfactory groove meningiomas (Fig. 20-5). When anosmia is caused by such tumors, optic atrophy results because the nearby optic nerve is compressed. Most important, if these tumors involve the frontal lobe, personality changes, seizures, and hemiparesis may accompany anosmia.

Anosmia may of course be a manifestation of a psychologic aberration. In such cases, patients are almost always unable to "smell" either irritative solutions, such as alcohol, or odorous substances, such as coffee. This complete loss would be possible only if the trigeminal as well as the olfactory nerve were impaired.

Sensations of smell not stemming from the environment may result from the irritation of the olfactory nerves or their cerebral connections. Sinusitis often causes a continual sensation of a putrid smell, headache, and impaired ability to perceive actual odors. Also, olfactory hallucinations may be a manifestation of seizures that originate in the medial-inferior surface of the temporal lobe, the *uncus.* Uncinate seizures, which last several seconds, are usually composed of episodes of ill-defined but often sweet smells associated with impaired consciousness and behavioral aberrations (see Psychomotor Seizures, Chapter 15).

Olfactory hallucinations, of course, can also arise from causes that are purely psychologic. In contrast to the odor sensation episodes of uncinate seizures, these odor sensations are almost always foul-smelling and continual.

THE OPTIC NERVE (SECOND CRANIAL NERVE)

The major function of the optic nerves is to transmit vision from the eye to the brain. The optic nerves originate in the retina of each eye. Continuing toward the brain, they intersect at the optic chiasm, where the medial fibers of each nerve cross, while the lateral fibers continue (Fig. 4-1). Thus, the optic *tracts* are formed from the temporal fibers of the ipsilateral eye and the nasal fibers of the contralateral eye. The optic tracts pass through the temporal and parietal lobes and terminate in the occipital lobe cortex.

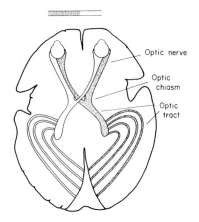

Fig. 4-1. The optic nerves extend from the retina to the optic chiasm, where they divide to form the optic tracts. The primary effect of this system is that the impulses from each visual field are brought to the cortex of the contralateral occipital lobe.

Another function of the optic nerve is to assist in the control of pupil size. Such adjustments are necessary both to focus the visual image on the retina (*accommodation reflex*) and also to permit the appropriate amount of light to fall on the retina (*light reflex*). For these reflexes, the optic nerves form the afferent limb and carry information regarding an object's proximity and brightness. After synapsing in the midbrain, the oculomotor nerve (third cranial nerve) forms the efferent limb and transmits impulses to the iris muscles. The pupils constrict with increasing light or with a change in focus from a distant to a close object and expand if the situation is reversed.

Routine testing of the optic nerve includes examination of (1) visual acuity, (2) the visual fields, and (3) the ocular fundus. Visual acuity is measured as the patient reads a hand-held card (see Fig. 12-2) or a wall chart. Each eye must be tested individually. The patient should wear glasses or contact lenses to correct purely ocular difficulties, such as astigmatism or myopia.

In visual field testing by the confrontation method, the patient looks at the examiner's nose and points to fingers moved within the four quadrants of the peripheral visual fields (Fig. 4-2). Each eye should be tested individually. (Only in this way will bitemporal hemianopsias be detected.) The examiner's fingers must be within his or her own visual fields and their views not obstructed by an enlarged nose or protruding eyebrows.

Children and patients unable to comply with this testing method may be examined in a more superficial but still meaningful manner by assessing their response to attention-catching objects brought into their field of vision from different directions. A dollar bill, a toy, or a glass of water usually attracts notice. Failure of such a stimulus to catch the patient's attention when presented to one side suggests that a hemianopsia is present.

Next, the examiner must observe the ocular fundus using an ophthalmoscope (Fig. 4-3). The examiner should note the color of the disk and the clarity of its margins and try to estimate the retinal arterial-to-venous diameter ratio, which should be 3:5. (As everywhere else in the body, the veins are larger than arteries.)

The tests just described for disturbances in visual acuity, patterns of visual loss, and changes in the ocular fundus usually suffice to localize the cause of visual impairment. It should be noted that the optic nerves as well as the entire visual system are subject to various disorders caused by ocular, neurologic, iatrogenic, and psychogenic illnesses. The frequency and complexity of these disturbances justify a separate chapter on visual disturbances (Chapter 12).

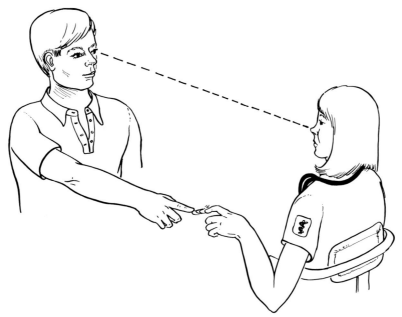

Fig. 4-2. In testing visual fields by the confrontation method, the physician wiggles his or her index finger as the patient points to it without deviating his or her eyes from the nose of the physician.

THE OCULOMOTOR, TROCHLEAR, AND ABDUCENS NERVES (THIRD, FOURTH, AND SIXTH CRANIAL NERVES)

The oculomotor, trochlear, and abducens nerves are considered as a group because they act together in a complementary manner to coordinate eye movement. The nerves and their interconnecting circuit, the *medial longitudinal fasciculus* (*MLF*), must be intact to permit depth perception and prevent diplopia (double vision).

The oculomotor nerves (third cranial nerves) originate in the midbrain. After passing through the red nucleus and corticospinal tract (Fig. 4-4), they leave the base of the brainstem and supply the pupil constrictor, the eyelid, and the adductor and

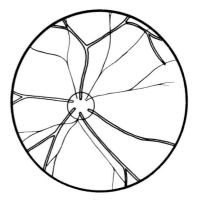

Fig. 4-3. As seen through an ophthalmoscope, the normal optic disk is yellow, flat, and well-demarcated from the surrounding red retina. The retinal veins, which are larger than the retinal arteries, pulsate. This can be seen by looking carefully at their segment overlying the optic disk.

MIDBRAIN

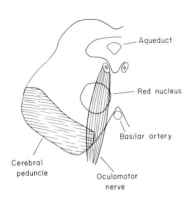

Fig. 4-4. The oculomotor nerve (third cranial nerve) arises as a pair of nerves from nuclei located in the dorsal portion of the midbrain. It descends through the red nucleus, which carries contralateral cerebellar outflow fibers, and the cerebral peduncle, which carries the corticospinal tract that will supply the contralateral trunk and limbs.

elevator muscles of the eyeball (medial rectus, inferior oblique, inferior rectus, and superior rectus). Impairment of this nerve leads to pupillary dilation, ptosis, and deviation of the eye downward and outward (Fig. 4-5). For example, a patient with an injury to the right oculomotor nerve would have diplopia, especially when looking to the left (see Fig. 12-9); outward deviation, i.e., abduction, of the right eye; dilation of the right pupil; and ptosis of the right eyelid.

Like the oculomotor nerves, the trochlear nerves (fourth cranial nerves) originate in the midbrain. They supply only the superior oblique muscle, which is responsible for depression of the eye when adducted (turned inward). Since this nerve is rarely injured, and since such complicated movements are difficult to assess, only specialists are responsible for recognizing injuries to it.

The abducens nerves (sixth cranial nerves) originate in the pons (Fig. 4-6). They pass through the brainstem near the facial nerve (seventh cranial nerve) and terminate entirely on the abductor (lateral rectus) muscle of the eye.

Abducens nerve impairment will lead to adduction of the eye (Fig. 4-7). For example, a patient with damage to the right abducens nerve would have diplopia,

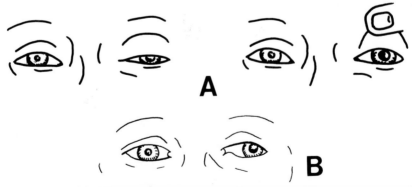

Fig. 4-5. (A) The patient with paresis of the *left oculomotor nerve* has ptosis and lateral deviation of the left eye, which has a larger and unreactive pupil. (B) In a milder case, close inspection reveals ptosis, lateral deviation of the eye, and dilation of the pupil.

PONS

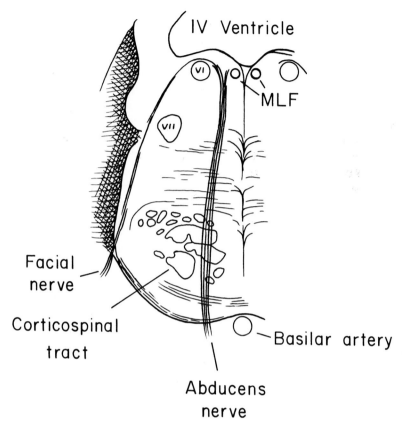

Fig. 4-6. The abducens nerve (sixth cranial nerve) arises as a pair of nerves from nuclei located in the dorsal portion of the pons. At its origin, the abducens nerve is adjacent to the medial longitudinal fasciculus (MLF) (see Chapter 15). As the nerve descends, it passes just medial to the facial nerve and nucleus and through the corticospinal tract.

especially when looking to the right, and deviation of the right eye toward the nose, that is, medially (see Fig. 12-10).

In summary, the lateral rectus muscle is innervated by the sixth cranial nerve, the superior oblique by the fourth, and all the rest by the third. A mnemonic captures this relationship: LR_6SO_4.

Examination of the oculomotor and abducens nerves involves testing pupillary reaction and extraocular muscle function. The pupils are inspected for their size,

Fig. 4-7. The patient with paresis of the *left abducens nerve* has medial deviation of the left eye.

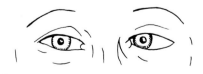

equality, and shape. Then a bright light is shone directly into one eye. Normally, the pupil receiving the light will constrict (*direct light reflex*), as will the other (*consensual light reflex*). Normally, the pupil will also constrict when the gaze changes from a distant to a close object (*accommodation reflex*).

The examination includes observing the position of the eyelids relative to the face and pupils. If ptosis is present, it is generally accompanied by elevation of the ipsilateral eyebrow and forehead muscles in an attempt to keep the pupil uncovered.

After observing the patient's face and eyes, the physician asks the patient to look at a light held off to each side laterally and then vertically. The patient should be able to maintain a gaze for 5 seconds in each direction, during which time diplopia or nystagmus (oscillation of the eyeballs) might be noted.

The oculomotor nerve on one side is complementary to the abducens nerve on the other. Therefore, diplopia in one direction of gaze is explainable by a lesion in either the oculomotor nerve on one side or the abducens nerve on the other. For example, if a patient has diplopia on looking to the left, either the left abducens nerve or the right oculomotor nerve may be paretic. Likewise, diplopia on right gaze suggests a paresis of either the right abducens nerve or left oculomotor nerve. Although elaborate diagnostic tests may be performed, the presence or absence of other signs of oculomotor nerve palsy (pupillary dilation and ptosis) will usually indicate if that nerve is responsible.

Midbrain lesions can cause diplopia when the oculomotor nucleus or nerve is damaged. In classic but rare cases, midbrain lesions also damage either the corticospinal tract, which carries motor function to the contralateral limbs, or the red nucleus, which carries cerebellar outflow to the contralateral limbs. Such injuries lead to syndromes in which oculomotor nerve palsy is combined with either contralateral hemiparesis or contralateral ataxia and tremor.

Pontine lesions, similarly, can cause diplopia when the abducens nucleus or nerve is damaged. They may also damage the corticospinal tract as well as the abducens nerve. Such a lesion would cause a syndrome of abducens nerve palsy and contralateral hemiparesis.

For example, a patient with a right-sided midbrain lesion might have right oculomotor nerve palsy, which would cause diplopia, and left hemiparesis (Fig. 4-8). Likewise, with a slightly different right-sided midbrain lesion, a patient might have right oculomotor nerve palsy and left-sided tremor (Fig. 4-9). With a right-sided pontine lesion, a patient may have right abducens nerve paresis, causing diplopia, and left-sided hemiparesis (Fig. 4-10). In almost all cases, such syndromes are the result of an occlusion of a small branch of the basilar artery (Chapter 11).

The medial longitudinal fasciculus (MLF) (Fig. 4-10) is a tract within the brainstem that coordinates impulses between the nuclei of the oculomotor and abducens nerves. Interruption of this communicating tract produces the MLF syndrome, which is a characteristic impairment of ocular motility. Also called *internuclear ophthalmoplegia,* this syndrome consists of nystagmus of the abducting eye and failure of the adducting eye to cross the midline (see Fig. 15-2).

Internuclear ophthalmoplegia is almost always a manifestation of either multiple sclerosis or a small cerebrovascular infarction of the brainstem. When it results from multiple sclerosis, the patient is usually a young or middle-aged adult who develops bilateral internuclear ophthalmoplegia long with other signs of CNS dysfunction.

MIDBRAIN

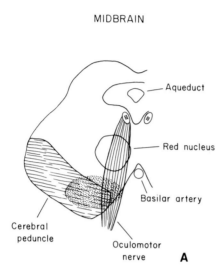

Aqueduct

Red nucleus

Basilar artery

Cerebral
peduncle

Oculomotor
nerve

A

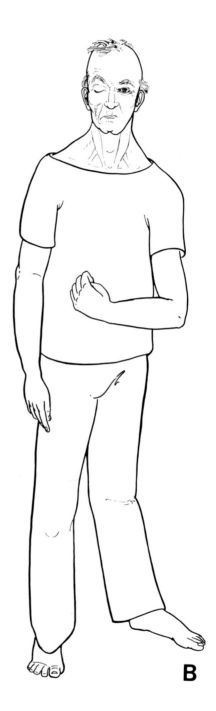

B

Fig. 4-8. The syndrome of oculomotor nerve palsy and contralateral hemiparesis. (A) A small right midbrain infarction may damage the oculomotor nerve that supplies the *ipsilateral eye* and the adjacent cerebral peduncle, which contains the corticospinal tract. That tract, which subsequently crosses in the medulla, supplies the *contralateral arm and leg*. (B) This patient has right-sided ptosis from a right-sided oculomotor nerve palsy and left hemiparesis.

MIDBRAIN

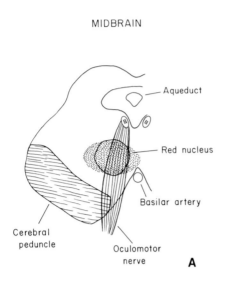

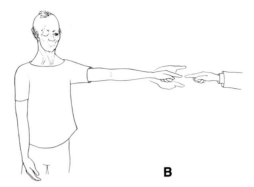

B

Fig. 4-9. The syndrome of oculomotor nerve palsy and contralateral ataxia. (A) A small right midbrain infarction may damage the oculomotor nerve and the *red nucleus*, which conveys left cerebellar hemisphere outflow to the left arm and leg by a "double-cross." (B) This patient has right ptosis from the oculomotor nerve palsy and left arm ataxia from the damage to the red nucleus.

When it results from a brainstem infarction, the patient is usually an older person suffering from unilateral internuclear ophthalmoplegia (see Chapters 12 and 15).

The most common cause of an oculomotor or abducens nerve palsy is diabetic infarction. Another frequently occurring cause is Wernicke's encephalopathy, which is the combination of one or both of these cranial nerve palsies with confusion, ataxia, and nystagmus. The oculomotor nerve is occasionally compressed by an aneurysm of the posterior communicating artery; oculomotor nerve palsy, in such cases, is one component of a subarachnoid hemorrhage.

Cerebral lesions generally do not affect the cranial nerves because, being in the brainstem, they are located a safe distance away from such injuries. Massive cerebral hemorrhages, subdural hematomas, and other intracranial mass lesions, however, often compress both the oculomotor nerve and the brainstem against the tentorium. In this syndrome, *transtentorial herniation,* a comatose patient's dilated pupil suggests the presence of a subdural hematoma or other mass lesion ipsilateral to the dilated pupil (see Fig. 19-3).

Several disorders that affect the neuromuscular junction of the ocular muscles mimic injuries of the cranial nerves themselves. Myasthenia gravis, the classic neuromuscular disorder, causes paresis of various extraocular muscles, although the pupils characteristically continue to have normal size, shape, and reactivity to light. Further evaluation in myasthenia patients will usually reveal facial and neck muscle weakness (Chapter 6).

Some conditions in which frank ocular muscular paresis is evident curiously fail to have diplopia. Intermittently dysconjugate, or "crossed," eyes are usually not associated with diplopia. If uncorrected in childhood, however, such muscle imbalances will lead to blindness of the deviated eye, *amblyopia.* In motor neuron diseases, such as ALS and poliomyelitis, the oculomotor nerves are spared despite destruction of almost all other motor neurons.

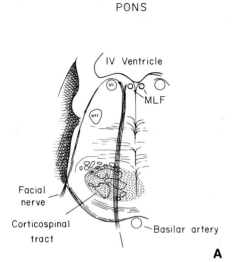

PONS

IV Ventricle

MLF

Facial
nerve

Corticospinal
tract

Basilar artery

A

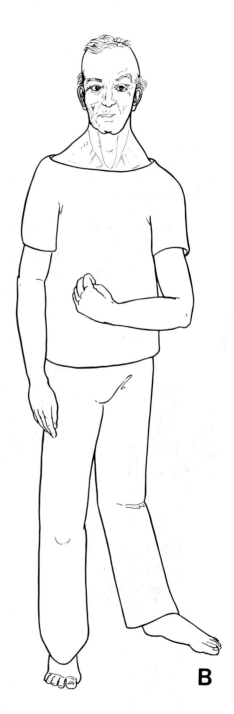

B

Fig. 4-10. Syndrome of abducens nerve palsy and contralateral hemiparesis. (A) A small right pontine infarction may damage the abducens nerve, which supplies the *ipsilateral eye*, and the adjacent corticospinal tract, which supplies the *contralateral arm and leg*. (This is analogous to midbrain infarctions; see Fig. 4-8.) (B) This patient has inward turning of the right eye from paresis of the right abducens nerve and left hemiparesis.

People can usually feign ocular muscle weakness only by staring inward with both eyes, as if looking at the tip of their nose. Children often do this playfully; however, adults with their eyes in such a position are easily recognized as displaying voluntary, although bizarre, activity. Some people who complain of diplopia have no objective sign of ocular muscle or nerve impairment. This problem, along with that of hysterical blindness, is discussed in Chapter 12.

THE TRIGEMINAL NERVE (FIFTH CRANIAL NERVE)

The main functions of the trigeminal nerves are to provide sensory innervation to the face and motor supply to the jaw muscles. Their motor nuclei are in the pons, but the sensory synapses are dispersed in an orderly manner from the midbrain to the medulla (see Fig. 2-5).

The sensory areas innervated by the nerve, designated as V_1, V_2, and V_3 and roughly described as the forehead, cheek, and jaw, respectively (Fig. 4-11), include the facial skin down to the angle of the jaw and the scalp as far back as the vertex. Within the V_1 distribution is the cornea.

The *corneal reflex* is an important reflex that is based upon the innervation of the cornea by the trigeminal nerve. Stimulation of the cornea, as with a wisp of cotton, will trigger a synapse in the brainstem, excite both facial (seventh cranial) nerves, and cause both eyes to blink.*

The trigeminal nerve also supplies the large, powerful muscles that close and protrude the jaw. Since their main function is to assist in chewing, they are often designated the "muscles of mastication."

The *jaw jerk reflex* is another important reflex. It is formed by the sensory fibers of the trigeminal nerve and a brainstem synapse, but unlike the corneal reflex, the jaw jerk reflex also utilizes the motor fibers of the trigeminal nerve. Here, stretching of the jaw muscles, as with a tap from a percussion hammer, will cause an involuntary jaw muscle contraction, so that tapping the partially opened jaw will prompt its normal reflex closing (Fig. 4-12). Hyperactivity and other alterations of this reflex are discussed below (see Bulbar and Pseudobulbar Palsy).

Examination of the trigeminal nerve begins with testing sensation in its three sensory divisions. A cotton wisp or applicator is brushed successively against each side of the forehead, cheek, and jaw. The patient is then asked if sensations are equal. Areas of reduced or no sensation, i.e., *hypalgesia,* are plotted. Their pattern should conform to anatomic outlines. The corneal reflex might be used in assessing the stuporous, uncooperative, or possibly hysteric patient.

After evaluating sensation, the physician would test jaw muscle strength by asking the patient to clinch, then protrude his or her jaw. In most patients, the jaw jerk should be tested.

---

* If the cotton tip is first applied to the right cornea and neither eye blinks, and then to the left cornea and both eyes blink, the interpretation would be that the right trigeminal nerve (the afferent sensory component) is impaired. If application of cotton to the right cornea fails to provide a right eye blink, but succeeds in provoking a left eye blink, the interpretation is that the right facial nerve (the efferent motor component) is impaired.

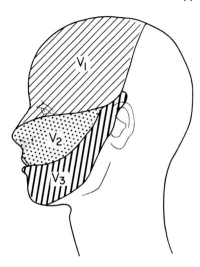

Fig. 4-11. The three divisions of the trigeminal nerve provide facial sensory innervation. The first division (V_1) supplies the forehead, the cornea, and the scalp up to the vertex; the second (V_2) supplies the malar area; and the third (V_3) supplies the skin of the lower jaw except for the angle.

Injury of the trigeminal nerve will cause facial hypalgesia, corneal reflex loss, jaw jerk hypoactivity, and weakness of the jaw muscles ipsilateral to the lesion. Such injuries, which are rare, may be caused by nasopharyngeal tumors, wounds, and tumors of the cerebellopontine angle.

Brainstem injuries characteristically impair facial sensation and the corneal and jaw jerk reflexes. Unilateral cerebral lesions, however, create little impairment of facial sensation, jaw strength, or reflexes. If bilateral cerebral lesions are present, pseudobulbar palsy develops, and jaw strength and reflexes are altered (see below).

Sometimes, as in *trigeminal neuralgia* (tic douloureux), the trigeminal nerve is irritated but not damaged. People with this condition have bursts of lancinating pain, usually in the cheek or jaw, i.e., the V_2 or V_3 areas. Likewise, patients with migraine headaches have throbbing periorbital and anterior skull (V_1 area) pain because the meninges is innervated by the first division of the trigeminal nerve. Another commonly encountered problem is *Herpes zoster infection*, which causes an excruciat-

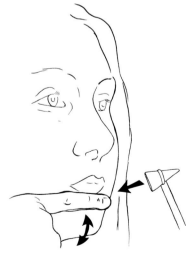

Fig. 4-12. In the jaw jerk reflex, the jaw will move slightly downward and then rebound softly. Abnormalities are mostly a matter of the rapidity and strength of the rebound. In a hypoactive reflex, as found in bulbar palsy, there is little or no rebound. In a hyperactive reflex, as in pseudobulbar palsy, there is a quick and forceful rebound.

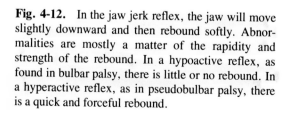

ingly painful skin eruption in the V_1 division or other divisions of the trigeminal nerve.

Finally, important causes of "lost" facial sensation are hysteria and related disorders. In these conditions, the sensory "loss" will usually encompass the entire face or will be one aspect of sensory "loss" of one half the body. In almost all cases, the following three nonanatomic features will be present: (1) The hysteric sensory loss will not involve the scalp (although its anterior portion is supplied by the trigeminal nerve); (2) despite the facial sensory loss, the corneal reflex will remain intact; and (3) when only one-half the face is affected, sensation will be lost sharply (rather than gradually) at the midline, i.e., the midline will be split.

THE FACIAL NERVE (SEVENTH CRANIAL NERVE)

The major functions of the facial nerves are motor supply of the facial muscles and the sense of taste. Cerebral impulses innervate the facial nerve motor nuclei of both the contralateral and ipsilateral pons. Ultimately, the upper facial muscles are innervated by both cerebral hemispheres, whereas the lower ones are innervated only by the contralateral cerebral hemisphere (Fig. 4-13).

The facial nerve itself originates in the pons and leaves the brainstem at the cerebellopontine angle. It supplies the ipsilateral temporalis, orbicularis oculi, and orbicularis oris muscles, which are responsible for a person's smile, frown, grimace, or raised eyebrows. The facial nerve, it is said, supplies the "muscles of facial expression."

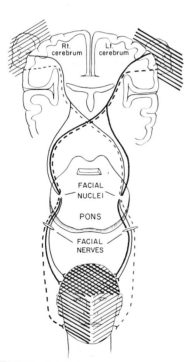

Fig. 4-13. The facial nerve is derived, in almost a unique arrangement, from corticobulbar tracts originating in the ipsilateral as well as in the contralateral cerebral hemisphere. Each facial nerve supplies the facial muscles, with the upper half of the face receiving cortical innervation from both hemispheres. With cerebral injuries, therefore, only the lower half of the contralateral face is deprived of innervation. With injury to the facial nerve itself, of course, both the upper and lower half of the facial musculature are deprived of innervation.

Taste receptor fibers of the anterior two thirds of the tongue are also conveyed in the facial nerve. (The glossopharyngeal nerve—the ninth cranial nerve—receives those from the posterior third.) Actually, taste sensation is limited. Receptors are able to detect only four fundamental sensations: bitter, sweet, sour, and salty. It is predominantly aroma, which is detected by the olfactory nerve, that gives food its flavor. Moreover, the olfactory system, not the facial nerve, is the one having extensive connections in the cerebral cortex and limbic system.

Routine facial nerve testing involves examining the strength of the facial muscles and, occasionally, assessing taste. The examiner observes the patient's face, first at rest and then during a succession of maneuvers relying on various facial muscles. He or she also asks the patient to look upwards, close his or her eyes, and smile.

If weakness is detected, the examiner should try to ascertain if both the upper and lower, or only the lower, facial musculature is paretic (Fig. 4-14). Upper and lower paresis suggests a lesion of the facial nerve itself. Other functions, such as taste, then are likely to be impaired as well.

In contrast, paresis of only the lower facial musculature suggests a lesion of the contralateral cerebral hemisphere. In such a case, paresis might also affect the ipsilateral arm and leg, and the deep tendon and plantar reflexes might be abnormal. With weakness of the right lower face, aphasia might be present. Taste sensation and other facial nerve functions will be preserved.

To test taste, the examiner applies either a dilute salt or sugar solution to the anterior portion of each side of the tongue, which must remain protruded to prevent the solution from spreading to its other parts. A patient will normally be able to identify salty, sweet, and other fundamental taste sensations, but not those "tastes" that depend on aroma, such as onion and garlic.

Facial nerve damage results in paresis of the entire ipsilateral side of the face with or without loss of taste sensation. *Bell's palsy*, an inflammatory injury, is probably the most commonly encountered facial nerve disorder, although lacerations and tumors of the nerve or adjacent structures are also common causes of nerve injury.

Patients with psychologic aberrations do not "develop" unilateral facial paresis, probably because such a posture is difficult to mimic. People who refuse to be examined, particularly children, might assume a posture in which their eyelids and mouth are forced closed. The willful nature of such "paresis" is evident when the examiner finds resistance on opening the eyelids and jaw, and that the eyeballs tend to retrovert as the eyelids are pried open (Bell's phenomena).

THE ACOUSTIC NERVE (EIGHTH CRANIAL NERVE)

Each acoustic nerve is actually composed of two nerves with separate courses and different functions. The *cochlear nerve*, one of the two components, transmits auditory impulses from the ear to the superior temporal gyri of both cerebral hemispheres (Fig. 4-15).

This bilateral cortical representation of sound means that whereas lesions of the acoustic nerve or damage to an ear itself may cause deafness in that ear, unilateral lesions of the brainstem or cerebral hemisphere will not cause any hearing impairment. Since most cerebral lesions do not impair hearing, patients with cerebrovascular accidents, tumors, and Alzheimer's disease typically have normal hearing.

Central   Peripheral

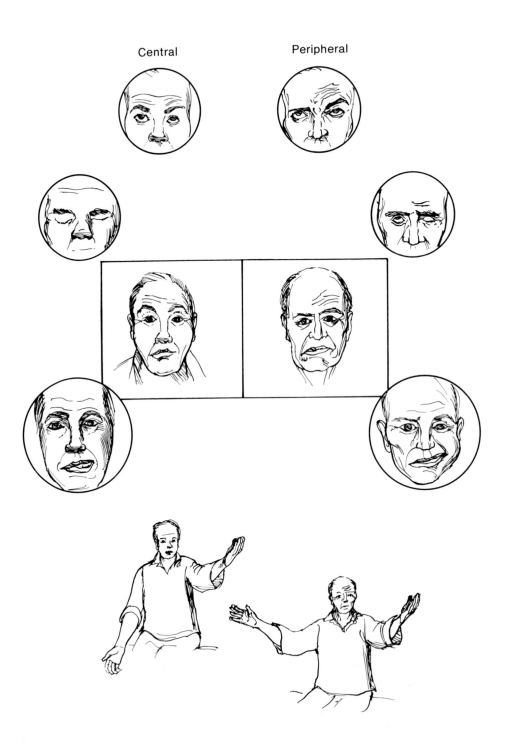

During the routine examination, hearing is tested by the examiner whispering into one of the patient's ears while covering the other. Although this method does not permit an objective measure, the experienced physician can use this simple test to detect a gross hearing loss.

Hearing impairment may result from damage to the middle ear, the inner ear, or the acoustic nerve. It is not, as already mentioned, usually a result of brain injury. The auditory nerve may be damaged by medications, such as aspirin or streptomycin, by fractures of the skull, or by nerve tumors, such as acoustic neuromas. Congenital damage is commonly found as a result of in utero rubella infections or kernicterus (Chapter 13).

When patients mimic deafness, the examiner may attempt to startle or awaken them from sleep with loud noises or have them look reflexly toward a noise (the *auditory-ocular reflex*). Factitious hearing loss may also be revealed by obtaining an EEG while the patient is subjected to particular noises; auditory evoked responses will be elicited when hearing mechanisms are intact (Chapter 15).

Such investigations are necessary not only in diagnosing malingering and hysteria, but also in the full evaluation of persons who cannot speak, especially children. In

---

Fig. 4-14. Weakness of the face from cerebral and facial (seventh cranial) nerve injuries. The patient on the left has weakness of his lower right face from thrombosis of the left middle cerebral artery. He might be said to have a central (CNS) paralysis. In contrast, the patient on the right has right-sided weakness of both the upper and lower face from a right facial nerve injury (Bell's palsy). He might be said to have a peripheral (cranial nerve) paralysis.

In the center, boxed sketches, the patients are pictured while at rest. The man with the central palsy, on the left, has flattening of the right nasolabial fold and sagging of the mouth downward to the right. This pattern of weakness indicates paresis of only the lower facial muscles. The man with the peripheral palsy on the right, however, has right-sided loss of the normal forehead furrows in addition to flattening of the nasolabial fold. This pattern of weakness indicates paresis of the upper and well as the lower facial muscles.

In the circled sketches at the top, the patients have been asked to look upwards—a maneuver that would exaggerate upper facial weakness. The man with central weakness has normal upward movement of the eyebrows and furrowing of the forehead. The man with peripheral weakness has no eyebrow or forehead movement, and the forehead skin remains flat.

In the circled sketches second from the top, the men have been asked to close their eyes—a maneuver that also would exaggerate upper facial weakness. The man with the central weakness has widening of the nasolabial fold, but he is able to close his eyelids and cover the eyeball. The man with the peripheral weakness is unable to close his eyelids, although his genuine effort is apparent by the retroversion of the eyeball (Bell's phenomenon).

In the lowest circled sketches, the men have been asked to smile—a maneuver that would exaggerate lower facial weakness. Both men have strength only of the left side of the mouth and thus it deviates to the left. If tested, the man with Bell's palsy would have loss of taste on the anterior two thirds of his tongue.

The bottom sketches show the response when both men are asked to elevate their arms. The man with the central facial weakness also has paresis of the adjacent arm, but the man with the peripheral weakness has no arm paresis.

In summary, the man on the left with the left middle cerebral artery occlusion has paresis of his right lower face and arm. The man on the right with right Bell's palsy has paresis of his right upper and lower face and loss of taste.

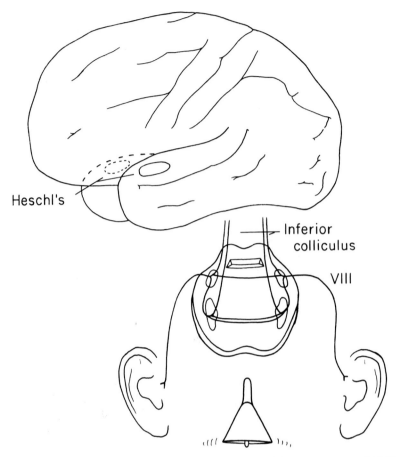

Fig. 4-15. The cochlear division of the acoustic nerve synapses extensively in the pons. Crossed and uncrossed fibers pass upward into the brainstem and terminate in the auditory (Heschl's) areas of both temporal lobes. In the dominant hemisphere, Heschl's area is adjacent to Wernicke's language area (see Fig. 8-1).

addition, the possibility of hearing impairment should be considered in all children with cerebral palsy, mental retardation, or autism.

Hearing loss may affect 25 percent of the elderly. In such cases, it usually results from middle or inner ear degeneration rather than auditory nerve damage. Whenever subject to the combination of visual, hearing, and intellectual impairments, the elderly are prone to develop thought and emotional disturbances. Hearing aids, which should be dispensed readily and even on a trial basis, may improve attentiveness and communication and avert psychologic problems.

A ringing or whistling sound in the ears, *tinnitus*, is another commonly occurring problem among the elderly. While it may be caused by damage to the inner ear by medications, tinnitus is most often caused by inner ear ischemia resulting from atherosclerotic cerebrovascular disease. Likewise, an audible heartbeat is often a manifestation of atherosclerotic cerebrovascular disease.

The other component of the acoustic nerve is the *vestibular nerve*. This nerve transmits labyrinthine system impulses to monitor equilibrium, orientation, and change in position.

The most characteristic symptom of vestibular nerve damage is *vertigo*, a sensation that one is spinning within the environment or that the environment is itself spinning. Dizziness, lightheadedness, giddiness, weakness, or unsteadiness are not equivalent to vertigo. Unfortunately, physicians mistakenly use the terms interchangeably. If vertigo is caused by vestibular dysfunction, then nystagmus, ataxia, and often auditory changes are usually present. When vertigo is severe, nausea and vomiting develop.

Viral infections of the inner ear, *labyrinthitis*, affect the origin of the vestibular nerve and cause incapacitating vertigo with nausea. Traumatic injuries and ischemia cause similar symptoms. In addition, vestibular nerve damage may result from some of the medications that also cause cochlear nerve damage.

Meniere's disease, an important chronic vestibular nerve disorder of unestablished etiology, causes episodes of vertigo, unilateral tinnitus, and often nystagmus. Beginning in middle age and occurring in women more often than men, it leads to progressive hearing loss. In typical cases, attacks of Meniere's disease are readily identifiable; however, in the elderly they may be indistinguishable from basilar artery transient ischemic attacks. Many cases are justifiably confused with anxiety, but anxious patients do not have clear-cut vertigo or nystagmus.

THE GLOSSOPHARYNGEAL, VAGUS, ACCESSORY, AND HYPOGLOSSAL NERVES (NINTH THROUGH TWELFTH CRANIAL NERVES)

The ninth through twelfth cranial nerves are considered together because all arise from the lower brainstem; have certain common functions, such as production of speech; and are affected by the same disorders. Their impairment leads to an important clinical syndrome, bulbar palsy. This disorder, which itself merits special attention, is most notable because of its superficial resemblance to pseudobulbar palsy.

Bulbar and Pseudobulbar Palsy

BULBAR PALSY

The *bulb, or medulla*,* contains the descending corticospinal tracts, the ascending sensory tracts, and the nuclei and initial portions of the ninth through the twelfth cranial nerves. These bulbar cranial nerves innervate the muscles of the soft palate, pharynx, larynx, and tongue. Their primary function is to implement cerebral commands to produce speech and to swallow food and saliva. They also control unconscious actions of the palate and pharynx, largely through swallowing and gag reflex mechanisms.

Injury to the bulbar cranial nerves, either within the brainstem or anywhere along

---

* For practical purposes, however, the bulb is often considered to be the pons as well as the medulla (see Figs. 20-1 and 20-13).

their course, leads to bulbar palsy. This commonly occurring disorder is characterized by speech impairment (*dysarthria*), difficulty in swallowing (*dysphagia*), and unresponsiveness of the gag reflex. The salient clinical features are summarized and compared with those of pseudobulbar palsy in Table 4-1.

The examiner should listen to the patient's speech first during the history taking and then during repetition of sounds. In most cases of bulbar palsy, patients have thickened speech with heavy nasal intonation; some patients can even be altogether mute. Even if a patient's speech is not strikingly abnormal during casual conversation, repetition of guttural consonants, such as "ga . . . ga . . . ga . . .," will usually evoke typically thickened, nasal sounds, uttered "gna . . . gna . . . gna. . . ."

In contrast to patients with aphasia, those with bulbar palsy, despite markedly impaired articulation, still employ normal syntax, express full meaning when speaking, and have normal understanding of verbal information. Moreover, their ability to express themselves in writing is preserved.

People with bulbar palsy who are severely dysarthric, for example, would not be able to repeat the phrase, "Pick up your hand." They would, however, be able to understand and follow the command and also be able to write the phrase correctly.

In contrast, patients with aphasia typically would be unable to repeat the command and also would fail to understand and execute it. Moreover, they probably would not be able to write it (see Aphasia, Chapter 8).

Examination of a patient with bulbar palsy will also reveal little or no palate elevation on attempts to say "ah." In contrast, a normal person's palate, during such an effort, will contract and rise in a tentlike fashion, with the uvula remaining in the midline.

The other cardinal sign of bulbar palsy is dysphagia. Because of pharyngeal and palatal paresis, food tends to lodge in the trachea or be forced upwards into the nasopharyngeal cavity. In fact, patients with advanced bulbar palsy nasally regurgitate liquids.

Though paucity of voluntary palatal movement and dysphagia are important characteristics of bulbar palsy, they do not by themselves distinguish bulbar from pseudobulbar palsy. Impairment of the gag reflex (Fig. 4-16), however, is distinctive.

What happens in bulbar palsy to impair the gag reflex is that damage to the ninth through twelfth cranial nerves or their intramedullary connections interferes with normal transmission of impulses produced by irritative stimulation of the posterior pharynx. Ordinarily, such impulses are transmitted along these nerves' afferent

Table 4-1

Comparison of Bulbar and Pseudobulbar Palsy

	Bulbar	Pseudobulbar
Dysarthria	Yes	Yes
Dysphagia	Yes	Yes
Movement of palate		
Voluntary	No	No
Reflex	No	Yes
Jaw Jerk	Hypoactive	Hyperactive
Emotional lability	No	Yes
Intellectual impairment	No	Yes

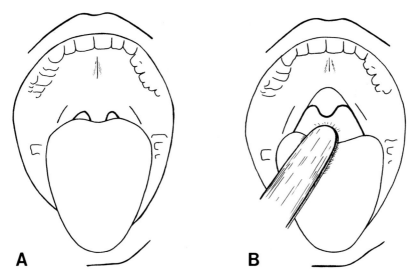

Fig. 4-16. (A) Normally, the soft palate forms an arch from which the uvula seems to hang. (B) When the pharynx is stimulated, the normal gag reflex causes pharyngeal muscle contraction; the soft palate elevates straight upward, the uvula remaining in the midline. With impairment of the bulbar nerves (bulbar palsy), there may be little, no, or an asymmetric movement of the palate. With impairment of the corticobulbar tracts (pseudobulbar palsy), there is a brisk, overly forceful reaction that causes retching, coughing, or crying.

branches to the medulla, then back along the efferent branches. Stimulation normally produces prompt elevation of the palate, contraction of the posterior pharyngeal muscles, and a sensation of gagging. In bulbar palsy, the reflex is absent because one or both reflex limbs are damaged. (In pseudobulbar palsy, as will be discussed shortly, the gag reflex, far from being impaired, is hyperactive.)

Depending on its cause, bulbar palsy is associated with still other physical findings. Since the twelfth cranial nerve is frequently impaired, the tongue is often immobile. Patients with bulbar palsy often have jaw and facial muscle weakness. When the jaw muscles are involved, the jaw jerk reflex (Fig. 4-12) will be notably depressed. When the brainstem is the site of neurologic disorder and the corticospinal tract is damaged, patients with bulbar palsy have hyperactive DTRs and Babinski signs.

Recognizing that a patient has bulbar palsy and determining whether the injury is within the brainstem or the cranial nerves in their course outside the brainstem will aid in establishing the neurologic illness. Conditions that commonly cause bulbar palsy by damaging the cranial nerves within the brainstem are ALS and thrombosis of a vertebral artery, although several decades ago, poliomyelitis was probably the most commonly encountered cause. Diseases likely to cause bulbar palsy by damaging the cranial nerves after they have exited the brainstem are Guillain-Barré syndrome, chronic meningitis, tumors that grow along the base of the skull or within the adjacent meninges, and myasthenia gravis and botulism, which are diseases that impair the neuromuscular junctions.

PSEUDOBULBAR PALSY

Although dysarthria and dysphagia are present in both bulbar and pseudobulbar palsy, the two conditions differ in the sites of anatomic abnormality, the quality of dysarthria and dysphagia, associated mental changes, and the spectrum of underlying causes. Pseudobulbar palsy is associated with damage to the frontal lobes and results from impairment of the corticobulbar tracts, which are upper motor neurons. Such damage is analogous to damage of the (adjacent) corticospinal tracts (Fig. 4-17).

In contrast, bulbar palsy results from damage to the lower brainstem or the bulbar cranial nerves along their course. This condition results from impairment of the nuclei of the nerves or of the nerves themselves, which are elements of lower motor neurons.

Clinical differences can be subtle. The speech in pseudobulbar palsy is character-ized by variable rhythm and intensity, and it is often said to have an "explosive" cadence. For example, when asked to repeat the consonant "ga," patients might blurt out "GA . . . GA . . . GA . . . ga . . . ga . . . ga." Their speech often has less of a nasal quality than is found with bulbar palsy. In general, the abnormal cadence is more striking than the abnormal articulation.

Although dysphagia is a characteristic manifestation of pseudobulbar palsy, liq-uids are swallowed relatively easily and nasal regurgitation is uncommon. This less severe dysfunction in pseudobulbar palsy is the result of preservation of the swallow-ing and gag reflexes.

A major difference in the two conditions, however, is the reactivity of the gag reflex (Fig. 4-16). When tested, pseudobulbar palsy patients have brisk elevation of the palate and contraction of the pharynx, often overreacting with coughing, crying, and retching. They have, however, little or no palatal or pharyngeal movement in response to voluntary effort, as when attempting to say "ah." By contrast, in bulbar palsy the palate and pharynx do not respond either to reflex stimulation or voluntary effort.

Another major difference between the two conditions is that while the jaw jerk reflex is depressed in bulbar palsy because the lower motor neurons of the cranial nerves are impaired, it is hyperactive in pseudobulbar palsy because the upper motor neurons of the corticobulbar tract are impaired. Also, in pseudobulbar palsy damage to the frontal lobes is so common that it almost always leads to signs of bilateral corticospinal tract damage, e.g., hyperactive DTRs and Babinski signs, whereas in bulbar palsy such signs of corticospinal tract damage are an uncommon feature.

The most prominent and generally well-known feature of pseudobulbar palsy is the accompanying alteration in the emotional state. The damage to the frontal lobes leads to inappropriate affect and fluctuation (lability) of emotions, as well as dysar-thria and dysphagia. Patients seem to cry, or less often, laugh in response to minimal provocation. Moreover, as a manifestation of their emotional lability, they appear to switch readily between euphoria and depression (Fig. 4-18).

The actual emotions of such patients, however, are certainly not as expansive as the crying and laughing would suggest. Patients most often describe themselves as being awash with tearfulness. Amitriptyline, in relatively low doses (eg, below 75 mg daily), and apart from its antidepressant effect, may suppress the unwarranted laugh-ing and crying.

A patient's tendency to cry and laugh is so dramatic that dysarthria and dysphagia may go unrecognized. Such emotionality is commonly, and, in general, correctly

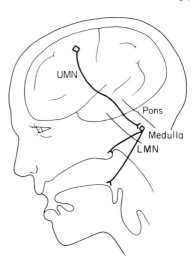

Fig. 4-17. The corticobulbar tract is an upper motor neuron (UMN) tract that innervates the bulbar cranial nerves (of the pons and medulla). These cranial nerves are essentially lower motor neurons (LMNs) Damage to them, which causes bulbar palsy, abolishes the jaw jerk and gag reflexes; such areflexia is typical of LMN injury (Fig. 2-2C). Although mental changes may be the most prominent feature of pseudobulbar palsy, it is characterized by hyperactivity of these reflexes; such hyperactivity is typical of UMN injury (Fig. 2-2B).

attributed to pseudobulbar palsy, even without testing for dysarthria and dysphagia. Therefore, the term *pseudobulbar palsy* has become the commonly accepted explanation for unwarranted emotional states in people with brain damage.

On the other hand, the tendency toward tearfulness should not always be ascribed to brain damage. A great deal of true sadness can reasonably be expected under the circumstances of extensive and progressive incapacity.

Pseudobulbar palsy is associated with intellectual impairment (dementia) as well as with emotional lability because the extensive cerebral damage that underlies pseudobulbar palsy also causes generalized intellectual dysfunction (Chapter 7). Likewise, when the left cerebral hemisphere is particularly damaged, pseudobulbar palsy may be associated with aphasia, usually of the nonfluent variety (Chapter 8). This association, seen in reverse, might account for the tendency of some aphasic patients to appear tearful at any provocation. In any case, patients with pseudobulbar palsy should be carefully evaluated for dementia and aphasia.

In pseudobulbar palsy, the emotional and intellectual disturbances generally

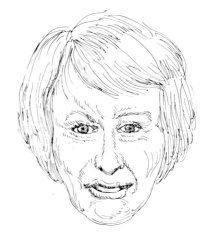

Fig. 4-18. Patients with pseudobulbar palsy, such as this woman who has suffered multiple cerebral infarctions, often sit with an open mouth, furrowed forehead, and somewhat vacant stare. The caricature of the mentally retarded person, with a deep voice (saying "dahh"), mouth open, and drooling is the popular, implicit recognition of such extensive cerebral damage.

appear in proportion to the extent of the cerebral injury. They do not appear in bulbar palsy because there is no underlying *cerebral* damage.

The conditions causing pseudobulbar palsy are those that damage both frontal lobes or, more often, the entire cerebrum. Although a wide variety of degenerative, structural, or metabolic disturbances may be responsible, pseudobulbar palsy is most often the result of Alzheimer's disease, multiple cerebrovascular infarctions, or multiple sclerosis. In childhood, congenital cerebral damage, i.e., cerebral palsy, causes pseudobulbar palsy along with bilateral spasticity and choreoathetotic movement disorders. Finally, since ALS causes both upper and lower motor neuron damage, it is associated with a mixture of bulbar and pseudobulbar palsy; however, since ALS is a disorder of motor neurons exclusively, it is not associated with either dementia or aphasia (Chapter 5).

THE HYPOGLOSSAL NERVE (TWELFTH CRANIAL NERVE)

The hypoglossal nerves innervate the ipsilateral tongue muscles, which move the tongue within the mouth and protrude it when people eat and speak. The muscles tend to push the tongue contralaterally when it is protruded. Since the pressure of each side is balanced, the tongue protrudes in the midline.

This nerve originates from paired nuclei near the midline of the medulla. After it leaves the base of the medulla, the nerve passes through the base of the skull and travels through the neck to innervate the muscles of the tongue.

If one hypoglossal nerve were injured, that side of the tongue would be weakened and, in time, it would atrophy. When protruded, the tongue would deviate toward the weakened side because the normal, strong musculature would overpower the effort at protrusion of the weakened side (Fig. 4-19). Such a finding illustrates the adage "the tongue points toward the side of the lesion."

If both nerves were injured, as in bulbar palsy, the tongue would become immobile. In cases of ALS, fasciculations as well as atrophy might be observed (see Fig. 5-4).

The most frequently occurring conditions in which one hypoglossal nerve is damaged are brainstem infarctions, penetrating neck wounds, and nasopharyngeal tumors. Both hypoglossal and other bulbar cranial nerves are injured in Guillain-Barré syndrome, myasthenia gravis, and ALS.

SUMMARY

Identification of damage to the individual cranial nerves is helpful in localizing lesions and diagnosing particular neurologic illnesses. Cranial nerves are often damaged in combination with other portions of the nervous system. Important examples are the syndromes that indicate brainstem lesions, such as cases of paresis of the oculomotor (III) or abducens (VI) nerve combined with contralateral hemiparesis; the lateral medullary syndrome; facial paresis, which may result from either cerebral or facial nerve damage; and lower cranial nerve dysfunction, which might be attributable to either bulbar or pseudobulbar palsy. The distinction between cranial nerve and CNS damage, which may appear clinically similar, may be made on the basis of readily

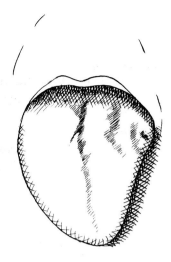

Fig. 4-19. With (left) hypoglossal nerve damage, the tongue deviates toward the weaker side, i.e., turns toward the side of the lesion, and the affected (left) side atrophies.

observable signs. When damage is restricted to cranial nerves and the brainstem, despite extensive motor and sensory impairment, patients do not have mental abnormalities.

QUESTIONS: CHAPTERS 1–4

1. A 68-year-old man has the sudden, painless onset of paresis of the right upper and lower face, inability to abduct the right eye, and paresis of the left arm and leg. Where is the lesion and what structures are involved?

2. What deficits would be produced with occlusion of the left internal carotid artery?

3. What symptoms and signs will a patient have with sudden occlusion of the right internal carotid artery?

4. A 20-year-old man has the subacute onset of complete loss of vision in the right eye, incoordination of the left hand, and moderate spastic paraparesis. What is the localization?

5. A 20-year-old woman complains of right eye "blindness," right hemiparesis, and right hemisensory loss. Pupillary and deep tendon reflexes are normal. Hoover's sign is present. Localize the lesion.

6. What diseases with movement disorders are associated with dementia?

7. What physical abnormalities are frequently found with cerebral degenerative conditions such as Alzheimer's disease?

8. A 45-year-old woman, who was entirely well previously, has the sudden onset of jargon speech and hysteria. She is admitted to the psychiatric ward with a diagnosis of schizophrenia. The physical examination reveals only a right Babinski sign and an equivocal right hemiparesis. This common neurologic condition frequently mimics psychiatric disturbances. What is her deficit and what is its origin?

9. An elderly man has left ptosis, a dilated and unreactive left pupil, external deviation of the left eye, a right hemiparesis, right-sided hyperreflexia, and a right Babinski sign. He does not have either aphasia or hemianopsia. Where is (are) the lesion(s)?

10. A person is found to have a left superior homonymous quadrantanopsia. Where might the lesion be located?

11. A 60-year-old man has seizures that begin with clonic activity of the left hand and spread to the left arm, then face, and then leg. Subsequently, he has transient paresis of the left arm. Where is the lesion?

12. A 50-year-old woman complains of gait difficulties and decreased hearing on the right for many years. The right corneal reflex is absent. The entire right side of her face is weak. Auditory acuity is diminished on the right. There is left-sided hyperreflexia with a Babinski sign and right-sided difficulty with rapid alternating movements. What structures are involved? Where is (are) the lesion(s)?

13. A 60-year-old man develops moderate interscapular back pain, paraparesis with hyperreflexia, loss of sensation below the umbilicus, and incontinence. Where exactly is the lesion?

14. A young man, having sustained an injury in a minor car accident, complains of being able to see an area of only 2 m², paralysis of the legs, and loss of sensation below the waist. On examination, he is found to have a constant visual loss of 2 m² at every distance, an inability to raise his legs or walk, brisk DTRs, and loss of pin and position sense in the legs and toes. Plantar responses are flexor, cremasteric and anal reflexes are present, and sensation of warm versus cold is intact. Formulate the case.

15. A 50-year-old man with mild dementia has absent reflexes, loss of position and vibration sensation, and ataxia. What nonstructural diseases must be considered?

16. A 55-year-old woman, thought to have depression, is then found to have right optic atrophy, papilledema on the left, and left hemiparesis. Where is the lesion?

17. A middle-aged man complains of impotence. He has been in excellent health except for hypertension. On examination, he has orthostatic hypotension and lightheadedness, but the neurologic examination is otherwise normal. What neurologic conditions may be the cause or a contributing factor?

18. A 60-year-old man with right upper lobe pulmonary carcinoma has the rapid development of lumbar spine pain, paraparesis with areflexia, loss of sensation below the knees, and urinary and fecal incontinence. Where is the lesion?

19. Subsequently, the man in question 18 develops a flaccid, areflexic paresis of the right shoulder and arm and a right Horner's syndrome. Where is the lesion?

20. A 60-year-old man has developed stiffness of his left leg. Examination reveals that he has a spastic paraparesis, DTR hyperreflexia in all extremities, and bilateral extensor plantar response. There are fasciculations in the left leg, both arms, and tongue. There is atrophy of most muscle groups of the left arm. All sensation, bladder and bowel function, and ocular movements are intact. What process is developing?

21. A 21-year-old woman has the mildly painful loss of vision in the left eye. She is found to have an acuity of 20/400 in the eye; a mild left hemiparesis with hyperreflexic DTRs and a Babinski sign; and right-sided ataxia. She had a similar episode 5 years before. Formulate the case.

22. A 40-year-old man has interscapular spine pain, paraparesis with hyperreflexia, bilateral Babinski signs, and a complete sensory loss below his nipples. Formulate the case and list the preliminary approach to the diagnosis.

23. Contralateral hemiparesis, hemisensory loss, and hemianopsia are found in lesions of either hemisphere. What higher cortical function deficits are specifically referable to the dominant or nondominant hemisphere?

24. An elderly man has right retro-orbital pain, vertigo, nausea, and vomiting. He has a right Horner's syndrome, loss of the right corneal reflex, and dysarthria because of paresis of the palate. What are the other features of this common eponymic syndrome? Which way does the palate deviate?

25. A 54-year-old woman complains of having experienced several episodes of shaking in her left leg beginning in the foot. There is hyperreflexia at the left knee and ankle and a left Babinski sign. What sensory abnormalities might be detected?

26. What area of the brain is the primary site of damage in Wilson's disease, Huntington's chorea, and choreiform cerebral palsy? What neurologic system is involved and what are the traditional manifestations of abnormalities there?

27. Name the frontal lobe release reflexes. Are they always pathologic?

28–39. Define these symptoms or signs and specify the location of associated lesions.

28. Anosognosia	**34.** Dementia
29. Aphasia	**35.** Dysdiadochokinesia
30. Astereognosis	**36.** Gerstmann's syndrome
31. Athetosis	**37.** Homonymous hemianopsia
32. Bradykinesia	**38.** Micrographia
33. Chorea	**39.** Homonymous superior quadrantanopsia

40. Which of the following neurologic diseases are genetically transmitted and, if so, in what manner?

a. Alzheimer's disease	i. Friedreich's ataxia
b. Amyotrophic lateral sclerosis (ALS)	j. Guillain-Barré syndrome
c. Cluster headaches	k. Huntington's chorea
d. Creutzfeldt-Jakob disease	l. Migraine headaches
e. Down's syndrome	m. Sturge-Weber disease
f. Duchenne's muscular dystrophy	n. Subacute sclerosing panencephalitis
g. Dystonia musculorum deformans	(SSPE)
h. Familial amaurotic idiocy (Tay-Sachs)	o. Wilson's disease

41. A young man sustains major head trauma. Afterwards, he has insomnia, fatigue, intellectual and personality changes, and claims that food tastes differently. What might have happened?

42. A middle-aged woman has increasing blindness in the right eye, where the visual acuity is 20/400 and the disk is white. The right pupil does not react directly or consensually to light. The left pupil reacts directly, although not consensually. All motions of the right eye are impaired. Where is the lesion? What cranial nerve(s) is (are) involved?

43. In what condition do pupils accommodate but not react to light?

44. In what condition is a patient in an agitated, confused state with abnormally large pupils?

45. In what condition is a patient in coma with pinpoint-sized pupils?

46. What are the most common causes of asymptomatic miosis?

47. After sustaining a severe head injury, a patient is admitted in coma. The right pupil is dilated and unreactive. There is right hemiparesis and bilateral Babinski signs. What well-known catastrophe is happening?

48. On looking to the left, a patient has diplopia. What nerve(s) may be paretic?

49. On looking to the left, the left eye fails to abduct fully. Which nerve is probably involved?

50. If the right third cranial nerve were injured, how would the eyes appear? In what direction of gaze would diplopia occur?

51. Nystagmus is observed bilaterally, horizontally, and vertically in a 15-year-old girl who is lethargic, disoriented, walks with an ataxic gait, and has slurred speech. What is the most likely cause of her findings?

52. A young man complains of vertigo, nausea, vomiting, and left-sided tinnitus. He has nystagmus to the right. Where is the lesion?

53. A soldier has vertical and horizontal nystagmus, mild spastic paraparesis, and ataxia of finger-to-nose motion bilaterally. What process has occurred?

54. A man who has diplopia looks to the left, but the right eye fails to adduct across the midline and the left eye has nystagmus. Both eyes, however, are forward while looking ahead and converge while reading. What process has occurred?

55. A 35-year-old man, who has been shot in the back, has paresis of the right leg and loss of position and vibration sensation at the right ankle. Sensation of pinprick is lost in the left leg. Where is the lesion?

56. A 25-year-old man develops impotence. He has been found previously to have retrograde ejaculation during an evaluation for sterility. Since age eight, he has had diabetes mellitus. Examination of his fundi reveal hemorrhages and exudates. He has absent DTRs at the wrists and ankles, loss of position and vibration sensation at the ankles, and no demonstrable anal or cremasteric reflexes. Why is he impotent?

57. A 27-year-old man has a bitemporal hemianopsia. He has had loss of libido for 2 years and mild frontal headaches for the previous 3 months. Examination of the optic disks shows them to be white. The pupils are large but react to light. The right eye fails to abduct fully. Aside from a eunuchoid habitus, the routine physical examination reveals no abnormalities. What is the neurologic basis of his symptoms and signs?

58. An 8-year-old boy with increasing difficulty in athletic activities and with headaches, nausea, and vomiting is found to have papilledema, tremor on intention, ataxia of gait, bilateral hyperreflexia, and bilateral Babinski signs. Where is the lesion and what are the possible causes?

59. Gait abnormalities are important signs of neurologic diseases. Match the abnormality of the gait with its description.

a. Short-stepped, narrow-based with a shuffle	1. Apraxic
b. Impaired alternation of feet and "magnetism" to floor	2. Astasia-abasia
c. Broad-based and lurching	3. Ataxic
d. Seeming to be extraordinarily unbalanced, but without falls	4. Festinating
e. Swinging one leg outward with excessive wear on the inner sole	5. Hemiparetic

60. Match the descriptions of gait abnormalities with the associated neurologic illnesses.

a. Cerebral infarction	1. Apraxic
b. Cerebellar degeneration	2. Astasia-abasia
c. Parkinsonism	3. Ataxic
d. Normal pressure hydrocephalus	4. Festinating
e. Hysteria	5. Hemiparetic

61. Match the pictures (1, 2, 3) with the associated characteristics.
   a. Cerebral infarction
   b. Loss of taste on one side of tongue
   c. Idiopathic inflammation
   d. Normal
   e. Overexposure and drying of eye
   f. Loss of the corneal reflex

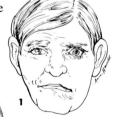

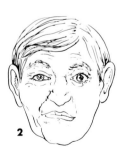

62–67. The patient who is pictured below is looking slightly to her right and attempting to raise both arms.

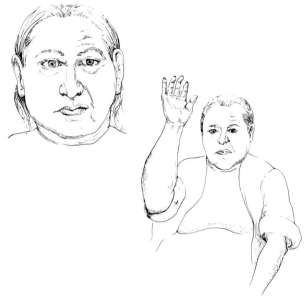

62. Paresis of which extraocular muscle prevents the affected eye from moving laterally?
    a. Right superior oblique
    b. Right abducens
    c. Left abducens
    d. Left lateral rectus
    e. Right lateral rectus

63. The left face does not seem to be involved by the left hemiparesis. Why might the left side of the face be uninvolved?
    a. It is. The left forehead and mouth are contorted.
    b. The problem is in the right cerebral hemisphere.
    c. The corticospinal tract is injured only after the corticobulbar tract has innervated the facial nerve.
    d. The problem is best explained by postulating two lesions.

64. On which side of the body would a Babinski sign be elicited?
    a. Right   c. Both
    b. Left   d. Neither

65. What is the most likely cause of this disorder?
    a. Bell's palsy   c. Cerebral infarction   e. Pontine infarction,
    b. Hysteria   d. Medullary infarction   f. Midbrain infarction

66. With which conditions might such a lesion be associated?
    a. Homonymous hemianopsia
    b. Diplopia
    c. Impaired monocular visual acuity
    d. Intellectual impairment
    e. Aphasia, if the patient were right cerebral dominant
    f. Various nondominant hemisphere syndromes

67. Sketch the region of the damaged brain, inserting the damaged structures and the area of damage.

ANSWERS

1. The damaged structures include the abducens and facial nerves on the right and the corticospinal tract that originates in the right cerebral hemisphere and passes through the right midbrain and pons before crossing in the medulla. Only a lesion on the right side of the pons could damage all these structures. Small infarctions are the most common cause of such lesions. (If the lesion pictured in Fig. 4-10 extended more laterally, it would create these deficits.)

2. Unless anastomoses are present, occlusion of the left internal carotid artery will impair function of the left hemisphere and cause right-sided hemiparesis, hemisensory loss, homonymous hemianopsia, and aphasia.

3. Like the previous case, the patient will have contralateral hemiparesis, hemisensory loss, and homonymous hemianopsia. Notably, since such patients frequently have anosognosia, they may not describe any deficit.

4. The patient probably has lesions in the right optic nerve, left cerebellum, and thoracic spinal cord. Such disseminated lesions are typically found in cases of multiple sclerosis.

5. The symptoms cannot be explained by a single lesion, cannot be confirmed by objective signs, and lack the usual accompanying symptoms such as aphasia. Moreover, she fails to exert maximum effort voluntarily with one leg while "trying" to lift the other against resistance (Hoover's sign). Neurologic disease may not be present. Rather, she might have a psychogenic disturbance.

6. Dementia is part of Wilson's disease, Huntington's chorea, and Creutzfeldt-Jakob disease, but not necessarily part of Parkinson's disease, Sydenham's chorea, or choreoathetotic cerebral palsy.

7. Signs of frontal lobe dysfunction that are usually present with cerebral degenerative conditions include corticospinal tract abnormalities (hyperreflexic DTRs and Babinski signs), corticobulbar signs (dysarthria, hyperactive gag reflex, briskly reactive jaw jerk), and frontal lobe release signs (snout, suck, rooting, palmomental, and grasp reflexes).

8. Schizophrenia rarely develops in middle age and almost never produces "word salad." More likely, the patient had a fluent aphasia and has subtle corticospinal tract signs from a left temporoparietal lesion.

9. The patient has a left oculomotor nerve palsy and right hemiparesis. Therefore, the lesion is in the left midbrain. As expected, he does not have a language or visual field deficit since the cerebrum is uninjured.

10. Such a defect is usually found with a lesion of the right temporal or inferior occipital lobes, but occasionally an optic tract lesion may be responsible.

11. The lesion is located in the right lateral cerebral cortex. It gives rise to focal motor seizures, which then have secondary generalization (a jacksonian march). Following the seizure, he has postictal (Todd's) paresis.

12. The right-sided corneal reflex loss, facial weakness, and hearing impairment all indicate damage to the trigeminal, facial, and acoustic cranial nerves, which emerge together from the brainstem at the right cerebellopontine angle. The right-sided dysdiadochokinesia, which indicates right-sided cerebellar damage, and the left-sided DTR abnormalities are also consistent with damage to the right cerebellopontine angle. Frequently occurring lesions in this region are acoustic neuromas and meningiomas.

13. The lesion is in the thoracic spinal cord at the T-10 level.

14. Many features of the examination indicate that the basis of his symptoms and signs is not neurologic. Hysteria or malingering is suggested by the following: (1) the constant area ($2m^2$) of visual loss at all distances—tunnel vision—is contrary to the optics of vision, in which a greater area of vision is encompassed at greater distances from the eye; (2) the sensory loss to pain (pin) is inconsistent with preservation of thermal (warm versus cold) sensation because both sensory systems follow the identical anatomic pathways; (3) despite his apparent para-paresis, the normal plantar response and intact anal and cremasteric reflexes indicate that both the upper and lower motor neuron systems are intact, while the DTRs are brisk because of anxiety.

15. This patient has dysfunction of the posterior columns of the spinal cord and the cerebellar system. Combined system disease (pernicious anemia), tabes dorsalis, spinocerebellar degenerations, and heavy metal intoxication should be considered first.

16. She has the classic Foster-Kennedy syndrome from a right frontal lobe tumor. The tumor compresses the underlying optic nerve, causing it to atrophy. The tumor also raises intracranial pressure, causing papilledema of the other optic nerve. Finally, the tumor causes contralateral hemiparesis because of the damage to the corticospinal tract of the frontal lobe.

17. Impotence, as well as orthostatic hypotension, may be the result of *autonomic* nervous system dysfunction. In this patient, antihypertensive medications, e.g., reserpine and guanethidine, may be responsible.

18. The paraparesis with absent DTRs, loss of sensation at the L-4 level, and *lumbar spine* pain suggest that the lesion is in the cauda equina.

19. This problem is from a brachial plexus injury, which involves the nerve roots of C-4–6 and the intrathoracic sympathetic chain. He has a Pancoast's tumor.

20. The patient has signs of corticospinal tract (upper motor neuron) disease in all extremities, as evidenced by the generalized hyperreflexia, stiffness (spasticity) in the legs, and Babinski signs. In addition, he has disease of the anterior horn cells (lower motor neurons), as evidenced by the fasciculations and atrophy. Notably, sensation and sphincter and ocular muscles are uninvolved. He has the motor neuron disease, amyotrophic lateral sclerosis (ALS).

21. Several areas of the nervous system are involved: the left optic nerve, the right corticospinal tract, and the right cerebellar hemisphere. Moreover, this is the second episode. Since she has lesions that are disseminated in space and time, she most likely has multiple sclerosis. Alternatively, while a single lesion in the midbrain might produce similar corticospinal tract and cerebellar (outflow tract) findings, vision would not have been affected.

22. The lesion clearly affects the spinal cord, at the T-4 level. Likely causes include benign and malignant mass lesions, e.g., a herniated thoracic intervertebral disk or an epidural metastatic tumor; infections, e.g., abscess or tuberculoma; and inflammations, e.g., transverse myelitis or multiple sclerosis. A complete history, physical examination, routine laboratory tests, and thoracic spine and chest x-ray films should all be performed before a myelogram or spine CT scan.

23. Aphasias and Gerstmann's syndrome are usually referable to dominant hemisphere lesions. Hemi-inattention, anosognosia, somatopagnosia, and constructional apraxia are found in nondominant hemisphere lesions. Perseverations, ideomotor apraxia, dementia, pseudo-bulbar palsy, and occasionally, constructional apraxia and fluent aphasia result from bilateral or diffuse cerebral disease.

24. The patient has a right-sided lateral medullary (Wallenberg's) syndrome. This will include crossed (right-facial and left-truncal) hypalgesia and right-sided ataxia. The palate will deviate to the left because of right-sided palatal weakness.

25. The lesion, which is causing focal motor seizures, is located on the right medial cerebral cortex. There might only be loss of cortical sensation, e.g., stereognosis and two-point discrimination. Sensation of pain and temperature may be preserved because they are perceived in the thalamus. Most likely the lesion is a tumor, e.g., a parasagittal meningioma or glioblastoma, but a scar from a cerebral infarction is another possibility.

26. These diseases, like Parkinson's disease, affect the basal ganglia, which is the basis of the extrapyramidal, i.e., noncorticospinal, motor system. Basal ganglia dysfunction causes tremor and other movement disorders, rigidity, and bradykinesia. In contrast, corticospinal tract dysfunction causes spasticity, DTR hyperreflexia, and Babinski signs.

27. The frontal release reflexes are those seen about the face (snout, suck, and rooting reflex) and those related to the palm (palmomental and grasp reflexes). Some neurologists would also include an increased jaw jerk. Almost all of them are normally present in infants and none of them reliably indicates the presence of a pathologic condition in adults. If, however, most are detected and especially if they are present unilaterally, a frontal lobe lesion or cerebral degenerative condition is likely to be present.

28. Anosognosia is the failure to recognize a deficit or disease. The most common occurrence is ignorance of a left hemiparesis from a right parietal lobe infarction or tumor.

29. Aphasia is the impairment of verbal and written communications, i.e., a language disorder, which usually results from lesions in the dominant cerebral hemisphere.

30. Astereognosis is the inability to identify objects by touch. It is found with lesions in the contralateral parietal lobe.

31. Athetosis is an involuntary movement disorder in which there is a slow writhing movement of the arm(s) or leg(s) that is more pronounced in the distal part of the extremity. Usually it is the result of basal ganglia damage from perinatal jaundice, anoxia, and prematurity.

32. Bradykinesia, i.e., slowness of movement, is seen with many basal ganglia diseases.

33. Chorea is involuntary intermittent jerking of one or more extremities, or of the trunk. Tardive dyskinesia and several medications, e.g., L-dopa, as well as basal ganglia disease, cause chorea.

34. Dementia is impairment of intellectual function. It usually results from diffuse cerebral damage or a single lesion that creates a generalized effect. In some cases, dementia is reversible.

35. Dysdiadochokinesia is impaired ability to perform rapid alternating movements. It is found with lesions of the ipsilateral cerebellar hemisphere.

36. Gerstmann's syndrome is the combination of agraphia, finger agnosia, dyscalculia, and inability to distinguish right from left. It is found with lesions of the parietal lobe in the dominant hemisphere.

37. Homonymous hemianopsia is a visual field defect in which one half of each eye field is lost. For example, in a right homonymous hemianopsia, the right half of the field is lost; it could be illustrated:

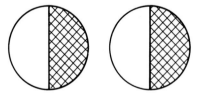

The lesion is in the contralateral optic tract or intrahemispheric radiations.

38. Micrographia is the writing of small letters. It is a characteristic of patients with parkinsonism.

39. *Homonymous* superior quadrantanopsia is the visual field defect in which the same top quarter is lost, i.e.,

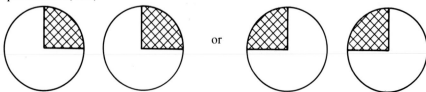

In *bitemporal* superior quadrantanopsia, neither eye appreciates the upper–outer quarter, i.e.,

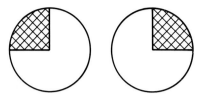

The former is found with lesions of the temporal or lower occipital lobe, while the latter is found with lesions of the optic chiasm.

40. a. Nongenetic, except in certain families.
b. Nongenetic*
c. Nongenetic
d. Nongenetic*
e. Nondysjunction (trisomy 21)
f. Sex-linked recessive disease
g. Autosomal recessive (in Jews), autosomal dominant, or sporadic
h. Autosomal recessive
i. Autosomal recessive in typical cases
j. Nongenetic*
k. Autosomal dominant
l. Frequently familial, especially in females, but not proven to be a genetic trait
m. Autosomal dominant, variable penetration
n. Nongenetic*
o. Autosomal recessive

41. He probably has had a contusion of both frontal lobes resulting in a postconcussive syndrome manifested by change in mentation and personality. In addition, the thin fibers of the olfactory nerve have probably been severed as they pass through the cribriform plate, accounting for his anosmia.

42. She evidently has right-sided optic nerve damage since she has right-sided impaired visual acuity, optic atrophy, and loss of direct light reaction. In addition, she has oculomotor, trochlear, and abducens nerve damage, since there is complete extraocular muscle paresis. Only a lesion located behind the eye would be able to damage all these nerves. Such a lesion is the relatively common meningioma of the sphenoid wing.

43. Tabes dorsalis with Argyll-Robertson pupils.

44. Atropine, scopolamine, and similar intoxications.

45. The combination of coma and miosis is found most often in heroin, barbiturate, and other overdoses. Pontine infarctions and hemorrhages are also frequent causes.

46. The most common causes of asymptomatic miosis are use of ocular medications for glaucoma and normal changes of old age.

47. He probably has herniation of the right temporal lobe through the tentorial notch, which leads to compression of the ipsilateral third cranial nerve and, more important, the brainstem, i.e., the transtentorial herniation syndrome.

48. Either the left sixth or right third cranial nerve is paretic.

49. The left sixth cranial nerve is responsible.

50. The right lid would be paretic, the right eye would be deviated laterally (abducted), and the pupil would be dilated. The patient would have diplopia on looking forward. It would increase on looking to the left.

---

*Probably infectious.

51. She is probably intoxicated with alcohol, barbituates, or other drugs of abuse, i.e., she is drunk. A cerebellar tumor is an unlikely possibility without signs of raised intracranial pressure or corticospinal tract damage. Multiple sclerosis is unlikely because of the lethargy, disorientation, and young age.

52. The unilateral nystagmus, hearing abnormality, nausea, and vomiting are most likely caused by left-sided inner ear disease rather than neurologic dysfunction.

53. This patient seems to have a lesion in the brainstem producing the nystagmus, a lesion in the cerebellum causing ataxia, and a lesion in the spinal cord causing paraparesis. The picture of disseminated lesions is typical of but not diagnostic of multiple sclerosis.

54. The patient has internuclear ophthalmoplegia, which is found as the result of small lesions in the brainstem from multiple sclerosis, vascular infarctions, or inflammatory conditions.

55. He suffers from a classical Brown-Sequard syndrome, i.e., hemitransection of the spinal cord. The lesion is at the right side of the thoracic spinal cord.

56. He has a combination of peripheral and autonomic system neuropathy because of diabetes mellitus. A peripheral neuropathy is suggested by the distal sensory and reflex loss and the absent anal and cremasteric reflexes. Autonomic neuropathy is suggested by the retrograde ejaculation. Other manifestations of autonomic neuropathy that might be sought are urinary bladder hypotonicity, gastroenteropathy, and anhidrosis.

57. A lesion near the optic chiasm will cause his optic atrophy and bitemporal hemianopsia. It might also damage the adjacent sixth cranial nerve by invading the cavernous sinus. Moreover, the eunuchoid appearance and the loss of libido may be referable to damage to the hypothalamus, which is directly above the optic chiasm. Therefore, the patient's symptoms and signs indicate that he has a large mass lesion pressing against both the optic chiasm and the hypothalamus. These lesions are commonly chromophobe adenomas of the pituitary gland, but other tumors, e.g., meningiomas, and aneurysms are sometimes responsible.

58. He has increased intracranial pressure, compression of the corticospinal tracts, and cerebellar dysfunction. Most likely he has obstructive hydrocephalus from a cerebellar tumor, which is a relatively common pediatric condition. Lead intoxication, which causes diffuse neurologic dysfunction and cerebral swelling, can mimic a cerebellar tumor in children.

59, 60.

59: a–4; b–1; c–3; d–2; e–5.

60: a–5; b–3; c–4; d–1; e–2.

Normal pressure hydrocephalus is characterized by dementia, incontinence, and, most strikingly, apraxia of gait, which is the inability to initiate alternating movements of the legs with appropriate shift of weight. The feet are often immobile because the weight is not shifted as the patient moves. Thus, the feet seem magnetized to the floor (see Fig. 7-7). Hysteria has various manifestations, but a pattern of walking in which the patient seems to alternate between a broad stance for stability and a narrow, tightropelike stance, with contortions of the upper torso is clearly hysteric and termed astasia-abasia (see Fig. 3-2). In cerebellar degeneration there is ataxia of the limbs and trunk that makes the patient place his or her feet widely apart, i.e., in a broad base, to maintain stability. Since coordination is also impaired in cerebellar disease, the gait and other movements have an uneven, unsteady, lurching pattern (see Fig. 2-13). A relatively minor feature of parkinsonism is the short-stepped gait with shuffling, which is now called festinating gait but has been called *marche á petits pas* (see Fig. 18-9). The hemiparesis and increased tone (spasticity) from cerebral infarctions forces the patient to lift the paretic leg by swinging it from its hip. This motion, i.e., circumduction, permits walking despite the paresis, if the hip and knee are extended. The weak ankle, however, lets the inner front surface of the foot drag (see Fig. 2-4).

61. a–2; b–1; c–1; d–3; e–1, f–1.

Patient No. 1, who has weakness of his left upper and lower facial muscles, probably has Bell's palsy. With damage to the facial nerve, taste sensation is usually lost in the ipsilateral, anterior two thirds of the tongue. Paresis of the eyelid muscles does not permit spontaneous or reflex eyelid closure when sleeping: dehydration and foreign body irritation can result. Patient No. 2 has weakness of his left lower facial muscles. This pattern of facial weakness is typical of contralateral cerebral injuries and is usually accompanied by arm and leg weakness, i.e., hemiparesis. Patient No. 3 is normal.

62–67. This patient has weakness of the right eye that prevents it from moving laterally, weakness of the right upper and lower face, and paresis of the left arm. She probably has damage of the right abducens (VI) and facial (VII) cranial nerves and the corticospinal tract before it crosses in the medulla. Such lesions are located in the base of the pons and are caused by occlusions of small branches of the basilar artery.

62. e. The right lateral rectus *muscle* is the extraocular muscle that has been damaged.

63. c.

64. b.

65. e. A right pontine infarction would produce this condition.

66. b. Diplopia would be present on right lateral gaze.

67. PONS

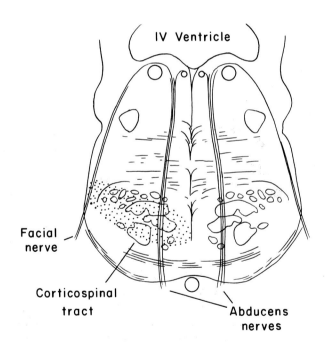

5

Peripheral Nerve Disorders

Clinical findings should permit peripheral nervous system (PNS) dysfunction to be distinguished from central nervous system (CNS) dysfunction and should allow the PNS damage to be localized. Disorders of the PNS, *neuropathies,* are the result of damage of the peripheral nerves singly, in groups, or entirely and are characterized by variable combinations of weakness, DTR loss, and sensory abnormalities.

Neuropathies are important because, besides causing neurologic deficits, some are associated with mental deterioration, indicate systemic illness, or have a fatal course. This chapter describes the anatomy and clinical aspects of peripheral nerve injuries and presents details of several important neuropathies. It then describes amyotrophic lateral sclerosis (ALS) and related motor neuron disorders. Last, it reviews the anatomy, signs, and treatment of nerve injury from herniated intervertebral disks and other orthopedic conditions.

ANATOMY

The corticospinal tracts, as discussed in Chapter 2, convey impulses from the motor cortex to the *anterior horn cells* of the spinal cord. These cells, the lower motor neurons (LMNs), give rise to the motor fibers of the peripheral nerves (Fig. 5-1).

Motor fibers leave the anterior spinal cord and most mingle within the cervical or lumbosacral plexuses to form the major peripheral nerves, such as the femoral and radial nerves. Since many of these nerves are quite long, especially in the legs, they must conduct electrochemical impulses without diminution over considerable distances. *Myelin,* a lipid-based sheath surrounding the nerve fiber, acts as insulation for the transmission of these impulses.

Where a nerve terminates against its appropriate voluntary muscle, the nerve ending contains packets of acetylcholine (ACh). When ACh is released across the neuromuscular junction, it binds onto ACh receptors, thereby triggering a muscle contraction (Chapter 6).

Sensory information is also transmitted along fibers within the peripheral nerves.

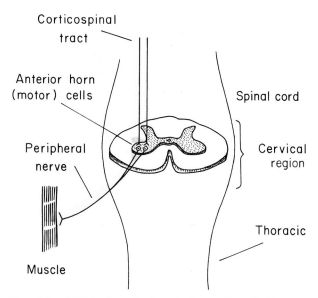

Fig. 5-1. Within the spinal cord, the corticospinal tract synapses onto the *anterior horn cells*. These are the motor cells whose axons, along with sensory fibers, join to form peripheral nerves.

Impulses from receptors in the skin, tendons, joints, and other areas flow toward the brain through peripheral nerves to the spinal cord. Virtually all major peripheral nerves carry both motor and sensory fibers.

CLINICAL CONDITIONS

Mononeuropathies are disorders of single peripheral nerves. With impairment of each major nerve, there will be a characteristic pattern of motor and sensory loss: paresis, DTR loss, and *hypalgesia* (loss of painful sensation) (Table 5-1).

The loss of an individual peripheral nerve is often the result of blunt trauma. Many nerves have long courses, during which they are protected in certain areas only by the overlying skin and subcutaneous tissue. At such points they are vulnerable to compression. For example, the radial nerve is subject to damage as it winds around the lateral humerus (Fig. 5-2), and the common peroneal nerve is apt to be injured as it winds around the lateral aspect of the fibula. Even leaning against the upper arm for several hours may therefore result in a "wrist drop," while pressure from continuous crossing of the knees or wearing a tight lower leg cast may result in a "foot drop." Likewise, some nerves pass through soft-tissue tunnels in which they are in danger of being compressed. For example, because the median nerve passes through the cramped carpal tunnel of the wrist, fluid retention before menses or during pregnancy can entrap this nerve in the wrist; median nerve damage within the carpal tunnel is called the *carpal tunnel syndrome*.

Peripheral nerve damage may also be the result of diabetes mellitus, vasculitis (e.g., lupus, polyarteritis nodosa) lead intoxication, and other systemic illnesses.

Table 5-1
Major Peripheral Mononeuropathies

| Nerve | Major Associated Deficits | | |
	Motor Paresis	DTR Loss	Sensory Loss
Median	Thumb and wrist flexor (thenar atrophy)	None	Thumb and index finger
Ulnar	Finger and thumb adduction ("claw hand")	None	Fourth and fifth fingers
Radial	Wrist and thumb extensors ("wrist drop")	Brachioradialis*	Dorsum of hand
Femoral	Knee extensors	Quadriceps (knee)	Anterior thigh
Sciatic	Ankle dorsi- and plantarflexors ("flail ankle")	Achilles (ankle)	Lateral calf and most of foot
Common peroneal	Ankle dorsiflexors and evertors ("foot drop")	None	Dorsum of foot and lateral calf

*When the radial nerve is damaged by compression in the spiral groove of the humerus, the triceps DTR is preserved.

Mononeuropathies, which are occasionally the first clinical manifestation of these conditions, are often quite painful at their onset.

Mononeuritis multiplex is the injury of a combination of two or more, but not all, individual peripheral nerves. Some cranial nerve involvement may also be found. For example, a patient with damage to the left radial, right sciatic, and right third cranial nerve would be said to have mononeuritis multiplex. This condition, which occurs much less frequently than simple mononeuropathies, is usually the result of diabetes mellitus, vasculitis, or, in Africa and Asia, leprosy.

Polyneuropathy, which occurs quite frequently, is the generalized, symmetrical involvement of all peripheral nerves. It usually affects nerves in proportion to their

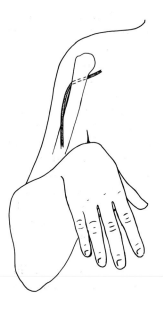

Fig. 5-2. As the radial nerve winds around the humerus, it is liable to be compressed when a person who is intoxicated by alcohol or drugs leans against the upper arm for several hours. When the radial nerve is damaged in this way, the wrist, finger, and thumb extensor muscles become paretic. Paralysis of extension of the wrist is called a "wrist drop."

length. Thus, the earliest symptoms are in the toes and feet, followed by ones in the fingers and wrists.

Complaints that patients offer usually reflect both sensory and motor impairment, although in some illnesses one or the other kind of disturbance may predominate. Patients generally do offer some description of abnormal sensations, *paresthesias,* in the distal part of their arms or legs. For example, they might describe "burning" or "tingling" in the fingers and toes. Patients, when examined, have absent or diminished sense of position and vibration. Sensory loss in the hands and feet, *stocking-glove hypalgesia* (Fig. 5-3), is characteristic of polyneuropathy and a reflection of nerves being affected in proportion to their length. Similarly, patients will have weakness in the distal portions of their limbs and therefore difficulty using their fingers to perform fine, skilled movements, e.g., buttoning a shirt. Also, since their ankle and toe muscles will be much weaker than their hip muscles, patients will have difficulty raising their feet when they walk or climb stairs.

Polyneuropathy leads to muscle atrophy and flaccidity and to loss of wrist and ankle DTRs because of interruption of the LMN in the peripheral nerve. Likewise, on attempts at eliciting a Babinski sign, there will be no response to plantar stimulation (Fig. 2-2).

Polyneuropathy may be caused by many conditions; however, the most common causes are Guillain-Barré syndrome,* diabetes mellitus, alcoholism, or ingestion of a toxic substance (Table 5-2).

Idiopathic or postinfectious polyneuropathy (Guillain-Barré syndrome) is a disorder of young and middle-aged adults in which patients develop paresthesias and sensory loss of their fingers and toes, often after a viral respiratory illness. Over the next several days they may go on to develop profound, areflexic paresis of the limbs, beginning in the feet and hands. Sometimes patients become transiently quadriplegic and apneic (from paresis of the phrenic and intercostal nerves). The illness generally resolves over three weeks to three months. From a strictly clinical viewpoint, Guillain-Barré syndrome is characterized by a much greater impairment in motor function than sensation.

Diabetes mellitus, on the other hand, is associated with a polyneuropathy that is predominantly sensory, as well as mononeuropathies, as discussed previously. Almost all patients with diabetes for more than 10 years have loss of sensation and DTRs in the feet and ankles. Diabetic polyneuropathy is characterized by painful paresthesias, which are especially distressing at night. In severe cases, sensation in the fingertips is also impaired, preventing those diabetics who are blind from "reading" Braille. For most patients, however, strength usually remains relatively normal.

Besides having extensive PNS injury, longstanding diabetics often also have autonomic nervous system injury. In such cases, patients will have impairment of gastrointestinal mobility, bladder muscle contraction, and ejaculatory function, i.e., impotence (Chapter 16). Unfortunately, even fastidious control of blood glucose does not prevent diabetic neuropathy.

The polyneuropathy associated with alcoholism is predominantly but not exclusively sensory. Alcoholics with neuropathy usually have normal strength but mild loss

---

*Patients with Guillain-Barré syndrome may receive assistance from the Guillain-Barré Syndrome Support Group. Write PO Box 262, Wynnewood, Pennsylvania 19096, or call (215)649-7837.

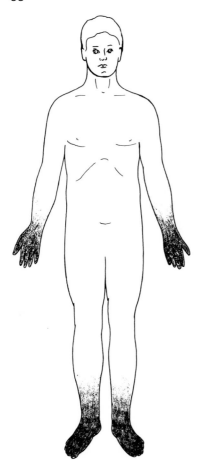

Fig. 5-3. In cases of polyneuropathy, sensation is lost symmetrically and most severely in the distal portions of the limbs, and the legs are more severely involved than the arms. Decreased pain sensation, hypalgesia, follows the pattern of someone wearing knee stockings and gloves. Patients with this disturbance are said to have "stocking-glove hypalgesia."

of position and other sensations in their feet and ankles. The sensory loss is usually asymptomatic except when they walk in the dark and must rely on position sense in their feet. Contrary to popular opinion, alcoholic neuropathy probably results not as much from alcohol or other toxins as from the "starvation" that occurs when alcoholics subsist on alcohol and carbohydrates rather than a balanced diet and thus deprive themselves of thiamine (vitamin B_1) and other vitamins. Alcohol is directly toxic to the brain, and alcoholism, of course, is associated with dementia as part of the Wernicke-Korsakoff syndrome.

Elderly people have sensory losses attributable to peripheral nerve degeneration. Almost all otherwise normal people who are 80 years of age or older have loss of some position and vibratory sensation in their toes and feet. This sensory loss, which is accompanied by loss of ankle DTRs, prevents elderly persons from standing with their feet placed closely together and, more importantly, contributes to their falling.

Self-Induced Nutritional Neuropathies

Inadequate nutrition is not only the cause of the polyneuropathy associated with alcoholism, but also causes polyneuropathy in two special circumstances to which young adults are prone. Patients with anorexia nervosa occasionally develop a typical

Table 5-2

Important Causes of Polyneuropathy

Endogenous toxins
Diabetes mellitus
Uremia*
Acute intermittent porphyria*
Nutritional deficiencies
Starvation: dieting, malabsorption, alcoholism*
Combined system disease/pernicious anemia*
Medicines
INH, nitrofurantoin, antineoplastic agents
Nitrous oxide (anesthesia)
Industrial toxins
Metals: lead, organic and inorganic mercury
Organic solvents: n-hexane and others
Infectious/inflammatory conditions
Vasculitis: systemic lupus, polyarteritis*
Postinfectious: mononucleosis, hepatitis, idiopathic (Guillain-Barré)
Leprosy
Syphilis*
Familial (genetic) diseases
Charcot-Marie-Tooth
Friedreich's ataxia and other spinocerebellar degenerations

*Associated with mental status abnormalities.

starvation-induced neuropathy that is predominantly sensory. However, possibly because these patients usually do have some selective food intake and often scrupulously take vitamins, there is a low incidence of clinically significant neuropathy.

The other special situation is where people take excessive quantities of vitamin B_6 (pyridoxine). Megavitamin treatment, which is usually self-administered, has led to profound sensory neuropathy. Although the normal adult requirement of pyridoxine is only 2 to 4 mg daily, affected patients have been consuming several grams daily.

Furthermore, whenever persons lose weight, the protective subcutaneous fat is removed from the nerves in the limbs. With loss of this protection, these people are susceptible to compression neuropathies. Thus, quite commonly, people on "crash diets" and those with anorexia from cancer develop a foot drop from peroneal nerve injury (Table 5-1).

CLINICAL CONSIDERATIONS

The distinction between signs of PNS disease and signs of CNS disease (Table 5-3) is crucial in deciding whether a patient with paraparesis or quadriparesis is suffering from severe polyneuropathy (PNS disease) or damage to the spinal cord (CNS disease). When the cause is polyneuropathy, the weakness involves the hands and feet more than the shoulders and hips, i.e., the weakness is predominantly distal. When the cause is a spinal cord injury, the extremities are weakened all along their length and, in addition, the trunk muscles below the site of injury are also weakened.

The tone and reflexes of the weakened muscles also differ. With polyneuropathy, the muscles are flaccid and the DTRs diminished or absent. With spinal cord injury, after a period of several weeks the muscles become spastic, deep tendon reflexes become hyperactive, and Babinski signs develop.

Table 5-3
Contrast of Central and Peripheral Nervous System Signs

	Central Nervous System	Peripheral Nervous System
Motor system	*Upper motor neuron*	*Lower motor neuron*
Paresis	Patterns*	Distal
Tone	Spastic†	Flaccid
Bulk	Normal	Atrophic
Fasciculations	No	Sometimes
Reflexes		
DTRs	Hyperactive	Hypoactive
Plantar	Babinski sign(s)	Absent
Sensation areas	Patterns*	Hands and feet

*Examples: motor and sensory loss of one side or lower half of the body, e.g., hemiparesis or paraparesis, and hemisensory loss.
†May be flaccid initially.

Sensation in polyneuropathy is impaired mostly in the hands and feet but preserved in the upper arms, thighs, and trunk, i.e., there is stocking-glove hypalgesia (Fig. 5-3). In spinal cord injury, sensation is lost below the level of involvement (see Fig. 2-15).

Finally, in polyneuropathies (except for diabetic polyneuropathy), bladder, bowel, and sexual function are preserved, probably because the nerves innervating these organs are so short. In contrast, loss of bladder and bowel control and sexual function develops almost immediately in cases of spinal cord injury.

Another important clinical consideration is the differences between demyelinating diseases of the CNS and PNS. Guillain-Barré syndrome exemplifies PNS demyelinating disease. Symptoms and signs of Guillain-Barré syndrome usually abate after several weeks, although occasionally patients may have initially become quadriplegic and apneic. Recovery takes place in virtually all cases because PNS myelin is regenerated.

Demyelination of the CNS in multiple sclerosis (see Chapter 15) results in recurring episodes of symptoms and signs referable to several discrete CNS areas, including the optic nerves. Despite performing a similar insulating function, CNS and PNS myelin differ in their cells of origin (oligodendrocytes and Schwann cells, respectively), chemical composition, and antigenic capacity. While damaged PNS myelin is regenerated and patients with polyneuropathy recover, damaged CNS myelin is not regenerated, and clinical impairments are often permanent. (The partial or even complete recovery that multiple sclerosis patients seem to achieve between episodes is probably the result of resolution of an inflammatory response rather than regeneration of myelin.)

Polyneuropathies Associated with Mental Status Abnormalities

A particular clinical problem with peripheral neuropathies is that of detecting one in a patient who has an abnormal mental status. Besides indicating the presence of a neurologic condition rather than an exclusively psychologic disturbance, the finding of a peripheral neuropathy can suggest several underlying illnesses (Table 5-2).

Acute intermittent porphyria (AIP).   This illness, which is rare in America, is an inherited disorder of porphyrin metabolism. Patients with AIP experience attacks in which they develop mental disturbances that have been so bizarre as to be called "psychosis" and a polyneuropathy that can result in quadriplegia. During attacks the urine turns red and the Watson-Schwartz test and other tests for urinary porphyrins will be positive. The attacks may be exacerbated if the patient is given barbiturates. Phenothiazines may be given for psychosis.

Alcoholism.   As noted before, polyneuropathy and dementia are frequent complications of alcoholism. Alcoholics often have peripheral neuropathy without the other aspects of Wernicke-Korsakoff syndrome (Chapter 2); however, if they have the dementia, they usually have neuropathy. Alcoholism may also cause degeneration of the cerebellum, damage to the pons (central pontine myelinolysis), and alcohol withdrawal seizures (Chapter 10).

Combined system disease (pernicious anemia or B_{12} deficiency).   Polyneuropathy is present in pernicious anemia, although it is overshadowed by signs of spinal cord dysfunction and dementia. Combined system disease, which is diagnosed by determining the serum B_{12} level or by performing a Schilling test, is treated with B_{12} injections. Since folic acid can reverse the hematologic aspects but permits the neurologic complications to worsen, it should not be included in over-the-counter vitamin preparations.

Syphilis.   Patients with tabes dorsalis, which is now a rare condition, often have signs of polyneuropathy, including lancinating, radicular pains and absent DTRs. Over 90 percent of such patients also have Argyll-Robertson pupillary abnormalities. The clinical diagnosis can be confirmed by a positive finding from a VDRL test on the cerebrospinal fluid.

Uremia.   Uremic polyneuropathy is commonplace in patients who are undergoing maintenance hemodialysis. If uremia becomes pronounced, the neuropathy increases and the patient can develop an encephalopathy.

Vasculitis.   Vascular inflammatory diseases, such as lupus or polyarteritis nodosa, often create infarctions in both the CNS and PNS arteries. When the arteries supplying the peripheral nerves are damaged, single or multiple mononeuropathies develop. Vascular inflammation in the brain, *cerebritis,* leads to the "3 S's of lupus": seizures, strokes, and psychosis.

On the other hand, in some persons damage to the PNS may result from psychiatric disturbances. Nutritional deficiency polyneuropathy may result from voluntary starvation, anorexia, or alcoholism. Mononeuropathies may result from unusual pressure against sensitive areas, as when patients remain too long in fixed positions because of drug or alcohol excess. Finally, a profound polyneuropathy can result from several weeks' use of nitrous oxide, a gaseous dental anesthesia that has been inhaled by thrill-seekers, including dentists, to produce a brief euphoria.

AMYOTROPHIC LATERAL SCLEROSIS AND OTHER MOTOR
NEURON DISORDERS

Amyotrophic lateral sclerosis (ALS)* a relatively uncommon disorder but one
that merits special attention, is the best known example of a *motor neuron disease*. In
ALS, both upper and lower motor neurons degenerate, but sensory systems are
unaffected. More important, despite the widespread CNS (motor neuron) destruction,
mental faculties are preserved. The etiology of ALS remains an enigma, but recent
work on similar diseases has shown that "slow virus" infections may cause this truly
fearful illness.

Amyotrophic lateral sclerosis is usually found only in people 45 years of age or
older. One exception, however, was Lou Gehrig, the famous baseball player who
developed ALS when he was about 37 years old and at the height of his career; thus,
for decades ALS was known as "Gehrig's disease."

Patients with ALS usually first notice weakness and subcutaneous muscular
twitching, *fasciculations,* in a single limb. Initially, examination of the affected limb
will also reveal paresis and atrophy—signs that together with the fasciculations reflect
damage to the anterior horn cells of the spinal cord. In time, signs tend to spread in an
asymmetric pattern to the other limbs (Fig. 5-4).

Characteristically, even atrophic muscles will have brisk DTRs. This surprising
finding of hyperactive DTRs with muscle atrophy probably is the result of the remaining lower motor neurons being supplied by damaged upper motor neurons. Babinski
signs, which are another manifestation of upper motor damage, are also characteristic.

As ALS advances, atrophy and fasciculations will be recognized in the facial,
pharyngeal, and tongue (bulbar) muscles as well as in the limb muscles. Patients will
then suffer from dysarthria and dysphagia, i.e., bulbar palsy. Pseudobulbar palsy
usually will also be present. It will be indicated by a hyperactive gag reflex and jaw
jerk. Being superimposed upon bulbar palsy, pseudobulbar palsy will eventually make
speech unintelligible and swallowing impossible. Despite extensive motor impairment, ocular muscle control and bladder-bowel function remain entirely normal.

Patients remain tragically alert and completely aware of their plight throughout
the course of their disease, which is untreatable. Death usually occurs within 2 to 4
years from respiratory complications.

There are, unfortunately, other motor neuron diseases. These diseases, which
also cause extensive loss of anterior horn cells, differ from ALS primarily in their lack
of upper motor neuron loss. Hereditary varieties of motor neuron disease in infants
(Werdnig-Hoffmann disease) and in adolescents (Kugelberg-Welander disease) are
both characterized by flaccid quadriplegia with atrophic, areflexic muscles.

Poliomyelitis (polio) was the most frequently occurring motor neuron disease
until development of the Salk vaccine. In this illness, viral infections damaged the
anterior horn (motor neuron) cells of different regions of the spinal cord or lower
brainstem (the bulb). Polio patients had paresis with muscle fasciculations and absent
DTRs. When more than one limb was involved, the paralysis was typically asymmetric. Patients who suffered bulbar polio had phrenic and intercostal nerve impairment

---

*Patients with ALS may receive assistance from the National ALS Foundation, 185 Madison Avenue,
New York, New York, 10016. (212)679-4016.

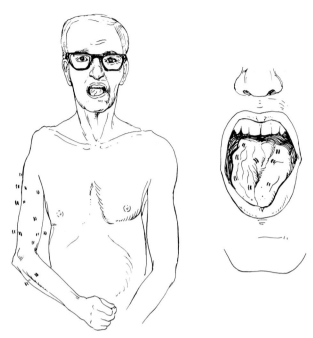

Fig. 5-4. This elderly gentleman, who suffers from ALS, has typical (right arm) asymmetric limb atrophy, paresis, and fasciculations. His tongue also has fasciculations and atrophy, as indicated by clefts and furrows.

that caused respiratory muscle paralysis; most of these patients had to be placed in the notorious "iron lung." As in ALS, mental, oculomotor, bladder, bowel, and sexual functions are normal in all forms of poliomyelitis.

Benign Fasciculations

Several innocent phenomena resemble motor neuron diseases. These conditions are transient and certainly not harbingers of neurologic disease. They are, nevertheless, frequently of great concern to medical students and others acquainted with ALS.

Many people have *benign fasciculations* in which muscle twitchings are not associated with weakness, atrophy, or reflex changes. They are usually precipitated by excessive physical exertion, psychologic stress, use of tobacco, excessive coffee intake, or exposure to some insecticides.

Myokymia, in which fasciculations are confined to the orbicularis oculi (eyelids), produces an annoying twitching or jerking movement around the eye. It also seems to be caused mostly by fatigue and anxiety.

ORTHOPEDIC DISTURBANCES

Cervical spondylosis may mimic ALS. In this far more common condition, osteoarthritic changes of the vertebrae lead to encroachment of the foramina and narrowing of the spinal canal. Cervical nerve roots are pinched and the spinal cord becomes compressed (Fig. 5-5). Thus, because of the cervical nerve compression, patients may have neck pain with arm and hand paresis, atrophy, hypoactive DTRs, sensory loss, and also fasciculations. If there is spinal cord compression, they will have spasticity, hyperreflexia, and Babinski signs in their legs.

Similarly, patients with *lumbar spondylosis* have lumbar nerve compression, and they will complain of low back pain, and sometimes have leg and feet paresis, atrophy, fasciculations, sensory loss, and paresthesias. Thus, spondylosis, unlike ALS, is associated with spine pain; sensory loss in the limbs; and normal facial, pharyngeal, and tongue musculature.

Herniated intervertebral disks (*"herniated disks"*) are one of the most common causes of low back pain. Low back pain from herniated disks and other causes is ubiquitous and the most expensive American work-related injury.

Herniated disks usually stem from prolonged pressure at the curve of the lower part of the spine. Strains, poor posture, or obesity squeeze the gelatinous intervertebral disk material that usually cushions the adjacent vertebral bodies and extrudes (herniates) it against the adjacent nerve root. Over 90 percent of disk herniations involve the intervertebral disk at either the L4-5 or L5-S1 interspace (Fig. 5-6).

Patients with herniated lumbar disks complain mostly of low back pain or paresthesias that often radiate to the buttocks and down the posterior or lateral aspect of the leg along the compressed nerve. Characteristically, buttock and leg pain as well as the low back pain is increased by coughing, sneezing, or elevating the straightened leg because these maneuvers press the herniated disk more strongly against the nerve root (Fig. 5-7).

If the herniation is large, it can lead to paresis and areflexia of ankle or toe muscles. Disk protrusions rarely affect the lower sacral nerve roots and cause bladder or sexual dysfunction.

Cervical intervertebral disks will sometimes be herniated by trauma, such as a "whiplash" automobile injury. These patients will have neck pain that radiates down the arm(s) and sometimes loss of a DTR.

In cases of acute lumbar or cervical disk herniation, the following treatment with analgesics and anti-inflammatory agents combined with resting the affected part of the spine will usually be successful. Pain and disability usually are alleviated after three weeks because the extruded disk material is absorbed.

- Give the patient mild analgesics, such as aspirin, codeine, or oral narcotics, e.g. Percocet, depending on the severity of the pain. Sometimes add an anti-inflammatory agent, although aspirin may provide this effect as well as analgesia. The new,

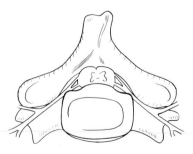

Fig. 5-5. When cervical spondylosis occurs, the cervical spinal cord is compressed by intervertebral ridges of bone, and the cervical nerve roots are compressed by bony constrictions at the foramina.

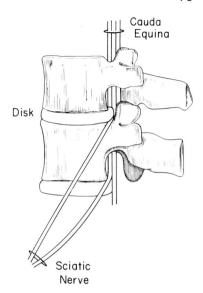

Fig. 5-6. As the cauda equina branches to form the lumbar and sacral nerves, the nerve roots leave the spinal canal through foramina, where they may be compressed by herniations of the intervertebral disks. Patients with herniated disks will often feel pain radiating along the distribution of the nerve as well as in their lower back. Their pains will be intensified by movements such as coughing, sneezing, or straining at stool, which transiently further herniate the disk.

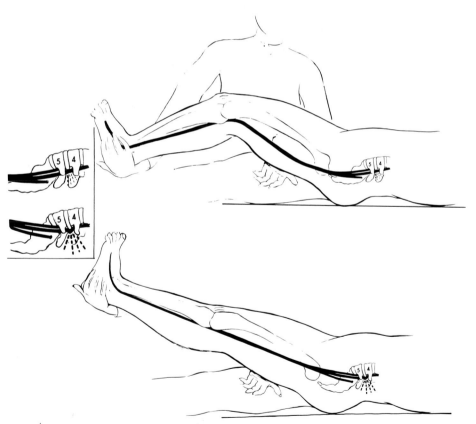

Fig. 5-7. In cases of herniated disks, the low back pain will be intensified and often radiates to the buttocks if an examiner raises the patient's *straightened* leg (Lasègue's sign). In this maneuver the nerve root is irritated because it is drawn tautly against the edge of the herniated disk.

nonsteroidal anti-inflammatory agents, e.g., Advil®, Clinoril®, Motrin®, Naprosyn®, may be beneficial.

• If the cervical spine is the affected region, immobilize the neck by urging the patient to wear a soft (foam rubber) cervical collar during the day. Instruct the patient to stop driving because it causes excessive neck rotation, stop working at a desk that forces excessive neck flexion, and use no more than one pillow at night to avoid prolonged neck bending. For severe or prolonged cases, cervical traction may provide relief.

• If the lumbar spine is the affected region, immobilize the low back by urging the patient to wear a lumbar support (a wide elastic belt), insert a bedboard, use well-contoured chairs, and sit on a supportive *car seat*. Strict bed rest is indicated if these simple measures do not help. Although lumbar traction keeps patients relatively immobile, it really does not exert sufficient force to separate the vertebrae and allow the herniated disk to be drawn back into its intervertebral space.

• Finally, this group of patients must reach relatively normal weight, avoid many physical activities, and maintain good posture.

Some patients with chronic low back pain are best approached by considering the pain itself a chronic illness that the physician can attenuate but not cure. In such cases, addictive analgesics must be avoided. Instead, antidepressants might be prescribed because they seem to have a particularly useful analgesic effect. Transcutaneous electrical nerve stimulation (TENS) also seems to be helpful, and this technique may be given as a short, harmless trial. Few patients, however, are said to respond for any length of time to biofeedback and other predominantly psychologic approaches.

Finally, the indications for surgery for herniated intervertebral disks must be strictly limited. Also, since patients involved in litigation over a painful accident may assert that they have intractable pain and permanent disability, all litigation should be settled before surgery can be expected to relieve their pain. The Minnesota Multiphasic Personality Inventory and other psychologic screening tests are also not reliable guides in distinguishing those patients who will have a good outcome.

SUMMARY

Mononeuropathies and the commonly occurring neuropathies, such as Guillain-Barré syndrome, diabetic polyneuropathy, and alcoholic polyneuropathy, are injuries to the PNS that can be contrasted to injuries of the CNS (Table 5-1). Mental aberrations are associated with acute intermittent porphyria and with uremic and alcoholic polyneuropathies (Table 5-2). Sometimes neurologic deficits are a manifestation of motor neuron disorders, such as ALS, although many benign conditions may mimic this fearful illness. Finally, nerve injury from herniated cervical or lumbar intervertebral disks leads to radiating neck or low back pain, respectively. The best treatment relies on medications and immobilization and eschews surgery.

REFERENCES

Ellenberg M: Diabetic neuropathy. In Ellenberg M, Rifkin H: Diabetes Mellitus: Theory and Practice, 3rd ed. New York, Medical Examination Publishing Co., 1983

Schaumberg H, Kaplan J, Windebank A, et al: Sensory neuropathy from pyridoxine abuse: A new megavitamin syndrome. N Engl J Med 309:445, 1983

Schaumburg HH, Spencer PS, Thomas PK: Disorders of Peripheral Nerves. Philadelphia, F. A. Davis Co., 1983

QUESTIONS

1. A 21-year-old heroin addict who overdoses awakens with an inability to extend his right wrist or fingers. All DTRs are intact, except for the right brachioradialis DTR. Where is the lesion and what is its cause?

2. An 18-year-old woman has fatigue, a low grade fever, and "tingling" in her fingers and toes. On examination, she has splenomegaly; paresis of the ankles, knees, and wrists; absent DTRs; and hypalgesia in the feet. What process is evolving?

3. A 40-year-old obese man has the sudden onset of low back pain, with inability to dorsiflex and evert his right ankle. Raising his straightened right leg produces back pain that radiates down the lateral leg. Sensation is diminished on the dorsum of the right foot. No alteration in DTRs is detectable. What is his problem?

4. A 54-year-old man with pulmonary carcinoma has two weeks of midthoracic back pain. He complains of the sudden onset of abnormal sensation in his legs and difficulty walking. Examination reveals marked weakness of both legs, areflexia of the legs, and hypalgesia from the toes to the umbilicus. What process is evolving?

5. A 27-year-old drug addict overdoses while sitting on a toilet. On awakening, he is unable to walk. Examination reveals paresis of the knee flexor (hamstring) muscles and all ankle and toe muscles. While the knee DTRs are normal, the ankle DTRs and plantar reflexes are absent. Sensation is absent below the knees. Where is (are) the lesion(s) and what is the cause?

6. A 58-year-old carpenter complains of weakness of his right arm and hand. Examination reveals fasciculations and atrophy of the hand and triceps muscles with no elicitable triceps reflex. There is mild sensory loss along the medial surface of his right hand. What process is occurring?

7. A 30-year-old pregnant woman complains of tingling and numbness of the thumb and adjacent finger of both hands. She frequently drops objects. Examination reveals hypalgesia in the area she described as "numb" and mild paresis of some of the thumb flexor and opposition muscles. Percussion of the wrist recreates the paresthesias. Reflexes are normal. Where is (are) the lesion(s) and what is the cause?

8. A young woman has confusion and hallucinations, flaccid paresis, and abdominal pain. Her urine is red. What disease does she have? What test should be done immediately?

9. A 21-year-old woman has the sudden onset of inability to elevate and evert her right ankle. While her DTR and plantar reflexes are normal, there is an area of hypalgesia on the lateral aspect of the calf and dorsum of the foot. Where is the lesion and what are possible causes?

10. Several workers in a chemical factory complain of tingling of the fingers and toes and weakness of the feet. Each seems to have stocking-glove hypalgesia and absent ankle DTRs. Which objective finding suggests that they suffer from a peripheral neuropathy? What are the common causes of industrial neuropathies?

11. A 29-year-old woman, recently found to have hypertension, rapidly develops a paresis of the dorsiflexors and evertors of the right foot, paresis of the extensors of the wrist and thumb of the left hand, and paresis of abduction of the right eye. Where is (are) the lesion(s) and what are the possible causes?

12. A 17-year-old man, after a (losing) fist fight, complains of inability to walk or feel anything below his waist. He has complete inability to move his legs, which have normally active DTRs and plantar responses. He has no response to noxious (pinprick) stimulation below his umbilicus, although sensation of position, vibration, and temperature is preserved. Where and what is the lesion?

13. A 68-year-old diabetic man has the sudden onset of pain in the anterior right thigh and difficulty walking. Examination reveals weakness of knee extension, an absent (quadriceps) knee DTR, and hypalgesia of the anterior thigh on the right. Where is the lesion and what is its cause?

14. A 34-year-old man with chronic low back pain has a sudden exacerbation while raking leaves. He has difficulty walking and pain that radiates from the low back down the left posterior thigh to the lateral ankle. He has paresis of plantar flexion of the left ankle and an absent ankle DTR. He has an area of hypalgesia along the left lateral foot. What has happened to him?

15. A 62-year-old man has the gradual onset of weakness of both arms and then the left leg. On examination he is alert and oriented but has dysarthria. His jaw jerk is overreactive, and gag reflex absent. There are atrophy and fasciculations of the tongue and muscles of both arms and left leg. DTRs are hyperactive and Babinski signs are present. Sensation is intact. What disease process is occurring and how extensive is it?

16. A 47-year-old watchmaker is unable to move his thumbs and fingers. He has sensory loss of the medial three fingers, but no change in reflexes. Where is (are) the lesion(s) and what is the cause?

17. An elderly man with chronic lumbar back pain radiating down both posterior thighs has paresis and atrophy of the calf muscles. Both ankle and plantar reflexes are absent. Fasciculations are observable in the calf muscles. The toes and dorsum of one foot are analgesic. Does he have ALS?

18. A 42-year-old school teacher has weight loss, burning dysesthesias of the feet, and a recent convulsion. Her sclerae are mildly icteric, and she had hepatosplenomegaly. She also has memory impairment, areflexia of the ankle and brachioradialis DTRs, and a stocking-glove hypalgesia. What areas of the nervous system are involved and what are the possible causes?

19. A 24-year-old man who makes and drinks moonshine develops a radial nerve palsy. What is the likely cause?

20. A 25-year-old man has gait difficulty, from which his older sister also suffers. He has an ataxic gait and tremor on finger–nose and heel–shin movements. He has atrophy of the foot, calf, and hand muscles with areflexia of the plantar reflex and DTRs. He has diminished position and vibratory sensation at the ankles. His speech is scanning. What areas of the nervous system are involved? What type of disease is it?

21–25. Which nerve roots subserve the following deep tendon reflexes?

21.	Triceps	a.	C2–3
22.	Biceps	b .	C4–5
23.	Brachioradialis	c.	C5–6
24.	Knee (quadriceps)	d.	C7–8
25.	Ankle (gastrocnemius)	e.	T5–6
		f.	L1–2
		g.	L2–4
		h.	L3–5
		i.	L5–S1

26–36. Which conditions are associated with fasciculations? (Yes or No)

26.	Guillain-Barré	**31.**	Fatigue
27.	Spinal cord compression	**32.**	Porphyria

28. Amyotrophic lateral sclerosis
(ALS)

29. Insecticide poisoning

30. Werdnig-Hoffmann

33. Psychogenic stress

34. Cervical spondylosis

35. Lumbar spondylosis

36. Poliomyelitis

37. A 42-year-old man with onset of severe depression is brought to the hospital in coma with cyanosis, hypotension, and bradycardia. He has miosis, but full extraocular movements are observed on oculocephalic testing. There is flaccid, areflexic quadriplegia with fasciculations of the muscles. With what chemical has he attempted suicide? What medication is a relatively specific therapy?

38. Which of the following conditions are associated with sexual dysfunction?

    a. Peroneal nerve palsy

    b. Carpal tunnel syndrome

    c. Diabetes

    d. Poliomyelitis

    e. Multiple sclerosis

    f. Alcoholism

    g. ALS

    h. Herniated disk with L-5 or S-1 root compression

39. A 40-year-old man with rapidly advancing Guillain-Barré syndrome develops confusion, overwhelming anxiety, and then agitation. Which of the following statements are correct?

    a. He should be treated with sedation.

    b. He should be treated with tranquilizers.

    c. He may be developing hypoxia, hypercapnea, or both because of chest and diaphragm muscle paresis.

    d. He probably has "ICU psychosis."

    e. Guillain-Barré syndrome is generally not associated with CNS complications early in its course.

40. A 43-year-old man admitted to the hospital for evaluation of several months of progressively severe polyneuropathy develops agitation, hallucinations, and disorientation. Of the various causes of polyneuropathy that are associated with mental status abnormalities, which one leads to mental changes during hospitalization?

41. A 19-year-old heroin addict was found in stupor sitting on a toilet seat. After being treated with Narcan for heroin overdose, he is unable to walk because of paresis of both feet. He has absent ankle DTRs and hypalgesia of both feet. He has no bladder or bowel impairment or spine pain. What is the nature of his neurologic injury?

    a. A peripheral neuropathy

    b. A low spinal cord injury

    c. A cauda equina injury

    d. A cerebral injury

    e. Bilateral sciatic nerve injuries

42–45. A 60-year-old man who has had mitral valve stenosis and atrial fibrillation suddenly developed quadriplegia with impaired swallowing, breathing, and speaking. He required tracheostomy and a nasogastric feeding tube during the initial part of his hospitalization. Four weeks after the onset of the illness, examination reveals that he seems to be alert, establishes eye contact, and, although his eyes are immobile, he blinks appropriately to questions. His vision in both visual fields is intact. He remains quadriplegic with hyperactive DTRs and Babinski signs.

42. A preliminary evaluation should determine if the neurologic condition is caused by CNS or PNS damage. Which are the findings that are helpful in this regard?

43. Is it possible to determine if the lesion is within the cerebral cortex or the brainstem?

44. Does the localization make a difference?

45. Which neurologic tests would help distinguish brainstem from extensive cerebral lesions?

46–60. Which conditions are associated with multiple sclerosis, Guillain-Barré syndrome, both, or neither?

46. Areflexic DTRs	a. Multiple sclerosis
47. Typically follows an upper respiratory tract infection	b. Guillain-Barré syndrome
	c. Both
48. Unilateral visual loss	d. Neither

49. Paresthesias

50. Internuclear ophthalmoplegia

51. Paraparesis

52. Mental changes early in the course of the illness.

53. Specific therapy available

54. Quadriparesis

55. Recovery through remyelination

56. Leads to pseudobulbar palsy

57. Leads to bulbar palsy

58. Where emotional lability of pseudobulbar palsy is frequently mistaken for "euphoria"

59. Typically a monophasic illness that lasts several weeks

60. Sexual dysfunction frequently is the only or primary persistent deficit

ANSWERS

1. The patient has a wrist drop from compression of the radial nerve as it winds around the humerus. This is a common event in drug addicts and alcoholics who lean against their arm while stuporous.

2. She has symptoms and signs of peripheral neuropathy: paresthesias, distal weakness, areflexia, and sensory loss. In view of her systemic illness, she may have the neuropathy because of mononucleosis.

3. He probably has a herniated invertebral disk at L4–5 compressing the L-5 nerve root. Identification of the particular root or disk, however, is not as important as recognition of this source of pain and occasional neurologic deficit.

4. He has an acute spinal cord compression from a metastatic tumor with paraparesis, sensory loss below T-12, and areflexia from "spinal shock." The absence of symptoms in the upper extremities, the presence of a sensory level, and localized back pain are inconsistent with polyneuropathy.

5. The patient has bilateral sciatic nerve injury resulting in paresis of the knee flexors and all foot muscles with loss of ankle reflexes. The sciatic nerves may be compressed while sitting on a toilet seat (toilet seat neuropathy). This is the lower extremity equivalent of the wrist drop, which is also commonly encountered in drug addicts (see question 1).

6. He has symptoms and signs of cervical spondylosis with nerve root compression, which is common among laborers. It resembles ALS because of the atrophy and fasciculations, but the sensory loss precludes that diagnosis.

7. She has bilateral carpal tunnel syndrome, i.e., median nerve compression at the wrist. She has the characteristic sensory and motor disturbances with a Tinel's sign (percussion over an injured nerve creating a tingling sensation distally).

8. She has classical acute intermittent porphyria. This may be confirmed with Watson-Schwartz test or total porphyrin test of the urine. Phenothiazines may be used for the mental aberrations, but barbiturates are contraindicated.

9. She has the sudden, painless onset of a peroneal nerve injury. Commonly, it is from compression by casts, crossing the legs, or leaning against furniture. The nerve is injured at the lateral knee where it is covered only by skin and subcutaneous tissue. Sometimes diabetes or a vascular disease is the cause.

10. The loss of ankle DTRs is objective. While the other symptoms and signs (e.g., hypalgesia) can be mimicked, areflexia cannot. Heavy metals, organic solvents, and other hydrocarbons are the industrial toxins most frequently associated with neuropathies.

11. She had developed injuries to the right common peroneal, left radial, and right abducens nerves. This is a case of mononeuritis multiplex, which usually results from vasculitis, diabetes, or leprosy. Since she is hypertensive, vasculitis is most likely.

12. While many injuries may affect the spinal cord, there is no objective evidence of neurologic disease in this patient. The apparent paraplegia is not accompanied by reflex changes. More important, he is able to feel temperature changes but not pinprick sensations, which are carried by the same pathways. He seems to have no neurologic abnormality.

13. He has had damage to the right femoral nerve, which has resulted in paresis of the quadriceps muscle and loss of its associated reflex. A diabetic infarction is the most likely cause.

14. He probably has a herniated L5–S1 intervertebral disk that compresses the S1 root on the left.

15. He has an obvious case of ALS with bulbar and pseudobulbar palsy, as well as wasting of the muscles of the extremities. There is involvement of the corticobulbar and corticospinal tracts, brainstem nuclei, and spinal anterior horn cells.

16. He has bilateral "tardy" (slowly developing) ulnar nerve palsies, probably from pressure on the ulnar nerves at the elbows. This is an occupational hazard of watchmakers and draftsmen, who lean on their elbows while working.

17. Clearly ALS should be considered because of the atrophy and fasciculations, but the back pain and sensory loss are inconsistent. Lumbar spondylosis, which is far more common than ALS, is the more likely disorder in this case because of the back pain and hypalgesia.

18. She has involvement of the cerebral cortex, as evidenced by the memory impairment and convulsion. She also has a peripheral neuropathy, indicated by the classical symptoms of dysesthesia, distal sensory loss, and areflexia. Since she has organomegaly, jaundice, and a history of weight loss, a systemic illness must be considered as a cause of the combination of CNS and PNS disease. Malignancies, hepatitis, and toxins are possible, but alcoholism is the most common cause of this combination of CNS and PNS findings.

19. Lead pipes used in illegal distillation cause lead intoxication. A compression neuropathy is also possible.

20. He has impairment of the cerebellum, peripheral nerves, and of posterior columns of the spinal cord, all of which indicate a spinocerebellar degeneration (e.g., Friedreich's ataxia).

21.	d	**29.**	Yes
22.	c	**30.**	Yes
23.	c	**31.**	Yes
24.	g	**32.**	No
25.	i	**33.**	Yes
26.	No	**34.**	Yes
27.	No	**35.**	Yes
28.	Yes	**36.**	Yes

37. He most likely has taken an insecticide that has marked anticholinesterase activity.

He should be treated with atropine, 2–4 mg intravenously, and with additional doses at frequent intervals thereafter.

38. a. No
   b. No
   c. Yes

   d. No
   e. Yes
   f. No

   g. No
   h. No

39. c. Hypoxia is a common complication of Guillain-Barré syndrome that often appears as anxiety and agitation.

   d. Most patients who are thought to have an "ICU psychosis" actually have underlying cerebral dysfunction.

   e. Guillain-Barré syndrome is rarely associated with central nervous system dysfunction.

   (a and b are incorrect: sedatives and tranquilizers might depress respirations.)

40. Alcoholic polyneuropathy is associated with delirium tremens (DTs) when hospitalized alcoholic patients do not receive alcohol. Such patients also may develop alcohol withdrawal seizures.

41. e. Drug addicts who overdose while sitting on a toilet seat, which is a common occurrence, press on their sciatic nerves with almost their full weight. Such sciatic nerve damage, called "toilet seat neuropathy," leads to paresis of lower leg muscles and loss of ankle DTRs. The bladder and bowel muscles are unaffected because their nerves are not involved. He would have had bladder and bowel dysfunction if he had had injury to the spinal cord, cauda equina, or cerebrum. A peripheral neuropathy was unlikely to have developed immediately.

42. The hyperactive DTRs and Babinski signs indicate the origin of the problem is CNS damage and that the PNS is intact.

43. A large pontine-medullary injury has caused oculomotor paresis as well as quadriparesis and apnea. While many such cases are difficult to diagnose and some may result from lesions in both regions, this patient seems to have a single lesion confined to the lower brainstem.

Despite the devastating paresis, his mental, visual, and upper brainstem functions are intact. Most important, he can communicate, albeit only by blinking his eyes. He has a well-known syndrome, "the locked-in syndrome" (Chapter 11). Patients who are locked-in may be mistaken for being comatose, demented, or vegetative.

Cerebral lesions do not cause either oculomotor paresis or apnea, even as part of pseudobulbar palsy. Also, cerebral lesions would generally not cause quadriparesis.

44. The localization of the lesion is important because if the damage is confined to the brainstem, as in this case, intellectual function is preserved. If the patient had suffered extensive cerebral damage, he would have had irreversible dementia. The presence or absence of mental function generally determines the appropriate nature and effort given to rehabilitation.

45. While a CT scan might be performed to detect or exclude a cerebral lesion, current CT technology is not sufficiently sensitive to detect many brainstem lesions. An EEG in this case would be the best available test because it would show a relatively normal pattern since the cerebral hemispheres are intact. Other suitable tests are also electrophysiologic studies. Visually evoked responses (VERs) will determine the integrity of the visual system, which is largely a function of the optic nerves and *cerebral hemispheres.* Brainstem auditory evoked responses (BAERs) will determine the integrity of the auditory circuits, which are predominantly *brainstem* functions.

46. b
47. b
48. a
49. c
50. a

51. c
52. d
53. d
54. c
55. b

56. a
57. b
58. a
59. b
60. a

6

Muscle Disorders

Patients with muscle diseases, including disorders of the neuromuscular junction, characteristically complain of weakness and may have findings that mimic CNS or PNS illness. These symptoms and signs, though relatively common, are easily overlooked or misinterpreted by the untrained examiner. Worse still, patients suffering from muscle diseases are frequently diagnosed erroneously as "neurotic." This chapter will present discussions of myasthenia gravis, which is a disease of the neuromuscular junction, and several diseases of the muscles themselves, *myopathies.* It will then review the relevant laboratory tests for diseases of nerve, neuromuscular junction, and muscle.

The pertinent anatomy and pathologic alterations of muscle disorders are simple. Dilations at the nerve endings contain packets of acetylcholine (ACh) that are released across the neuromuscular junction. When ACh contacts and depolarizes a muscular ACh receptor site, a muscular contraction is initiated. Diseases may be due to abnormalities in the functioning of the neuromuscular junction or the muscle itself (myopathies) (Fig. 6-1).

Generally, whenever muscle disorders occur, the muscles will be weak and their DTRs hypoactive. Various disorders primarily affect combinations of ocular, facial, bulbar, and *proximal* limb muscles. The muscular sphincters of the bladder and bowel, however, are practically never affected.

In contrast to PNS disorders, the distal limb muscles in muscle diseases are, with rare exceptions, relatively unaffected and there is never sensory loss. Also, with several exceptions, muscular diseases are not associated with mental impairment. (The similarities and differences between CNS, PNS, and muscular diseases are outlined in Table 6-1.)

MYASTHENIA GRAVIS*

Myasthenia gravis, which affects the neuromuscular junction, is usually a disease of young women and older men that is characterized by intermittent, asymmetrical

---

*Patients with myasthenia gravis may receive assistance from the Myasthenia Gravis Foundation, Suite 304, 711 South Broadway, White Plains, New York 10601, (914) 328-1717.

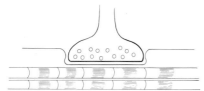

Fig. 6-1. At the neuromuscular junction, the nerve ending contains packets of acetylcholine (ACh). When released across the junction, ACh depolarizes specific receptor sites, triggering a muscle contraction.

weakness of the facial, extraocular, and bulbar muscles. While myasthenia usually occurs alone, it sometimes is associated with hyperthyroidism or mediastinal thymomas. The underlying problem seems to be that abnormal antibodies adhere to the neuromuscular ACh receptor, blocking normal deplorization and causing paresis (Fig. 6-2).

Almost 90 percent of myasthenia patients will first complain of diplopia and ptosis because of paresis of the ocular muscles. Characteristically, a patient with myasthenia will grimace when attempting to smile because of weakness of the facial muscles (Fig. 6-3). Speech will have a nasal quality because of nasopharyngeal muscle paresis. Ocular, facial, and vocal weakness will be exaggerated if the patient makes the sustained effort either voluntarily or on the request of the examiner. For example, ocular weakness will worsen with prolonged upward gaze, and speech will sound even more nasal during long conversations. In moderately advanced cases, the neck, shoulder, and respiratory muscles will become weak, while in severe cases apnea and quadriplegia may develop.

Several negative findings are important. Although extraocular muscles may be severely involved, intraocular muscles are spared. Therefore, despite paresis of the eyelids and eyeball motion, the pupils are equal, of normal size, round, and reactive to light. Even though there may be quadriparesis, the bladder and bowel sphincters will be unaffected. Of course, there is no sensory loss.

The physician's clinical diagnosis of myasthenia gravis can be confirmed by use of a Tensilon test in which 10 mg of edrophonium chloride (Tensilon) is administered intravenously. Saline is injected before or after as a control. Patients with myasthenia will have a dramatic reversal of ocular and facial weakness that lasts for several minutes. This will occur because Tensilon inhibits degradation of ACh by acetylcholinesterase, causing an increased ACh concentration that is better able to depolarize the remaining muscle ACh receptor sites.

Treatment of myasthenia gravis has rested on long-acting oral preparations that, like Tensilon, impede degradation of ACh. Recently, the administration of steroids

Table 6-1
Signs of CNS, PNS, and Muscle Disorders

	CNS	PNS	Muscle
Paresis	Pattern*	Distal	Proximal
Muscle tone	Spastic	Flaccid	Sometimes tender or dystrophic
DTRs	Hyperactive	Hypoactive	Normal or hypoactive
Babinski signs	Yes	No	No
Sensory loss	Pattern	Stocking-glove	None

* Hemiparesis, paraparesis, etc.

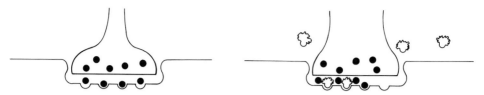

Fig. 6-2. (Left) Normally, packets of acetylcholine (ACh) (darkened circles) cross the neuromuscular junction, bind onto muscle ACh receptors, and initiate muscle contraction. The ACh is then metabolized by the enzyme *acetylcholinesterase.* (Right) In myasthenia gravis, abnormal antibodies (tufted circles) adhere to many ACh receptors and prevent ACh binding. However, remaining ACh receptor activity can be enhanced by inhibiting ACh metabolism with *anticholinesterases,* such as edrophonium (Tensilon) and physostigmine. (Physostigmine is also used experimentally to raise the abnormally low cerebral ACh concentrations in Alzheimer's disease [see Chapter 7]).

and the use of plasmaphersis have been found to help patients with myasthenia gravis, presumably by removing the antibodies from the ACh receptors. Of course, elimination of hyperthyroidism or mediastinal thymomas will improve or even eliminate myasthenia.

Several diseases have clinical findings similar to those of myasthenia gravis. One commonly encountered is psychogenic "easy fatigability," in which patients, generally middle-aged women, complain of dyspnea on exertion, or inability to walk, weakness of their arms, and even intermittent double vision. On manual muscle testing, they may seem to have "weakness" of the arms and wrists. They will, however, have full functional ability and be able to walk, climb stairs, and dress. Moreover, they will not have asymmetric weakness or extraocular muscle palsy.

Diagnosis of other conditions that affect the ocular, facial, and bulbar muscles requires astute observation. Lesions of the third cranial nerve from midbrain infarctions or compression by aneurysms of the posterior communicating artery can cause extraocular muscle paresis similar to that observed in myasthenia. The difference,

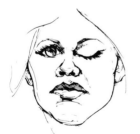 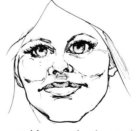

Fig. 6-3. (Left) This young woman with myasthenia gravis developed a weakened left eyelid following several days of double vision. Besides the ptosis, she has little facial expression because of facial muscle weakness. In particular, she has loss of the contour of the right nasolabial fold and a sagging lower lip. (Right) After edrophonium (Tensilon), 10 mg, is administered intravenously, she has a brief but dramatic restoration of eyelid, ocular, and facial strength.

which is subtle, is that in these disorders, the pupil will be widely dilated and unreactive to light because the intraocular (pupillary) muscles are also affected. Nevertheless, ALS, in particular, will still continue to present diagnostic difficulties. Amyotrophic lateral sclerosis may be diagnosed because it is a more extensive illness than myasthenia and does not involve either the intraocular or extraocular muscles. In any case, of all the diseases causing ocular, facial, or bulbar palsy, only myasthenia gravis responds to the Tensilon test.

MUSCLE DISEASES (MYOPATHIES)

Numerous patients will have *myopathies*. As would be expected, they will usually complain primarily of weakness. In most myopathies, the shoulder and hip girdle muscles, i.e., the proximal muscles, will be affected first, most severely, and often exclusively. These muscle groups, which have the greatest bulk, are indispensable for standing, climbing stairs, combing hair, and reaching upwards; however, even when their weakness is extensive and severe, patients will have no oculomotor or sphincter paresis.

Patients with inflammatory myopathies will have muscle aches, *myalgias,* along with weakness. When affected muscles are palpated, patients usually have tenderness. When myopathies lead to loss of muscle bulk, the atrophy is called *dystrophy.*

The DTRs are hypoactive roughly in proportion to the degree of paresis of the muscle. Babinski signs, of course, would not be elicitable. Finally, with rare exceptions (two of which are described below), mental aberrations are not associated with myopathies.

Clinically Important Myopathies

While there are many causes of myopathies, the physician should be particularly aware of those that occur frequently, are associated with mental aberrations, or indicate a systemic illness.

*Duchenne's muscular dystrophy** is a frequently occurring, sex-linked genetic illness with expression in childhood, i.e., it develops in boys. This muscular dystrophy begins as weakness of the thighs and shoulders. Therefore, boys who have it have trouble with athletic activities, especially riding bicycles. Since the muscles are infiltrated with abnormal cells, they appear bulky, *pseudohypertrophied,* so that the weakness appears paradoxical, occurring as it does in conjunction with apparently excellent development (Fig. 6-4). By the end of childhood, as the dystrophy evolves, these children become wheelchair-bound and have respiratory insufficiency.

On careful evaluation, Duchenne's dystrophy has been found to be accompanied by mild mental retardation, making it one of the few myopathies associated with mental impairment. Techniques have been introduced to identify female carriers of the trait and to detect the disease in utero.

---

*Patients with muscular dystrophy and related disorders may receive assistance from the Muscular Dystrophy Association of America, 810 Seventh Avenue, New York, New York 10019, (212) 586-0808.

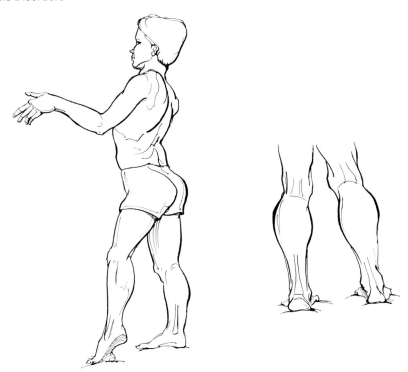

Fig. 6-4. This 10-year-old boy with typical Duchenne's muscular dystrophy has a waddling gait and inability to raise his arms above his head because of weakness of the shoulder and pelvic girdle muscles. His calves and other weakened muscles are characteristically enlarged, *pseudohypertrophied,* because of cellular infiltration. There is also a typical exaggeration of the normal inward curve of the lumbar spine, *hyperlordosis.* Such children with Duchenne's muscular dystrophy have frequently been pictured on fund-raising posters.

Myotonic dystrophy is a myopathy inherited as an autosomal dominant trait. Unlike Duchenne's muscular dystrophy and most other myopathies, in this illness facial and proximal limb muscles become dystrophic. More striking, muscles have persistent contractions, *myotonia,* for several seconds. For example, patients are unable to release their grip after opening a door or shaking hands.

Various nonneurologic abnormalities are associated with the dystrophy and myotonia. Loss of temple hair, i.e., frontal balding, is combined with facial muscle atrophy, leading to a facial appearance that is sunken, elongated, and characterized by ptosis and a prominent forehead (Fig. 6-5). Other associated abnormalities include cataracts, cardiac conduction system disturbances, and endocrinologic abnormalities, such as testicular atrophy, diabetes, and infertility.

Besides Duchenne's dystrophy, myotonic dystrophy is the only frequently occurring myopathy associated with mental status abnormalities. Patients are often described as having personality disorders, blunted affect, and limited intelligence and initiative, but they do not tend to develop psychosis.

Polymyositis is a muscle inflammation or infection characterized by myalgias and tenderness. Weakness is usually mild, although occasionally it can be severe enough

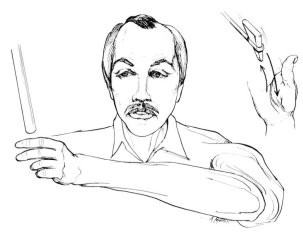

Fig. 6-5. This young man with myotonic dystrophy has the typically elongated face caused by temporal and facial muscles wasting, hairline recession, and ptosis. Because of myotonia, when his thenar eminence is struck with a percussion hammer, it undergoes a forceful, sustained contraction that pulls the thumb against his palm for 3 to 10 seconds. Also, he cannot rapidly release his grasp after clutching any object.

to be transiently debilitating. Unlike other myopathies, polymyositis is usually accompanied by signs of systemic illness, typically fever and malaise. Most often it is caused by a benign, self-limited systemic viral illness. In older adults, unlike children, polymyositis is often associated with underlying pulmonary or gastrointestinal malignancies.

Trichinosis is a special variety of polymyositis that is caused by *Trichinella* infection from eating insufficiently cooked pork or game.

Finally, polymyalgia rheumatica, polyarteritis nodosa, and other systemic inflammatory diseases are routinely complicated by polymyositis.

Steroid myopathy is caused by the prolonged use of oral or parenteral steroid medications. Aside from the lack of pain, it is similar to other myopathies. Discontinuing the steroids restores muscle strength after several months. Another iatrogenic disorder, *hypokalemic myopathy,* is usually caused by taking diuretics without potassium supplements. It is painless and readily reversible if the medication is stopped.

Some rare myopathies are noteworthy. Patients with *periodic paralysis,* which is an inherited condition, suffer one-hour to eight-hour episodes of quadriparesis because of transient hypokalemia. In *hyperthyroid myopathy,* weakness develops as part of an obvious systemic illness. Finally, muscle weakness and, frequently, cramps are hallmarks of Pompe's disease and McArdle's disease, rare inherited glycogen-storage diseases that are "important" biochemically rather than medically.

The Neuroleptic Malignant Syndrome

The neuroleptic malignant syndrome (NMS) is a rarely occurring disorder that is characterized by muscular rigidity so intense that it leads to *rhabdomyolysis* (muscle necrosis), hyperpyrexia (fevers of 103°F to 106°F), and, usually, obtundation. Those patients who remain alert are mute and seemingly cataleptic. Most have tachycardia, diaphoresis, and tremulousness. Their course is often complicated by renal failure, because of myoglobinemia, and cardiovascular collapse, which produces a mortality rate of 20 percent to 40 percent for the illness.

Neuroleptic malignant syndrome follows administration of medications that block dopamine transmission. It has been described most often in patients after they have received haloperidol (Haldol) and various phenothiazines, particularly fluphenazine (Prolixin). Those people with pre-existing brain damage, young men, and all people with physical exhaustion and dehydration are more susceptible. The underlying cause is unknown, but it is postulated to be an idiosyncratic reaction in which dopamine blockade in the basal ganglia produces muscular rigidity that is so extraordinarily intense that muscle tissue is crushed.

Laboratory studies typically show an elevated BUN level (reflecting dehydration, renal failure, or both) and a markedly elevated CPK level (because of rhabdomyolysis). The EEG is normal or has only mild, diffuse slowing, which is indicative of either a toxic disorder or use of psychotropic medicines (Chapter 10). Treatment includes stopping the neuroleptic medicine and providing fluids and antipyretics. The use of bromocriptine, dantrolene (Dantrium), or cogentin has been suggested.

Neuroleptic malignant syndrome is similar to malignant hyperthermia, which is an inherited muscle disorder in which general anesthesia leads to widespread rhabdomyolysis, hyperpyrexia, and brain damage. Likewise, hallucinogen ingestion, delirium tremens (DTs), alcohol intoxication, and catatonia all may be associated with muscle necrosis, elevated CPK levels, fever, and altered mental states; however, in these cases the muscle necrosis is less severe and the fever less elevated.

LABORATORY TESTS FOR NERVE AND MUSCLE DISEASE

Nerve Conduction Velocity (NCV) Studies

Determining the NCV can isolate the site of nerve damage, confirm a clinical diagnosis of polyneuropathy, and distinguish polyneuropathy from myopathy. The NCV is normally 50–70 m/sec (Fig. 6-6). If a nerve is damaged or trapped, the NCV will be slowed at the point of injury, which can be located by proper placement of the electrodes, e.g., across the carpal tunnel. In diabetic polyneuropathy, the NCV of all nerves will be slowed, typically to between 20 and 30 m/sec. In contrast, with a myopathy, the NCV will be normal. The cost of this test (1985) is about $50 for each nerve studied.

Electromyography (EMG)

Electromyographic studies are performed by inserting fine needles into selected muscles. The examiner observes the consequent electrical discharges on an oscilloscope during complete muscle rest, voluntary contractions, and stimulation of the innervating peripheral nerve.

Electromyographic abnormalities almost always occur whenever a myopathy is

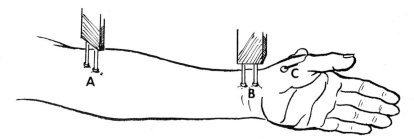

Fig. 6-6. In determining nerve conduction velocity (NCV), a stimulating electrode that is placed at points (A and B) along a nerve excites the appropriate muscle (C). The distances between the electrode and the responding muscle and the time intervals between nerve stimulation and muscle response are calculated to provide the NCV, which is normally 50–70 m/sec.

present. Virtually all the muscles will have abnormal, *myopathic,* EMG patterns. In addition, with several diseases, e.g., myasthenia gravis, ALS, and myotonic dystrophy, distinctive patterns are observable.

Abnormal EMG patterns may also be found with mononeuropathies and peripheral neuropathy because muscles develop changes if their nerves are damaged. Thus, EMGs will assist in determining which peripheral nerve or nerve root, if any, is damaged. This test is particularly useful in cases of low back pain when attempting to document nerve damage from herniated disks.

Electromyography studies cost between $250 and $500, depending on how many muscles are studied.

Serum Enzyme Determinations

Creative phosphokinase (CPK), lactic dehydrogenase (LDH), and serum glutamic-oxaloacetic transaminase (SGOT) are enzymes concentrated within muscle cells that escape into the bloodstream when muscles are damaged. Increases in their serum concentration are roughly proportional to the severity of muscle damage, being highest in NMS and similar disorders. Patients with peripheral neuropathy, of course, will have normal enzyme concentrations. Therefore, for patients with unexplained, ill-defined weakness, as well as ones with an apparent myopathy or NMS, the first specific laboratory test should be a determination of serum CPK, LDH, and SGOT levels. The cost is $15 to $50.

Muscle Biopsy

In expert hands, microscopic examination of muscle is useful when muscular atrophy might be the result of a neuropathy, ALS, or myopathy. Specific muscle disorders that might be diagnosed in this way include polymyositis, trichinosis, collagen-vascular diseases, and the rare glycogen-storage diseases. Nerve biopsy, on the other hand, is not performed routinely, since it is useful in uncovering only a few rare diseases.

SUMMARY

Muscle disorders are characterized by weakness. In many acute cases there is also myalgia and tenderness. In chronic cases, dystrophy develops.

Myasthenia gravis, a neuromuscular junction disorder, is characterized by ocular and facial weakness that responds briefly to the Tensilon test. Duchenne's dystrophy and myotonic dystrophy are relatively common inherited muscle disorders accompanied by mental impairments. Polymyositis and steroid myopathy, two frequent conditions in adults, are often manifestations of systemic illness and excessive medication, respectively. Neuroleptic malignant syndrome (NMS) and similar disorders are characterized by muscle necrosis (rhabdomyolysis) that is so severe that myoglobinemia may cause renal failure.

Various tests are readily available. Electromyograms are used mostly to detect myopathies and ALS; NCV studies are used mostly for confirming polyneuropathy, detecting the site of nerve damage, and differentiating nerve damage from herniated discs; and determinations of serum CPK, LDH, and SGOT concentrations are used to confirm muscle injuries, such as polymyositis and NMS.

REFERENCES

Granato, GE, Stern BJ, Ringel A: Neuroleptic malignant syndrome: Successful treatment with dantrolene and bromocriptine. Ann Neurol 14:89, 1983

Guze, BH, Baxter, LR: Neuroleptic malignant syndrome. N Engl J Med 313:163, 1985

Rodriguez M, Gomez MR, Howard FM, et al: Myasthenia gravis in children: Long-term follow-up. Ann Neurol 13:504, 1983

Smego RA, Durack DT: The neuroleptic malignant syndrome. Arch Intern Med 142:1183, 1983

QUESTIONS

1–3. A 17-year-old woman who complains of occasional double vision while looking to the left, has no headache or loss of acuity in either eye. She has right-sided ptosis and difficulty keeping her right eye adducted. Her pupils are 4mm, round, and reactive. Her speech is nasal and her neck flexor muscles are weak. There is no paresis of the limbs or corticospinal tract findings.

    1. Which diseases might explain the ocular abnormalities?

        a. Multiple sclerosis
        b. Psychogenic weakness
        c. Myasthenia gravis
        d. Right posterior communicating artery aneurysm

    2. Which test is most likely to be helpful?

        a. EEG
        b. NCV
        c. EMG
        d. Tensilon test
        e. Muscle enzymes: CPK, LDH, SGOT

3. Which conditions may also be present?
    a. Hypothyroidism
    b. Hyperthyroidism
    c. Bell's palsy
    d. Thymoma

4–5.   Another 17-year-old woman, who is a dancer, develops progressive weakness of the toes and ankles. On examination, she has only mild paresis in those areas, loss of only the ankle reflex, unresponsive plantar reflex, and decreased sensation in the toes and feet.

4. Which diseases might explain her symptoms and signs?
    a. Myasthenia
    b. Toxic polyneuropathy
    c. Polymyositis
    d. Guillain-Barré syndrome
    e. Thoracic spinal cord tumor

5. Which tests would be most likely to be helpful in making a diagnosis?
    a. EEG
    b. Nerve conduction velocities
    c. EMG
    d. Tensilon test
    e. Muscle enzymes: CPK, LDH, SGOT

6–11.   A 6-year-old boy is beginning to have difficulty standing upright. He has to push himself up on his legs in order to stand. He has not been able to run since the age of four. A cousin of the same age has a similar problem. The patient is well built and has a normal examination aside from paresis of his upper leg muscles and decreased quadriceps (knee) reflexes.

6. What disease is the patient likely to have?
    a. Porphyria   d. Duchenne's muscular dystrophy
    b. Peripheral neuropathy   e. A psychogenic disorder
    c. Spinal cord tumor   f. Kugelberg-Welander disease

7. What tests will help diagnose the case?
    a. EEG
    b. Nerve conduction velocities
    c. Electromyograms
    d. Tensilon test
    e. Muscle enzymes

8. What is the sex of the cousin?
    a. Male
    b. Female
    c. Either

9. Who is the carrier of the condition?
    a. Mother
    b. Father
    c. Either

10.   How can a sister of the patient know if she is a carrier?

11.   What percentage of a carrier's children will also be carriers or have the disease?

12–15.   A 68-year-old man has aches and tenderness of the shoulder muscles. He is unable to lift his arms above his head. There is a blotchy red rash about his head, neck, and upper torso.

12. What diseases should be considered?

    a. Steroid myopathy
    b. Dermatomyositis
    c. Polyneuropathy
    d. Periodic paralysis
    e. Myasthenia
    f. Trichinosis

13. Which tests are most likely to confirm the diagnosis?

    a. EEG
    b. Nerve conduction velocities
    c. EMG
    d. Tensilon test
    e. Muscle enzymes
    f. Skin and muscle biopsy
    g. Nerve biopsy

14. Which conditions are associated with dermatomyositis in the adult?

    a. Congestive heart failure
    b. Pulmonary malignancies
    c. Diabetes mellitus
    d. Gastrointestinal malignancies
    e. Tuberculosis
    f. Polyarteritis nodosa

15. Which of the above conditions are associated with polymyositis in the child?

16–24. Which medications are associated with myopathies or neuropathies?

16. Prednisone

17. Chlorpromazine

18. Nitrofurantoin
    a. Neuropathy
    b. Myopathy
    c. Neither
    d. Both

19. Isoniazid (INH)

20. Hydrochlorothiazide

21. Amitriptyline

22. Thyroid extract

23. Lithium carbonate

24. Phenytoin (Dilantin)

25–27. A 50-year-old man develops low back pain and difficulty walking. He has mild weakness in both legs, a distended bladder, diminished sensation to pinprick below the umbilicus, and equivocal plantar and DTRs. He has tenderness of the midthoracic spine.

25. With which conditions are his symptoms and signs most consistent?

    a. Polymyositis
    b. Herniated lumbar intervertebral disk
    c. Idiopathic polyneuropathy
    d. Thoracic spinal cord compression

26. If the routine history, physical examination, and laboratory tests, including a chest x-ray film, were normal, which of the following tests should be performed next?

    a. CT scan of the head
    b. X-ray studies of the lumbosacral spine
    c. Myelogram
    d. Tensilon test
    e. Muscle enzyme determination

27. The above test confirms the clinical impression. If such conditions do not receive prompt, effective treatment, which complications might ensue?

    a. Sacral decubitus ulcers

    b. Urinary incontinence
    c. Permanent paraplegia
    d. Hydronephrosis and urosepsis

28. Which of the following are complications of excessive or prolonged use of steroids?
    a. Obesity, especially of the face and trunk
    b. Steroid myopathy
    c. Lumbar spine compression fractures causing severe low back pain
    d. "Psychosis"
    e. Opportunistic lung and CNS infections
    f. Gastrointestinal bleeding
    g. Easy bruisability

29. A 31-year-old woman, who suffers from systemic lupus erythematosis (SLE) and has been treated for 10 months with prednisone (40 mg daily), develops agitation, hallucinations, and confusion. Aside from a temperature of 100.5°F, routine history, general physical and neurologic examination, and laboratory tests do not reveal a cause for the mental changes or a source of the fever. Which of the following tests or procedures should be attempted and in which order?
    a. Stop the steroids
    b. Begin haloperidol or another major tranquilizer
    c. Do a CT scan of the head
    d. Perform a lumbar puncture
    e. Raise the steroid dosage

30. A 75-year-old woman is hospitalized for congestive heart failure and placed on a low salt diet and given a potent diuretic. Although her congestive heart failure resolves, she develops somnolence, disorientation, and generalized weakness. What is the most likely explanation of her mental status change?
    a. Hypokalemia (low potassium)
    b. A cerebrovascular infarction
    c. A subdural hematoma
    d. Cerebral hypoxia from congestive heart failure
    e. Dehydration, hyponatremia, and hypokalemia

31. Which myopathies are associated with mental impairment?
    a. Polymyositis
    b. Duchenne's muscular dystrophy
    c. Carpal tunnel syndrome
    d. Myotonic dystrophy
    e. Periodic paralysis

32–37. Match the illness with its probable or usual cause:

32. Polymyositis in childhood		a.	Autosomal inheritance
33. Myotonic dystrophy		b.	Sex-linked recessive inheritance
34. Hypokalemic myopathy		c.	Parisitic infection
35. Trichinosis		d.	Viral illness
36. Duchenne's muscular dystrophy		e.	Underlying malignancy
37. Myasthenia gravis		f.	ACh receptor antibodies
		g.	Midications

38–50. Match the illness or condition with the appropriate diagnostic test(s):

38. Carpal tunnel syndrome	a.	Nerve conduction velocities
39. Spinal cord compression		(NCVs)

40. ALS
41. Porphyria (acute intermittent)
42. Polymyositis
43. Optic neuritis
44. Herniated lumbar intervertebral disk
45. Left hemiparesis from a cerebrovascular accident
46. Uremic polyneuropathy
47. Myotonic dystrophy
48. Duchenne's muscular dystrophy
49. Guillain-Barré syndrome
50. Poliomyelitis

b. Electromyograms (EMG)
c. CPK, LDH, and SGOT serum concentrations
d. Myelogram
e. None of the above

51–56. Match the phenomenon with the myopathy:

51. Unilateral ptosis
52. Facial rash
53. Waddling gait
54. Inability to release a fist
55. Pseudohypertrophy of calf muscles
56. Premature balding and cataracts

a. Myasthenia gravis
b. Duchenne's dystrophy
c. Myotonic dystrophy
d. Polymositis

57. Myasthenia gravis is a disorder in which antibodies damage the postsynaptic neuromuscular ACh receptor. Which of the following therapies are helpful?

a. Giving steroids to reduce the abnormal immunologic reaction
b. Performing plasmapheresis to draw ACh antibodies out of the bloodstream
c. Giving medications that enhance the effectiveness of acetylcholinesterase
d. Giving medications that impair the effectiveness of acetylcholinesterase
e. Giving medications that cross the blood–brain barrier
f. Performing a thymectomy if a thymoma is detected.

ANSWERS

1. This is a classical case of myasthenia gravis with ocular, pharyngeal, and neck flexor paresis, but no pupil abnormality(c).

a. No. This pattern of neck flexor paresis, ocular muscle weakness, and ptosis does not occur in multiple sclerosis (MS). Internuclear ophthalmoplegia, which does occur frequently in MS, is manifested by nystagmus in the abducting eye as well as paresis of the adducting eye.
b. No. It is virtually impossible to mimic either paresis of one ocular muscle or ptosis.
c. Yes
d. Very unlikely. Aneurysmal compression of the third cranial nerve does produce ptosis and paresis of adduction, but it has a painful onset and the pupil becomes large and unreactive to light. Furthermore, the bulbar palsy could not be explained by an aneurysm.

2. d
3. b, d

   4. She has distal lower extremity paresis, areflexia, and hypalgesia, which indicate a polyneuropathy (b or d).

   a. No. She has sensory loss. Furthermore, myasthenia rarely affects the legs alone.
   b. Yes. A toxic cause, e.g., alcohol or chemical, is possible.
   c. No. There is sensory loss, which precludes pure muscle disease as well as neuromuscular disorders.
   d. Yes. An inflammatory process is statistically most likely.
   e. No. The ankle reflexes are not hyperactive and Babinski signs are not present. Besides the absence of corticospinal tract signs, there is no "sensory level."

   5. a. No
   b. NCVs will confirm the presence of a peripheral neuropathy, although they will not suggest a particular cause.
   c. No
   d. No
   d. No
   c. No

   6. This is a typical case of Duchenne's muscular dystrophy. The patient and his cousin have Gower's sign: standing upright by pressing against one's legs. Characteristically, the muscles are apparently hypertrophic in the early stages (d).

   a. and b. No. The patient's paresis is proximal, and he has no sensory loss.
   c. No. The course is too long, deep tendon reflexes are hypoactive, and pathological reflexes are not present.
   d. Yes
   e. No. The loss of reflexes and the pattern of weakness rule against a psychogenic origin.
   f. No. Kugelberg-Welander disease is a rare hereditary form of motor neuron disease, similar to ALS, which affects infants and young boys and girls. The muscles are characteristically atrophied early in the course, unlike Duchenne's muscular dystrophy.

   7. a. No
   b. Possibly. NCVs might exclude peripheral nerve diseases.
   c. Yes. The affected muscle in muscular dystrophy will have abnormal (myopathic potential) patterns.
   d. No
   e. Yes. The CPK, LDH, and SGOT will be elevated.

   8. Male. It is a sex-linked (recessive) trait.

   9. The mother.

   10. She can have the serum CPK level measured. An elevation will suggest she is a carrier.

   11. One half of the boys and one half of the girls will receive the disease-linked X chromosome. The boys who receive it will develop the disease, whereas the girls who receive it will only be carriers. Therefore, 25 percent of the children (one half of the boys) will have the disease and 25 percent of the children (one half of the girls) will be asymptomatic carriers.

   12. The muscle pain, tenderness, and paresis suggest an inflammatory myopathy (b, f).

   a. No. Steroid and most other metabolically induced myopathies are painless.
   b. Yes. He has a florid rash as well as clinical signs of polymyositis.
   c. No
   d. No. This man has persistent, painful symptoms.

    e. No

    f. Yes. The rash and muscle symptoms and signs can be found in both dermatomyositis and trichinosis.

13. a. No

    b. No

    c. Yes. But the EMG would only confirm an overly apparent diagnosis.

    d. No. While patients with myasthenia may have weakness of the shoulder muscles, it is not painful or associated with a rash.

    e. Yes. There will be a marked elevation in concentrations of serum CPK, LDH, and SGOT.

    f. Yes. This will confirm the diagnosis of dermatomyositis and would identify vasculitis and Trichinella as possible causes.

    g. No

14. b, d, f

15. None. In children, polymyositis is usually associated only with viral illnesses or remains unexplained.

16. b

17. c

18. a

19. a

20. b (via hypokalemia)

21. c

22. b (hyperthyroid myopathy)

23. c

24. a

25. d. The patient has symptoms and signs of spinal cord compression at T-10, as indicated by the sensory "level" at the umbilicus. Metastatic tumors are the most frequent cause of spinal cord compression, but herniated *thoracic* intervertebral disks, multiple sclerosis, tuberculous abscesses, and trauma might also cause such a spinal cord injury. Polymyositis is an incorrect answer because this condition affects the arms as well as the legs and does not involve bladder muscles or cause loss of sensation. Also, while it causes myalgias, polymyositis does not cause spine pain or tenderness.

26. c. A myelogram would be performed to confirm spinal cord compression, determine its exact location, and indicate its nature. In the future, however, CT scans of the spine will probably replace myelography as the appropriate diagnostic test.

27. a, b, c, d. Thoracic spinal cord compression causes urinary and bladder obstruction, because of sphincter paresis, as well as paraplegia. Urinary catheters, despite the risk of obstruction and sepsis, might be used. Also, even with good nursing care, pressure from every bony prominence leads to ankle, knee, and hip as well as sacral decubitus ulcers.

28. a–g.

29. b, e, c, d. The main diagnostic problem in this case is to determine whether the patient suffers from too much steroid medication, i.e., steroid psychosis, or too little medication, i.e., lupus cerebritis. Alternatively, the use of steroids may have been complicated by an opportunistic CNS infection, such as tuberculosis or cryptococcal meningitis. While diagnostic tests are being undertaken, the psychosis must be controlled since it interferes with testing and is troublesome itself. Such patients should be given major tranquilizers (b). The question of stopping or raising steroids is best answered by raising them (e) because lupus cerebritis is statistically more likely to be present than steroid psychosis and prednisone at only 40 mg daily is not likely to have caused steroid psychosis. Moreover, since the patient is under physical and psychiatric stress, she might develop adrenal crisis if the steroids were stopped abruptly.

A CT scan (c) should be performed, if feasible, to exclude the possibility of an intracranial mass lesion, such as an abscess or a subdural hematoma. After a CT scan is done and if no mass lesion is detected, then a lumbar puncture (d) should be performed to examine the CSF, especially for indications of infection.

30. e. Administration of potent diuretics to patients on low salt diets eventually leads to hyponatremia and dehydration, which cause obtundation and confusion, especially in the elderly. Low potassium concentrations alone, however, do not cause mental abnormalities. The other possibilities are very unlikely.

31. b, d.

32. d	**34.** g	**36.** b
33. a	**35.** c	**37.** f

38. a. NCV studies will show a block of the affected wrist.

39. d.

40. b. EMG studies will reveal fibrillations, which are, roughly, the electrical counterpart of fasciculations.

41. e. Although NCVs might show slowed conduction, that finding is relatively nonspecific. The definitive test would be a Watson-Schwartz test or other test for urinary porphobilinogens.

42. c. Also, sometimes a muscle biopsy is performed to confirm the diagnosis of polymyositis.

43. e. VERs (visual evoked responses) would be helpful.

44. b or d or both. While the diagnosis of herniated disk is made on clinical evaluation, equivocal cases are confirmed with EMG studies, which ought to show dysfunction of certain muscles, or myelography, which should outline the herniated disk. Myelography is always a preoperative test that is used to confirm and localize the herniated disk(s). In the future, CT scans of the spine might become the procedure of choice.

45. e. None of these tests would be helpful. A CT scan of the head would be the best diagnostic test for a cerebrovascular accident.

46. a. NCVs will reveal slowing of the nerves of the limbs.

47. b. EMGs will reveal characteristic electrical discharges associated with myotonia.

48. b and c.

49. a. Guillain-Barré syndrome is a clinical diagnosis confirmed by an elevated CSF protein concentration, but nerve conduction studies would probably show some slowing.

50. e. CSF examination would show lymphocytes, slightly raised protein, and depressed glucose.

51. a	**53.** b	**55.** b
52. d	**54.** c	**56.** c

57. a. Giving steroids in large doses is a powerful, effective treatment.
    b. Plasmapheresis can be effective even when all other modalities have failed.
    c. No.

    d. By reducing the effectiveness of cholinesterase, the quantity of ACh would increase and therefore muscle strength would increase because all available ACh receptors become stimulated to their fullest extent.

    e. Being a disorder of the neuromuscular junction, myasthenia gravis does not involve the brain. The anticholinesterases in common use, e.g., Mestinon (pyridostigmine), do not cross the blood–brain barrier, and even in excessive quantities do not precipitate mental abnormalities.

    f. Removal of thymomas or even persistent thymus tissue improves the condition of patients with myasthenia gravis.

SECTION 2

Major Neurologic Symptoms

Introduction

The second half of this book deals with how to evaluate the most common symptoms encountered by neurologists, such as headache or dementia. While each may be an indication of serious illness or a medication side-effect, many are merely minor annoyances for which patients only seek reassurance that they are not manifestations of serious illness. Familiarity with all these symptoms will facilitate a prompt, appropriate, and reliable evaluation. It will also give psychiatrists greater expertise if they are apt, knowingly or unknowingly, to evaluate patients with neurologic illness.

Each chapter will review the clinical features of a symptom, results of routine laboratory tests, and the differential diagnosis. It will then review the various neuropsychologic aspects of these conditions, related nonneurologic conditions, and basic neurologic anatomy and biochemistry. Although recommendations are often made regarding therapies, especially medications, the physician must consult the package insert and other references for all indications, dosage, and potential complications.

7

Intellectual Deterioration

Intellectual deterioration affecting several areas, including memory, that is severe enough to interfere with social or occupational functioning is called *dementia*.* This descriptive definition is used in the DSM III, has been adopted by neurologists, and pinpoints the essential distinction between dementia and related disorders.

Dementia must be distinguished from *mental retardation*, in which intellectual impairments have resulted from congenital cerebral injuries (Chapter 13). In mental retardation, impairments are present since childhood, relatively stable, and usually accompanied by the physical stigmata of cerebral injury, such as seizures and hemiparesis. Although most cases of mental retardation are readily identifiable, several special situations must be recognized. In one, Down's syndrome, persons in their third decade develop dementia superimposed on mental retardation. In another, children and adolescents may develop dementia that can mimic mental retardation or a psychiatric disorder.

Dementia is also different from specific intellectual impairments. For example, memory impairment, i.e., *amnesia*, which is a cardinal feature of the Wernicke-Korsakoff syndrome, does not necessarily cause social or occupational impairments or generalized intellectual dysfunction. Likewise, *aphasia, anosognosia,* and several related disorders are limited impairments and, unlike most cases of dementia, result from discrete lesions of the cerebral hemisphere (Chapter 8). Skillful testing is necessary to identify these disorders and to detect cases where they coexist with dementia.

Dementia also differs from conditions in which intellectual deterioration is associated with clouded consciousness, stupor, or other altered state of awareness, i.e., situations where patients are not fully awake. These conditions, often called *delirium* or the *acute confusional state,* usually result from a *toxic-metabolic encephalopathy.* They are particularly severe in the elderly, especially those with dementia. Moreover, all of these conditions must be differentiated from the *locked-in syndrome,* in which

---

*Patients with dementia may receive assistance from the Alzheimer's Disease and Related Disorders Association, 360 North Michigan Avenue, Chicago, Illinois 60601, (312) 853-3060.

patients are mute and completely immobilized by brainstem infarctions but have preserved intellectual function (Chapters 10 and 11).

NORMAL AGING

Most important, dementia must be distinguished from *benign senescence* or *forgetfulness,* which normally begins at age 65 years, when people are considered "old," and becomes pronounced after age 80 years. Studies have shown that as persons age, they normally develop impaired memory for recent events and for people's names. They also have decreased attention span, slower learning (acquisition of new information), and decreased ability to perform complex tasks. Although the Wechsler Adult intelligence Scale (WAIS or, since 1981, its revised edition, WAIS-R) shows that their general intelligence is decreased, they have no significant loss of vocabulary, language ability, or general information.

Certain physical alterations also normally occur with old age. Sleep is fragmented, sleep and awakening times are phase advanced, and there is less stage 4 NREM sleep (Chapter 17). Visual and auditory impairments occur and accentuate all other impairments (Chapter 2). Also, older people usually lose ankle deep tendon reflexes (DTRs), vibration sensation in their legs, and sense of balance. All these deficits, combined with musculoskeletal changes, lead to a nonspecific gait impairment (senile gait) and a tendency to fall.

The electroencephalogram (EEG) typically shows slowing of the background alpha activity (Chapter 10). Computed tomography (CT) may be normal, but more often it shows atrophy of the cerebral cortex, expansion of the sylvian fissure, and dilatation of the lateral and third ventricles (see Figs. 20-2 and 20-3). These changes are associated with increasing age but, except for widening of the third ventricle, not necessarily with dementia.

Brain weight, which falls with increasing age, eventually reaches about 85 percent of normal. Histologic changes include the loss of large cortical neurons, and the presence of lipofuscin granules, granulovacular degeneration, neuritic (senile) plaques containing amyloid, and neurofibrillary tangles.

MENTAL STATUS TESTING

Screening Tests

Several tests are used to detect and roughly quantitate cognitive deficits. However, while these tests are generally valid, they are limited in several respects. They cannot indicate the origin of a dementia. They tend to indicate dementia in people who have been poorly educated or have been isolated. Most important, they are not particularly helpful in distinguishing mild dementia from benign forgetfulness and depression-induced cognitive impairments *(pseudodementia).*

One standard screening test is the *Blessed Mental Status Test* (Fig. 7-1). It has shown that increasing cognitive deficits are associated with greater senile plaque concentration. Of the various tests available, this one has been the one most validated in clinical-pathologic dementia research.

(1) Observation Date

Month / Day / Year

(2) Patient Study Number

Score each item 0 if correct, 1 if wrong.   Starting Time _____

☐ Name _____

Correct Name, if wrong _____

☐ Age _____ (D.O.B. _____)

☐ When born? _____ (Month, Year)

☐ Where born? _____ Say: Some questions will be easy, some will be hard.

☐ Name of this place _____

☐ What street is it on? _____

☐ How long are you here? _____ (How long today?)

☐ Name of this city? _____

☐ Today's date? _____ (Within a day)

☐   Month _____

☐   Year _____

☐   Day of Week _____

☐   Part of Day _____

☐   Time? (best guess) _____ (Time:) (Within 1 hour)

☐   Season _____

Something to remember (Score: immediate repetition-0; phrase by phrase-1; word by word-2; no repetition-3)

☐ ___ John   ___ Brown   ___ 42   ___ Market St.   ___ Chicago   Repetition Score _____

☐ Mother's first name _____ (Any sensible response)

☐ How much schooling did you have? _____

☐ Name of one specific school _____

☐ What kind of work have you done? _____

☐ Who is the president now? _____

☐ Who was the last president? _____

☐ Date of WW I (1914-18) _____ ☐ Date of WW II (1938-45) _____

Next 3 items: For uncorrected errors, score 2; for corrected errors, score 1.

☐ Months of the year, backwards. Start with December . . . .

    D   N   O   S   A   Jl   Jn   M   Ap   Mch   F   Ja

☐ Count 1-20

☐ Count 20-1 (20 19 18 17 16 15 14 13 12 11 10 9 8 7 6 5 4 3 2 1)

☐ Recall name & address ___ J ___ B ___ 42 ___ M ___ C (Cue with "John Brown" only. Score up to 5 errors.)

TOTAL BLESSED ☐   Finishing Time _____

Fig. 7-1. Blessed Mental Status Test. (Note that the dates of World Wars I and II are those of Britain's participation.) Each incorrect answer adds one point to the Blessed dementia score. The scores for normal middle-aged adults are 3 points or less. When people have scores of 8 points or more, they are diagnosed as having dementia. Those persons who die are found to have increased numbers of senile plaques. People with scores of 4 to 7 points may have senescence, benign forgetfulness, or early dementia. The critical questions are those requiring the repetition of the John Brown phrase and saying the months backwards. [Reprinted from Blessed G, Tomlinson BE, Roth M: The association between quantitative measures of dementia and senile change in the cerebral gray matter of elderly subjects. Br J Psychiatry 114:797, 1968. With permission of Dr. Blessed and The British Journal of Psychiatry.]

Another screening test is the *Mini-Mental State* (Fig. 7-2). It includes visuospatial relation and language function tests in addition to routine cognitive capacity tests. Its results are consistent with those of the Blessed Test. Besides detecting dementia, the Mini-Mental State is also reportedly helpful in distinguishing between pseudodementia and dementia.

A newer, more concise screening test is *The 6-Item Orientation-Memory-Concentration Test* (Fig. 7-3). It is probably able to distinguish between mild, moderate, and severe cognitive deficits. Many of the questions on this test were derived from the Blessed Test, and it too has shown that mental deficits correlated positively with histologic changes.

Psychometric Tests

Extensive testing is required if, after screening tests, a diagnosis of dementia remains uncertain, a quantitative measure of the severity of dementia is required, or the coexisting aphasia or another specific deficit is suspected. The standard test is the WAIS (or now the WAIS-R), which typically shows spotty results, but, overall, performance scales are relatively lower than verbal scales and intelligence decreased from estimated premorbid levels. An aphasia battery, such as the *Boston Diagnostic Aphasia Examination,* is also performed to identify and categorize language impairments. When a visuospatial disturbance is suspected, as is often the case, the *Benton Visual Retention Test* is recommended.

One study, which claimed to classify correctly 98 percent of Alzheimer's disease patients and a control group, suggested that the best test battery is the logical memory and mental control subtests of the *Wechsler Memory Scale,* Form A of the *Trailmaking Test,* and word fluency for letters S and P (Storandt). Other investigators found that Alzheimer's disease could be identified and distinguished from other forms of dementia by using age-corrected WAIS subtests (Fuld).

Although investigators have found that the Wechsler Memory Scale is not useful because it combines verbal and nonverbal testing, revised tests are being evaluated. The *Halsted-Reitan Test* battery, despite (or because of) its comprehensive nature, is not used in its complete form. Only its Trailmaking test is incorporated into standard, clinically useful batteries.

Several tests have been specifically designed to detect dementia in elderly people. The *London Psychogeriatric Rating Scale* (LPRS) is reported to be useful as a measure of mental status and also as a guide to appropriate placement and treatment programs (Hersch, 1978). Similarly, the *Clinical Dementia Rating* (Hughes) and the *Global Deterioration Scale* (Reisberg) have been used to detect early or mild dementia.

Mattis' *Dementia Rating Scale,* which is one of the most widely used tests in the United States, measures six areas of cognitive functioning in elderly people (Vitaliano). It was refined into the *Extended Scale for Dementia* (Hersch, 1979), which was correlated positively with the LPRS.

Cortical and Subcortical Dementias

Mental status testing, combined with analysis of certain physical features, had been purported to allow classification of dementias into two groups: "cortical" and "subcortical." Cortical dementias were characterized by the presence of aphasia and

```
                                        Patient . . . . . . . . . . . . . . . . . . . . . . . . . . .
                                        Examiner  . . . . . . . . . . . . . . . . . . . . . . . .
                                        Date . . . . . . . . . . . . . . . . . . . . . . . . . . . .
Maximum
 Score   Score
                                           ORIENTATION
   5     ( )    What is the (year)(season)(date)(day)(month)?
   5     ( )    Where are we: (state)(county)(town)(hospital)(floor).
                                           REGISTRATION
   3     ( )    Name 3 objects:  1 second to say each. Then ask the patient all 3 after you have said them.
                                 Give 1 point for each correct answer. Then repeat then until he learns all 3.
                                 Count trials and record.
                                 Trials
                                   ATTENTION AND CALCULATION
   5     ( )    Serial 7's. 1 point for each correct. Stop after 5 answers. Alternatively spell "world" back-
                wards.
                                           RECALL
   3     ( )    Ask for the 3 objects repeated above. Give 1 point for each correct.
                                          LANGUAGE
   9     ( )    Name a pencil, and watch (2 points)
                Repeat the following "No ifs, and, or buts." (1 point)
                Follow a 3-stage command:
                  "Take a paper in your right hand, fold it in half, and put it on the floor" (3 points)
                Read and obey the following:
                                   CLOSE YOUR EYES (1 point)
                Write a sentence (1 point)
                Copy design (1 point)
    _____   Total score
                ASSESS level of consciousness along a continuum_____
                                        Alert      Drowsy      Stupor      Coma
                          INSTRUCTIONS FOR ADMINISTRATION OF
                             MINI-MENTAL STATE EXAMINATION
                                       ORIENTATION
```

1. Ask for the date. Then ask specifically for parts omitted, e.g., "Can you also tell me what season it is?" One point for each correct.

2. Ask in turn "Can you tell me the name of this hospital?" (town, county, etc.). One point for each correct.

REGISTRATION

Ask the patient if you may test his memory. Then say the names of 3 unrelated objects, clearly and slowly, about one second for each. After you have said 3, ask him to repeat them. This first repetition determines his score (0–3) but keep saying them until he can repeat all 3, up to 6 trials. If he does not eventually learn all 3, recall cannot be meaningfully tested.

ATTENTION AND CALCULATION

Ask the patient to begin with 100 and count backwards by 7. Stop after 5 subtractions (93, 86, 79, 72, 65). Score the total number of correct answers.

If the patient cannot or will not perform this task, ask him to spell the word "world" backwards. The score is the number of letters in correct order, e.g. dlrow = 5, dlorw = 3.

RECALL

Ask the patient if he can recall the 3 words you previously asked him to remember. Score 0–3.

LANGUAGE

Naming: Show the patient a wrist watch and ask him what it is. Repeat for pencil. Score 0–2.

Repetition: Ask the patient to repeat the sentence after you. Allow only one trial. Score 0 or 1.

3-State command: Give the patient a piece of plain blank paper and repeat the command. Score 1 point for each part correctly executed.

Reading: On a blank piece of paper print the sentence "Close your eyes" in letters large enough for the patient to see clearly. Ask him to read it and do what it says. Score 1 point only if he actually closes his eyes.

Writing: Give the patient a blank piece of paper and ask him to write a sentence for you. Do not dictate a sentence, it is to be written spontaneously. It must contain a subject and verb and be sensible. Correct grammar and punctuation are not necessary.

Copying: On a clean piece of paper, draw intersecting pentagons, each side about 1 in., and ask him to copy it exactly as it is. All 10 angles must be present and 2 must intersect to score 1 point. Tremor and rotation are ignored.

Estimate the patient's level of sensorium along a continuum, from alert on the left to coma on the right.

Fig. 7-2. Mini-mental State Examination. Points are assigned for correct answers. Scores of 20 points or less indicate dementia, delirium, schizophrenia, or affective disorders alone or in combination. Such scores are not found in normal elderly people or those with neuroses or personality disorders. Note that this test assesses language and visuospatial ability. [Reprinted from Folstein MF, Folstein SE, McHugh PR: "Minni-mental state": A practical method for grading the cognitive state of patients for the clinician. J. Psychiatr Res 12:189, 1975. With permission.]

Items		Maximum Error	Score	Weight
1	What *year* is it now?	1	_____	× 4
2	What *month* is it now?	1	_____	× 3
Memory phrase	Repeat this phrase after me: John Brown, 42 Market Street, Chicago			
3	About what *time* is it? (within 1 hour)	1	_____	× 3
4	*Count* backwards 20 to 1	2	_____	× 2
5	Say the months in reverse order	2	_____	× 2
6	Repeat the memory phrase	5	_____	× 2

Score of 1 for each incorrect response; maximum weighted error score = 28.

Fig. 7-3. The 6-Item Orientation-Memory-Concentration Test. A higher score indicates progressively severe cognitive impairment. In this test, the critical question involves repeating the test phrase. Normal people, including elderly persons, have a weighted error score of 6 points or less. Persons whose weighted error scores are more than 10 points are considered to have dementia. [Modified from Katzman R, Brown T, Fuld P, et al: Validation of a short orientation-memory-concentration test of cognitive impairment. Am J Psychiatry 140:734, 1983. With permission of the American Journal of Psychiatry.]

related abnormalities, such as agnosia and apraxia (Chapter 8). Although patients had dementia and aphasia, they were alert, healthy, and ambulatory. The prime example of cortical dementia was that associated with Alzheimer's disease.

In contrast, subcortical dementia was supposedly typified by slowed mental processing and apathy, and accompanied by gait abnormalities. The prime examples were the dementias found in normal pressure hydrocephalus, Huntington's chorea, and Parkinson's disease.

This classification is now losing credibility. The intellectual, language, and physical abnormalities were found inconsistently. Moreover, most illnesses that cause dementia are now known to cause both cortical and subcortical histologic changes.

CAUSES OF DEMENTIA

The most common causes of dementia, which may occur in combination, are Alzheimer's disease, multiple infarctions (multi-infarct dementia), and, although probably not alcohol itself, alcoholism ("alcoholic dementia") (Table 7-1). Some conditions are identifiable because they are associated with peripheral neuropathy (see Table 5-2), involuntary movement disorders (see Table 18-4), or onset in adolescence (Table 7-2).

In several illnesses, dementia is familial. It is transmitted genetically in Wilson's disease, Huntington's chorea, and, rarely, Alzheimer's disease. In cases of Pick's disease and most cases of Alzheimer's disease, the illness has a tendency to affect several family members.

Dementia is occasionally "reversible;" however, in practice, few such cases are ever found. Most are associated with only mild dementia of less than two years' duration, and either hypothyroidism, use of several medicines, or depression. Also, many patients with theoretically reversible conditions, such as subdural hematomas or

Table 7-1

Commonly Cited Causes of Dementia and
Their Incidence

Disease	Incidence (%)
Alzheimer's disease	40–70
Multiple infarctions	7–10
Alcoholism	6–11
Medications	0–8
Normal pressure hydrocephalus	4–12
Cerebral mass lesions	2–4
Pseudodementia*	7–12
Other, usually rare causes	
Huntington's chorea†	
Infections	
Neurosyphilis	
Creutzfeldt-Jakob	
Encephalitis‡	
Metabolic abnormalities	
Hyper- or hypothyroidism	
Hepatic failure	
Pulmonary failure	
Combined system disease	
Drug abuse	

*Depression and other psychiatric conditions that cause
cognitive impairment.
†Also Parkinson's and Wilson's diseases (Chapter 18).
‡Including subacute sclerosing panencephalitis (SSPE).

normal pressure hydrocephalus, still have dementia after treatment, most likely
because they had pre-existing Alzheimer's disease.

Laboratory Evaluation

Diagnostic tests must be chosen by a physician with a good understanding of the
clinical situation. When no cause is obvious, a series of screening laboratory tests is
usually performed (Table 7-3).

A routine EEG (which costs about $150 in 1985) will be abnormal in most cases
of dementia. However, EEG slowing in early Alzheimer's disease may be indistin-

Table 7-2

Commonly Cited Causes of Dementia
that Affects Adolescents

Metabolic abnormalities
Wilson's disease
Drug and alcohol abuse
Degenerative illnesses
Huntington's chorea
Metachromatic leukodystrophy
Other rare, usually genetically transmitted illnesses
Infections
Subacute sclerosing panencephalitis (SSPE)

Table 7-3

Screening Laboratory Tests for Dementia

Routine tests
  Chest-ray
  EKG
  Complete blood count
  Chemistry profile (e.g., SMA 6 and 12)
Specific blood tests
  Syphilis test*
  Thyroid function (e.g., T_4)
  B_{12} level
Neurologic tests
  Electroencephalogram (EEG)
  Computed tomography (CT)

*In testing for neurosyphilis, either the FTA-ABS or MHA-TP test is preferred to the VDRL (see text).

guishable from that commonly found in normal old age. Also, when the EEG is clearly abnormal, it will rarely be of help in establishing the cause of the dementia.

The few illnesses in which the EEG is particularly helpful are Creutzfeldt-Jakob disease and subacute sclerosing panencephalitis (SSPE)—conditions in which the EEG shows virtually diagnostic "periodic complexes" (see Fig. 10-6). It is also helpful in diagnosing pseudodementia, where the EEG is normal or shows slight background slowing.

The CT scan (which costs about $300 in 1985) is the definitive diagnostic test for brain tumors, subdural hematomas, and other mass lesions. It is also helpful in diagnosing multiple infarctions and normal pressure hydrocephalus. However, it cannot be diagnostic in Alzheimer's disease. Cerebral atrophy, which is the most common CT finding in Alzheimer's disease, is also present in normal elderly persons and those with Down's syndrome, alcoholic dementia, some varieties of schizophrenia, and other conditions.

Lumbar puncture (which costs about $250 in 1985) should be performed to inspect the cerebrospinal fluid (CSF) when patients are suspected of having neurosyphilis, chronic meningitis, or SSPE; however, it need not be routinely performed. If adolescents or young adults develop dementia, additional tests would include serum ceruloplasmin determination and a slit-lamp examination (for Wilson's disease), urine for "toxicology screens," and possibly urinanalysis for metachromatic granules and arylsulfatase-A (for metachromatic leukodystrophy). Likewise, folate level determination, systemic lupus erythematosus (SLE) procedures, and other specific tests should be reserved for those cases in which there are specific indications.

ALZHEIMER'S DISEASE

Although a "definite" diagnosis of Alzheimer's disease requires histologic examination of brain tissue, a diagnosis is considered probable and acceptable for practical purposes when adults have the insidious onset of progressive intellectual deterioration, and other neurologic and systemic illnesses have been excluded by clinical and laboratory evaluation.

Clinical Features

Alzheimer's disease typically has a progressive course with some plateaus, but its rate of progression and its manifestations are somewhat variable. Nevertheless, three "stages," based on the severity of intellectual deterioration, have been described. In the "early" stage, the most common problems are impaired judgment and impaired recent memory (an "amnestic syndrome"). Patients are easily distracted, unable to complete complex tasks, and relatively apathetic. These harbingers, which are often only identified in retrospect, are frequently misinterpreted because they mimic depression or benign senescence.

The "middle" stage is marked by greater memory loss, further decline in judgment, and difficulties in performing almost all intellectual functions. Language impairments cause word-finding difficulties, e.g., *anomia* (Chapter 8). Patients in the middle stage may be confused, especially at night or whenever they are moved to new surroundings. They also tend to have depression, hallucinations, paranoid ideation, and physical, emotional, or sexual outbursts. These mental disturbances are not only troublesome symptoms but can overwhelm remaining cognitive ability.

In the early and middle stages, patients may have frontal release signs (Fig. 7-4), increased jaw jerk reflex (see Fig. 4-12), and Babinski signs, but they do not have gross paresis, sensory loss, or incoordination. Although myoclonus (Chapter 18) may be found rarely in Alzheimer's disease, it is more indicative of Creutzfeldt-Jakob disease.

In the "late" stage, patients become mute, unresponsive to verbal requests, and eventually bedridden in a decorticate (fetal) posture. Until this stage, unlike nearly all other illnesses that cause dementia, Alzheimer's disease does not cause *major* physical impairments.

Tests

The CT scan usually, but not always, shows atrophy of the cerebral cortex with widening of the third ventricle. However, this atrophy is not peculiar to Alzheimer's disease: Many normal or highly intelligent people have CT scans that show cerebral atrophy. Moreover, when cerebral atrophy is present in Alzheimer's disease, it has no predicative value.

The EEG may also be normal in the early stage, when the clinical diagnosis is most difficult. Although over 80 percent of Alzheimer's disease patients eventually have EEG slowing, it is not diagnostic. In the future, more sophisticated electrophysiologic testing, such as spectral frequency analysis and evoked responses (Chapter 15), may be able to identify this disease.

Positron emission tomography (PET) in Alzheimer's disease patients, compared with age-matched controls, shows that cerebral oxygen and glucose metabolism are symmetrically decreased in proportion to the severity of dementia. Since oxygen extraction is known to be normal, the hypometabolism is thought to be a result rather than a cause of Alzheimer's disease. In addition, in cases where language impairment is disproportionately severe, left frontal, temporal, and parietal hypometabolism is detected, and in those with disproportionately severe visuoconstruction impairments, right parietal hypometabolism is found (Chapter 8).

Since the histologic findings in Alzheimer's disease are more quantitatively than qualitatively different from age-related changes, cerebral cortex biopsy specimens examined in only a routine fashion will yield incorrect diagnoses. Nevertheless, a

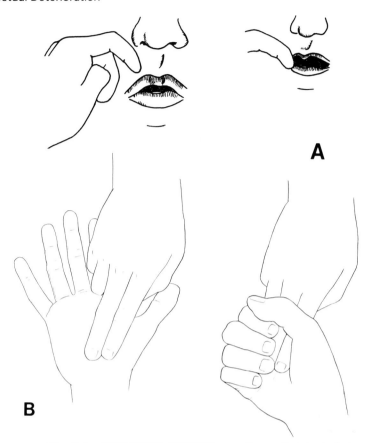

Fig. 7-4. The frontal lobe release reflexes that have been found more frequently by some authors in demented than in nondemented old people are the snout and grasp reflexes. (A) The snout reflex is elicited by tapping the patient's upper lip with a finger or a percussion hammer. This reflex causes the patient's lips to purse and the mouth to pout forward. (B) The grasp reflex is elicited by the examiner's fingers stroking the patient's palm crosswise or the fingers lengthwise. The reflex consists of the patient's grasping the examiner's fingers and failing to let go despite requests.

cerebral cortical biopsy is occasionally an appropriate diagnostic test. In particular, if enzyme studies (see below) can be performed on the specimen, a biopsy can be diagnostic of Alzheimer's disease. Also, specimens examined with electron microscopy as well as with standard methods can be diagnostic of Creutzfeldt-Jakob disease.

Pathology

Compared with age-matched controls, the brains of patients with Alzheimer's disease are more atrophied and have greater cortical neuron loss and increased senile plaque concentrations. However, the neuron loss is predominantly in the frontal and temporal lobes, and neurofibrillary tangles are concentrated in the hippocampus.

More important, the brains of persons with Alzheimer's disease have pronounced neuron loss in the *substantia innominata,* also called the *nucleus basalis Meynert.* This structure is a group of large neurons located in the septal region beneath the globus pallidus (see Fig. 18-1). These neurons project upward to the cerebral cortex and provide extensive cholinergic innervation. In Alzheimer's disease, their loss is closely associated with reductions in cerebral cortex concentrations of *acetylcholine (ACh)* and the enzyme required for its synthesis, *choline acetyltransferase (CAT).* Acetylcholine is synthesized from acetylcoenzyme-A (acetylCoA) and choline:

$$\text{acetyl CoA} + \text{choline} \xrightarrow{\text{CAT}} \text{ACh}$$

Concentrations of intraneuronal somatostatin, substance P, and other putative neurotransmitters have been reported to be decreased. However, the most consistent abnormality has been the CAT deficit, which is proportional to the severity of the dementia and the concentration of histologic changes. These findings have given rise to the "cholinergic hypothesis," which states that Alzheimer's disease dementia results from reduced cholinergic activity. This hypothesis is supported by studies showing that scopolamine, a drug that has central anticholinergic effects, induces brief Alzheimer-like cognitive impairments, which can be reversed with physostigmine (Fig. 7-5) (Fuld).

Pronounced CAT deficits are also found in the cortex of brains of patients with Down's syndrome from trisomy 21 and patients with Parkinson's disease that has resulted in dementia, but not with Huntington's chorea (Chapter 18).

Etiology

Many statistically significant associations, but not causal relationships, have been noted between Alzheimer's disease and other conditions. For example, head trauma,

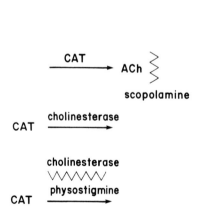

Fig. 7-5. (Top) Choline acetyltransferase (CAT) is the enzyme for acetylcholine (ACh) synthesis. Scopolamine, unlike most other anticholinergic substances, can cross the blood-brain barrier to block ACh. Atropine also blocks ACh but, unless large quantities are administered, it does not cross the blood–brain barrier. (Middle) CAT is metabolized or inactivated by cholinesterases. Either decreased CAT synthesis or increased CAT metabolism leads to decreased ACh. (Bottom) Anticholinesterases, or cholinesterase inhibitors, preserve CAT and thus increase ACh concentrations. Anticholinesterases such as edrophonium (Tensilon) and pyridostigmine (Mestinon) are used in treatment of myasthenia gravis, where they preserve neuromuscular junction ACh (see Fig. 6-2). For this reason, anticholinesterases are also widely used in insecticides, which cause paralysis by creating prolonged ACh activity at neuromuscular juntions. Physostigmine, which can cross the blood–brain barrier, is used in attempts to correct purported ACh deficits in tardive dyskinesia (Chapter 18) and Alzheimer's disease dementia. It is also used to counteract the profound anticholinergic activity in cases of tricyclic antidepressant overdose.

hyperthyroidism, and increased aluminum concentrations in the cerebral cortex have been found more frequently in Alzheimer's disease patients than in age-matched controls.

Recently, *prions*, which are unusual infectious agents, have been suggested to be the cause of Alzheimer's disease. Unlike viruses, prions are *slow* to produce symptoms, contain no nucleic acid (e.g., DNA and RNA), and appear on electronmicroscopy to be senile plaque amyloid. These agents are considered to be responsible for at least two infectious degenerative neurologic illnesses: scrapie, an illness of sheep and goats, and Creutzfeldt-Jakob disease (see below).

Genetic abnormalities have also been implicated as etiologic factors. In many families there are multiple cases of Alzheimer's disease or, occasionally, an autosomal dominant genetic inheritance pattern. In these families the illness begins in patients younger than 65 years and has a rapid course. Overall, siblings and children of Alzheimer's disease patients have a 33 percent chance of developing it.

Even more striking is a markedly increased incidence of Alzheimer's disease in people with Down's syndrome from trisomy 21. About 50 percent of such people who are older than 40 years develop typical Alzheimer-like intellectual deterioration, gross and histologic brain changes, PET metabolic abnormalities, and loss of CAT.

Therapy

Clinicians are unable to correct the basic abnormality of Alzheimer's disease. They can only suggest ways to reduce the psychological and behavioral aberrations. Most suggestions are applicable to all illnesses that cause dementia. Those that relate to the daily care of the patient and to long range psychosocial issues are discussed in a thorough, practical, and empathetic manner in Mace and Rabins (see references).

Patients may benefit from tranquilizers for anxiety or thought disorders. However, medicines with a sedative effect should be avoided because they can slow remaining cognitive processes, cause a paradoxical reaction, and disrupt sleep (Chapter 17). Sometimes major tranquilizers need to be given only at night when nocturnal hallucinations and paranoid ideation are most apt to occur.

Some patients will have pseudodementia, but many more will have depression superimposed on dementia. Several authorities have suggested giving antidepressants in diagnostic-therapeutic trials to identify patients with pseudodementia. Patients with depression, which may then be diagnosed in retrospect, and also those with both depression and dementia, benefit if the depression is treated. Although tricyclic antidepressants, which possess anticholinergic properties, would theoretically intensify the ACh deficiency of Alzheimer's disease, they have not been shown to be deleterious.

Attempts to correct a possible ACh deficit based on the cholinergic hypothesis have included the administration of choline or lecithin (phosphatidyl choline), physostigmine, or a combination. Physostigmine did produce some memory improvement, but it was only for long-term recall and only briefly and inconsistently. Other attempts at increasing ACh activity have been attempted administering ACh agonists, such as arecoline and oxotremorine, but they have not been helpful.

Trial administration of substances that have been shown to be depleted, such as somatostatin, has been unsuccessful. Likewise, two popular treatments, naloxone and vasodilators, do not improve memory.

OTHER CONDITIONS THAT CAUSE DEMENTIA

Aside from Alzheimer's disease, most conditions that cause dementia usually can be diagnosed from the patients' history, physical findings, and laboratory tests. However, psychometric tests cannot identify specific conditions with sufficient reliability to obviate a complete evaluation, and several standard laboratory tests, such as the Venereal Disease Research Laboratory (VDRL) test, may yield inaccurate results.

Multi-Infarct Dementia

Unlike people with Alzheimer's disease, those who sustain multiple cerebral infarctions develop a stepwise intellectual deterioration accompanied by prominent physical abnormalities, including spasticity, ataxia, pseudobulbar palsy, and unilateral or bilateral paresis. These persons usually have renal and cardiac disease as well as hypertensive cerebrovascular disease (Chapter 11).

Although the EEG is almost always abnormal, changes are nonspecific. The CT scan, which is a more reliable diagnostic test in this condition, usually shows multiple lucencies and cerebral atrophy. The PET scan has been able to distinguish multi-infarct dementia from Alzheimer's disease by revealing discrete hypometabolic areas.

Antihypertensive medications will diminish the likelihood of cerebral infarction. However, they must be used cautiously in the elderly, in whom they can produce or exacerbate cognitive deficits.

Alcoholism

Continual alcohol use is associated with a combination of intellectual deterioration, physical signs, and histologic changes; this is usually called the *Wernicke-Korsakoff syndrome*. Since similar changes are found in people who have undergone starvation or have been in dialysis programs, the syndrome may be the result of nutritional deprivation rather than any toxic effect of alcohol.

The outstanding characteristic of the Wernicke-Korsakoff syndrome is amnesia combining impaired recall of previously known facts (retrograde amnesia) with an inability to learn new ones (antegrade amnesia). Although confabulation has often also been considered a hallmark, it is rarely present. Besides amnesia, most patients have other intellectual impairments, such as impaired judgment. For example, the WAIS test reveals abnormalities in digit-symbol, block design, and other tasks that may be nonspecific but are beyond memory impairment.

Physical signs of the Wernicke-Korsakoff syndrome are cerebellar dysfunction (Chapter 2), peripheral neuropathy (Chapter 5), and, at the onset of the illness, conjugate gaze paresis, abducens nerve paresis, and nystagmus (Chapters 4 and 12). Nevertheless, the CT scan may be normal or show atrophy, and the EEG is usually normal. Examination of the brain reveals evidence of hemorrhage into the mamillary bodies and periaqueductal gray area, which are portions of the limbic system—the cornerstone of memory.

With proper nutrition, especially thiamine administration, the majority of patients do have some improvement in their dementia. However, only 20 percent enjoy a complete recovery.

Alcoholics are also vulnerable to several other conditions that cause cognitive impairment. Being susceptible to trauma, they frequently harbor subdural hematomas. Those with Laennec's cirrhosis are liable to develop hepatic encephalopathy after a high protein meal or gastrointestinal bleeding. Rarely, but interestingly, alcoholics have degeneration of the corpus callosum (Marchiafava-Bignami syndrome, Chapter 8). They can also have behavioral disturbances from rage attacks or alcohol-withdrawal seizures, which are much less likely to be partial complex (e.g., psychomotor) than generalized tonic-clonic seizures.

Medication-Induced Dementia

Overall, medication-induced dementia is one of the most common and readily reversible dementias. In evaluating a patient with intellectual deterioration, the physician should suspect every medicine. Many medicines can also induce excitement, depression, or other mental abnormalities. Some, such as reserpine and levodopa, cause impairments routinely, while others, such as cimetidine (Tagamet), do so infrequently and unpredictably.

Medicines prone to induce mental changes are antidepressants, hypnotics, and antihypertensives. Of the antihypertensives, the "false neurotransmitters," such as methyldopa (Aldomet), may be the most troublesome. In addition to mental changes, excessive use of antihypertensives can lead to orthostatic hypotension and syncope. Also, diuretics, even in routine doses, can cause dehydration, electrolyte imbalance, and toxic concentrations of other medicines.

Normal Pressure Hydrocephalus

A cause of dementia that is supposedly common, diagnosable, and reversible is normal pressure hydrocephalus (NPH). This is a condition in which meningitis, subarachnoid hemorrhage, or, most often, an unknown cause impedes CSF reabsorption through the arachnoid villi overlying the brain, causing continued CSF production to result in hydrocephalus (Fig. 7-6).

In NPH, dementia is characterized more by psychomotor retardation than cognitive impairments and is less prominent than physical symptoms. Also, despite treatment that results in resolution of physical symptoms, improvement of dementia is inconsistent.

Gait apraxia is usually the initial and most prominent symptom (Fig. 7-7). Severity is proportional to the degree of hydrocephalus but not the severity of dementia. With treatment, gait apraxia is also the first and most likely symptom to improve. Urinary incontinence is the other major symptom, however, in older persons, it may be due to many other causes.

The CT scan, in classic cases, shows ventricular dilatation and minimal or no cerebral atrophy (see Fig. 20-4); however, since this pattern is similar to cerebral atrophy with resultant hydrocephalus, *hydrocephalus ex vacuo* (see Fig. 20-3), diagnosis from the CT scan can be erroneous. The CSF pressure and its protein and glucose concentrations are normal.

Cisternography, which is a frequently used diagnostic test, consists of injection of radioactive albumin, indium, or other substance into the subarachnoid space through a lumbar puncture and tracing the radioactive material as it diffuses toward the brain. Normally, and in most cases of Alzheimer's disease, the radioactive mate-

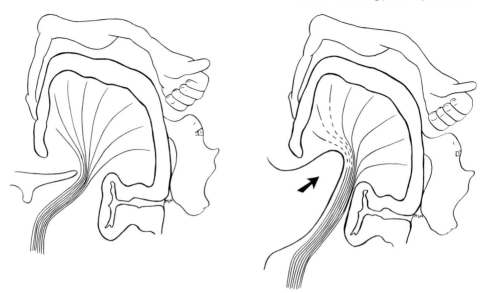

Fig. 7-6. Ventricular expansion, i.e., hydrocephalus, results in compression of brain paren-chyma and stretching of the corticospinal tracts of the internal capsule (see Fig. 18-1). Pressure on the frontal lobes and other portions of the brain leads to dementia and psychomotor retarda-tion. Since the tracts that are most stretched are the ones that govern the legs and the voluntary muscles of the bladder, gait impairment (apraxia) and urinary incontinence are usually the initial and most prominent symptoms of normal pressure hydrocephalus.

rial can be followed as it goes upward over the cerebral hemispheres, where it is absorbed along with the CSF through the arachnoid villi. By contrast, in most cases of NPH, radioactive material accumulates within the ventricles.

Another test is a therapeutic trial of CSF withdrawal by repeated lumbar punc-tures to reduce the hydrocephalus. Overall, clinical, psychometric, and laboratory diagnostic criteria are unreliable.

Not only is diagnosis problematic, therapy is inconsistently effective. Hydro-cephalus can usually be relieved by the placement of a thin plastic tube (shunt) into a lateral ventricle to divert CSF into the chest or abdominal cavity for absorption. However, only about 50 percent of patients are reported to recover partially and only 25 percent completely. Moreover, the neurosurgical complication rate is about 25 percent.

Infections

NEUROSYPHILIS

Neurosyphilis, which is caused by persistent *Treponema pallidum* infection, is often initially asymptomatic. If it is left untreated, patients may develop dementia that is initially nonspecific and unaccompanied by prominent physical signs. Delusions of grandeur, despite their notoriety, occur rarely. When neurosyphilis is advanced, patients have profound dementia and Babinski signs, dysarthria, tremulousness, Argyll-Robertson pupils (Chapter 12), and a CT scan showing cerebral atrophy.

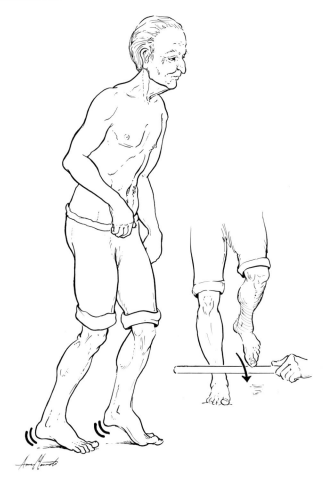

Fig. 7-7. Patients with gait apraxia walk slowly, deliberately, and with short steps. They tend to move asynchronously, failing to shift their weight to the forward foot. In severe cases, their inability to alternate their weight immobilizes their feet, which appear to stick to the floor: these people are said to have a "magnetic gait." Nevertheless, since their stepping reflex is preserved, they can walk over a stick or climb stairs. Gait apraxia is one of several characteristic gait abnormalities (see Table 2-4).

Dementia may be combined with other forms of neurosyphilis, including tabes dorsalis, optic atrophy, and myelitis, which almost always begins as syphilitic meningitis. Treatment with penicillin may improve cognitive impairments and reverse CSF abnormalities. However, complete clinical recovery is rare.

A blood VDRL test (which costs $10 in 1985) is the standard screening test for syphilis. However, false-positive results are common.* More important, as many as

---

*Old age, addiction, and autoimmune diseases, the "3 A's," are the most common causes of false-positive blood VDRL tests.

50 percent of neurosyphilis cases have a negative blood VDRL result because of natural resolution of serologic abnormalities or prior, sometimes inadequate, treatment. In contrast, the blood *fluorescent treponemal antibody absorption (FTA-ABS) test* (which costs $30) and the *treponema microhemagglutination assay (MHA-TP)* (which costs $35) are much more specific and are positive in more than 95 percent of neurosyphilis cases. Therefore, despite the greater expense of these tests, they are more appropriate when screening for neurosyphilis.

A lumbar puncture should be performed for CSF testing when people, with or without symptoms, have a positive FTA-ABS or MHA-TP test, but not solely on the basis of a positive blood VDRL test. In about 60 percent of neurosyphilis cases, the CSF has an elevated protein concentration (45 to 100 mg/100 mL). In addition, a lymphocytic pleocytosis (5 to 200 cells per millimeter) is found; however, there are 10 or fewer cells per millimeter in 90 percent of cases.

A positive CSF VDRL test, which can be found in the presence of a negative blood VDRL test, is almost always diagnostic of neurosyphilis, i.e., the CSF VDRL test is virtually never false-positive. More important, the CSF VDRL test is false-negative in as many as 40 percent of neurosyphilis cases (Hooshmand). Still, the FTA-ABS test cannot be used to test CSF because it can be false-positive, possibly because protein markers exude into the CSF from the blood. Nevertheless, a diagnosis of neurosyphilis can be made despite a negative CSF VDRL on the basis of the clinical situation, CSF protein elevation, and minimal pleocytosis. Even in equivocal cases, patients should be treated for neurosyphilis.

SUBACUTE SCLEROSING PANENCEPHALITIS

Subacute sclerosing panencephalitis (SSPE) is possibly the most common cause of dementia that begins in childhood. In this disease, children have insidious onset of dementia, which may appear initially as behavioral disturbances, accompanied by myoclonus (Chapter 18). The average age of onset is 10 years and those children most susceptible are boys from rural, low income families.

Subacute sclerosing panencephalitis is diagnosed by finding an elevated CSF measles antibody titer and, during the initial stage of the illness, periodic EEG complexes (see Fig. 10-6). The CT scan shows nonspecific ventricular dilatation and cerebral atrophy that are more pronounced the longer the duration and the greater the severity of the illness.

Although the infectious agent has not been discovered, several observations suggest it is probably a measles virus variant. The most important observation is that the incidence of SSPE is markedly reduced in children who have been vaccinated against measles.

CREUTZFELDT-JAKOB DISEASE

Creutzfeldt-Jakob disease, like SSPE, causes dementia, myoclonus, and periodic EEG complexes. However, it only affects people older than 65 years. Compared with Alzheimer's disease, it has a rapidly fatal course, lasting about 6 months. Cerebral cortex biopsy specimens, which are often obtained to diagnose this illness, reveal a characteristic *spongyform encephalopathy.*

The clinical and histologic features of Creutzfeldt-Jakob disease have been produced in animals by inoculating them with brain tissue from human victims. The disease apparently has also been accidentally transferred to humans by corneal transplantation, intracerebral EEG electrodes, and human growth hormone injections. The infectious agent is not measles or another common virus but probably a prion.

ACQUIRED IMMUNE DEFICIENCY SYNDROME

Acquired immune deficiency syndrome (AIDS) is believed to result from a virus, such as the human T-lymphotropic virus type III (*HTLV-III*), that damages the immune system's T cells and infects the brain. It is probably transmitted by male homosexual contact, blood transfusions, and, when needles or syringes are shared, drug abuse.

Patients are prone to develop CNS and nonCNS opportunistic infections, including toxoplasmosis and cryptococcosis, and lymphomas. They often have seizures, hemiparesis, and other signs of discrete cerebral lesions (see Chapter 15), and many eventually develop dementia.

The dementia is nonspecific and it may not be associated with physical neurologic abnormalities. However, by the time patients develop dementia, they usually have cachexia, fevers, and infections in several nonCNS organs. Even though many of AIDS' complications may be successfully treated, the dementia is progressive and associated with a fatal outcome.

About 90 percent of all AIDS' victims have serum antibodies to *HTLV-III*. Those who have neurologic illness should have a CT scan and, if it does not reveal a mass lesion, a lumbar puncture should be performed to search for signs of fungal and other unusual infections (see Chapter 20). Also, male homosexuals with neurologic illness should be evaluated for CNS syphilis. In the many cases where a diagnosis is not made by routine tests, a brain biopsy may be necessary.

Pseudodementia

Patients with typical pseudodementia have been described as being 45 to 64 years old and having affective and vegetative signs, emotional distress because of memory loss, fluctuations in their symptoms, and previous depressive episodes. Also, their Mini-Mental State Test may indicate depression and WAIS tests, unlike those for Alzheimer's disease patients, usually show comparably abnormal performance and verbal scales. However, when psychomotor retardation is present, the performance scales may be severely depressed. In addition, the EEG is normal.

Accepting that typical cases are readily identifiable, the clinician's real problem is to diagnose pseudodementia when it occurs in people older than 65 years who also have Alzheimer's disease. Here pseudodementia can be overlooked because of typical benign forgetfulness or mild dementia, EEG slowing, and a CT scan showing cerebral atrophy in these patients. Moreover, many variables are unreliable: the psychometric test results of patients vary between examinations, with patients often having no history or florid signs of depression.

Since pseudodementia is frequent and reversible, clinicians should attempt to diagnosis it in equivocal cases and where Alzheimer's disease is already suspected. Antidepressant medications can be prescribed on a trial basis. As noted previously, although the tricyclic and many newer antidepressants have anticholinergic properties, these medicines have been used for years apparently without exacerbating cognitive Alzheimer's disease impairments.

Miscellaneous

Pick's disease, which has a strong familial tendency, is characterized by atrophy of the frontal and anterior temporal lobes, but not the parietal lobe, and the presence of argentophilic intraneuronal (Pick's) bodies. As in Alzheimer's disease, there is neuron loss in the nucleus basalis Meynert.

It is included surprisingly often in discussions of dementia even though it is rare, untreatable, and virtually indistinguishable clinically from Alzheimer's disease. The clinical differences are only that, in Pick's disease, visuospatial ability is relatively preserved because the parietal lobe is spared and there are occasional language impairments and elements of Klüver-Bucy syndrome (Chapters 12 and 16) because of temporal lobe atrophy.

The *punch-drunk* syndrome, "dementia pugilistica," is a consequence of boxing in which progressive intellectual deterioration begins at, or precipitates, the end of a boxer's career. Dementia develops in proportion to the number of lost fights, especially as a result of knockouts. It is most apt to occur in small men and alcoholics. In addition to dementia, these retired boxers usually have corticospinal tract signs and parkinsonism (Chapter 18).

TOXIC-METABOLIC ENCEPHALOPATHIES

Patients with delirium, which neurologists call toxic-metabolic encephalopathy or acute confusional state, are usually lethargic, disoriented, and inattentive. Although they are usually bedridden, many are physically and mentally agitated, hallucinatory, and delusionary. Toxic metabolic encephalopathy evolves over hours to days and, because of the underlying illness, either progresses into coma, clears completely, or resolves into a state where the patients are alert but have residual brain damage.

Young children and old people, especially those with Alzheimer's disease, are especially susceptible to toxic-metabolic encephalopathy. They can develop it from relatively minor disturbances. A common example is that in elderly persons slight dehydration causes impaired consciousness and behavioral abnormalities.

Signs of systemic illness, such as fever and tachycardia, are common, but physi-

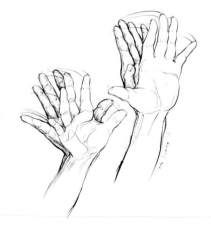

Fig. 7-8. Asterixis is elicited by asking patients to extend their arms and hands, as though they were a policeman stopping traffic. Asterixis consists of the hands making a rapid, quick downward movement and a slow return to their extended position, as though someone were waving "goodbye." Asterixis indicates that patients have a toxic-metabolic encephalopathy, the most common ones being uremic and hepatic encephalopathy.

Table 7-4
Commonly Cited, Frequent Causes of Toxic-Metabolic
Encephalopathy

Drug, alcohol, or medication intoxication
Hepatic or uremic encephalopathy
Fluid or electrolyte imbalance, especially dehydration
Pneumonia or other nonneurologic infection

cal neurologic signs are usually subtle, not lateralized, and apparent only after mental aberrations have appeared. In most toxic-metabolic encephalopathy cases, patients have symmetric or asymmetric DTRs and Babinski signs. Otherwise, with several exceptions, neurologic abnormalities are nonspecific.

In Wernicke-Korsakoff syndrome, patients have oculomotor palsies, nystagmus, ataxia, and polyneuropathy (Chapters 5 and 12). Patients with hepatic or uremic encephalopathy have *asterixis* (Fig. 7-8). Some patients with uremia, penicillin intoxication, and other toxic conditions have myoclonus (Chapter 18).

Although hundreds of conditions may cause toxic-metabolic encephalopathy, several account for the majority of cases in acute care hospitals (Table 7-4). In addition, several common neurologic conditions may have the clinical stigmata of toxic-metabolic encephalopathy, but neurologists do not consider them to be either toxic-metabolic encephalopathy or delirium: examples are subarachnoid hemorrhage, postictal confusion (Chapter 10), and transient ischemic attacks including transient global amnesia (Chapter 11).

The diagnosis is usually revealed in the patient's history, routine physical examination, or laboratory tests. Depending on the clinical situation, blood and urine tests are the procedures most likely to reveal the exact diagnosis. As preliminary measures, blood can be tested for the white blood cell count, chemistry profiles, and alcohol and drug content. Urine can also be tested for drugs, bacteria, and signs of infection.

Whatever the cause, the EEG is practically always abnormal. In hepatic and uremic encephalopathy, it is likely to reveal triphasic waves (see Fig. 10-5). It will usually be abnormal as soon as mental changes develop, even before physical signs are present.

A CT scan is performed to exclude structural lesions, such as subdural hematomas, that can mimic toxic-metabolic encephalopathy. The CSF is inspected when meningitis, encephalitis, or subarachnoid hemorrhage is suspected. However, a CT scan should ideally be performed before a lumbar puncture when structural lessions might be present to avoid precipitating a transentorial herniation with a lumbar puncture (see Fig. 19-3).

REFERENCES

Berg L, Danziger WL, Storandt M, et al: Predictive features in mild senile dementia of the Alzheimer type. Neurology 34:563, 1984

Black PM: Idiopathic normal-pressure hydrocephalus: Results of shunting in 62 patients. J Neurosurg 52:371, 1980

Blessed G, Tomlinson BE, Roth M: The association between quantitative measures of dementia and of senile change in the cerebral gray matter of elderly subjects. Br Psychiatry 114:797, 1968

Coyle T, Price DL, Delong MR: Alzheimer's disease: A disorder of cortical cholinergic innervation. Science 219:1184, 1983

Cummings JL, Duchen LW: Klüver-Bucy syndrome in Pick disease: Clinical and pathologic correlations. Neurology 31:1415, 1981

Fisher CM: Hydrocephalus as a cause of disturbances of gait in the elderly. Neurology 32:1358, 1982

Folstein MF, Folstein SE, McHugh PR: "Mini-Mental State:" A practical method for grading the cognitive state of patients for the clinician. J Psychiatr Res 12:189, 1975

Fuld PA: Test profile of cholinergic dysfunction and of Alzheimer-type dementia. J Clin Neuropsychol 6:380, 1984

Hersch EL: Development and application of the extended scale for dementia. J Geriatr Soc 27:348, 1979

Hersch EL, Kral VA, Palmer RB: Clinical value of the London psychogeriatric rating scale. J Geriatr Soc 26:348, 1978

Hooshmand H, Escobar MR, Kopf SW: Neurosyphilis: A study of 241 patients. JAMA 219:726, 1972

Hughes CP, Berg L, Danziger WL, et al: A new clinical scale for the staging of dementia. Br J Psychiatry 140:566, 1982

Hyman BT, Van Hoesen GW, Damasio AR, et al: Alzheimer's disease: Cell-specific pathology isolates the hippocampal formation. Science 225:1168, 1984

Jaffe WH, Kabins SA: Examination of cerebrospinal fluid in patients with syphilis. Rev Infect Dis 4(suppl):S842, 1982

Katzman R, Brown T, Fuld P, et al: Validation of a short orientation-memory-concentration test of cognitive impairment. Am J Psychiatry 140:734, 1983

Katzman R, Terry R: The Neurology of Aging. Philadelphia, F.A. Davis Co., 1983

Koller WC, Glatt S, Wilson RS, et al: Primitive reflexes and cognitive function in the elderly. Ann Neurol 12:302, 1982

Mace NL, Rabins PV: The 36-Hour Day: A Family Guide to Caring for Persons with Alzheimer's Disease, Related Dementing Illnesses, and Memory Loss in Later Life. Baltimore, The Johns Hopkins University Press, 1981

Mattis S: Mental status examination for organic mental syndrome in the elderly patient. In Bellak L, Karasu B: Geriatric Psychiatry: A Handbook for Psychiatrists and Primary Care Physicians. New York, Grune & Stratton, 1976, pp 77–121

Mawdsley C, Ferguson FR: Neurologic disease in boxers. Lancet 2:795, 1963

Mayeux R, Stern Y, Rosen J, et al: Is "subcortical dementia" a recognizable clinical entity? Ann Neurol 14:278, 1983

McKann G, Drachman D, Folstein M, et al: Clinical diagnosis of Alzheimer's disease: Report of the NINCDS-ADRDA Work Group under the auspices of Department of Health and Human Services Task Force on Alzheimer's Disease. Neurology 34:939, 1984

McDowell FH (ed): Managing the Person with Intellectual Loss (Dementia or Alzheimer's Disease) at Home. White Plains, New York, The Burke Rehabilitation Center, 1980

Nakano I, Hirano A: Parkinson's disease: Neuron loss in the nucleus basalis without concomitant Alzheimer's disease. Ann Neurol 15:415, 1984

Prusiner SB: Prions. Sci Am 251:50, 1984

Prusiner SB: Some speculations about prions, amyloid, and Alzheimer's disease. N Engl J Med 310:661, 1984

Reisberg B, Ferris SH, De Leon MJ, et al: The global deterioration scale for assessment of primary degenerative dementia. Am J Psychiatry 139:1136, 1982

Sinex FM, Merrill CR: Alzheimer's Disease, Down's Syndrome, and Aging. New York, New York Academy of Sciences, 1982

Soininen B, Partanen JV, Puranen M, et al: EEG and computed tomography in the investigation of patients with senile dementia. J Neurol Neurosurg Psychiatry 45:711, 1982

Storandt M, Botwinick J, Danziger WL, et al: Psychometric differentiation of mild senile dementia of the Alzheimer type. Arch Neurol 41:497, 1984

Terry RD, Katzman R: Senile dementia of the Alzheimer type. Ann Neurol 14:497, 1983

Tweedy J, Reding M, Garcia C, et al: Significance of cortical disinhibition signs. Neurology 32:169, 1982

Vitaliano PP, Breen AR, Albert MS, et al: Memory, attention, and functional status in community-residing Alzheimer-type dementia patients and optimally healthy aged individuals. J Gerontol 39:58, 1984

Winstead DK, Mielke DH: Differential diagnosis between dementia and depression in the elderly. In Green JB (ed): Borderland Between Neurology and Psychiatry. Neurology Clinics. Philadelphia, W.B. Saunders, 1984, pp 23–35

Zilber N, Rannon L, Alter M, et al: Measles, measles vaccination, and risk of subacute sclerosing panencephalitis (SSPE). Neurology 33:1558, 1983

QUESTIONS

1. What are the cardinal neurologic features of the following cases of dementia or delirium?

a. CNS lupus	h. Porphyria
b. Normal pressure hydrocephalus	i. Wernicke's encephalopathy
c. Obstructive hydrocephalus	j. Myxedema madness
d. Wilson's disease	k. Tuberous sclerosis
e. Huntington's chorea	l. Hepatic encephalopathy
f. Bromism	m. SSPE
g. Arsenic poisoning	n. Creutzfeldt-Jakob disease

2. Name the single initial laboratory test that would indicate the following causes of dementia.

a. Myxedema	i. Bromism
b. Combined system disease (PA)	j. Subarachnoid hemorrhage
c. Porphyria	k. Subdural hematomas
d. Arsenic poisoning	l. Creutzfeldt-Jakob's disease
e. Lead poisoning	m. Wilson's disease
f. Tabes dorsalis	n. Sphenoid wing meningioma
g. SSPE	o. Hepatic encephalopathy
h. Water intoxication	p. Cryptococcal meningitis

3. In which causes of dementia is the EEG usually of diagnostic assistance?

a. Alzheimer's disease	i. Bromism
b. SSPE	j. Frontal lobe tumors
c. Olivopontocerebellar atrophy	k. Valium intoxication
d. Lead poisoning	l. Pseudodementia
e. Uremia	m. Parkinson's disease
f. Hepatic encephalopathy	n. Herpes encephalitis
g. Creutzfeldt-Jakob disease	o. Subdural hematomas
h. Neurosyphilis	

4. The diagnosis of normal pressure hydrocephalus (NPH) has received much attention in the literature because installation of a ventricular-peritoneal shunt is said to correct the dementia.

a. What conditions predispose a patient to NPH?
b. What tests are used in an attempt to establish this diagnosis?

5. Is a cerebral cortex biopsy routinely indicated for the diagnosis of Alzheimer's disease?

6. Match the electrolyte pattern (1–6) with the disturbances that are associated with metabolic encephalopathy:

a. Water intoxication   d. Inappropriate ADH secretion
b. Water deprivation (dehydration)   e. Bromism
c. Uremia   f. Diabetic ketoacidosis

	Na	K	Cl	CO_2	BUN	Cratine
1.	140	4.0	100	24	15	1.0
2.	140	4.0	125	20	20	1.2
3.	125	2.8	80	15	5	0.5
4.	138	4.8	100	20	60	4.9
5.	152	4.9	100	19	58	1.8
6.	130	5.1	102	10	35	1.9

7. What medication or therapy (column B) is appropriate for severe intoxications of the following (column A)?

[A]

1. Lithium
2. Bromide
3. Heroin
4. Methadone
5. Phenobarbital
6. Imipramine (Tofranil)
7. Valium
8. Water
9. Lead
10. Belladona alkaloids
11. Methanol
12. Arsenic
13. Organic phosphates
14. Phenothiazines
15. Mercury
16. LSD
17. Isoniazid (INH)
18. Scopolamine
19. L-dopa
20. Thyroxine

[B]

a. Physostigmine
b. Hypertonic saline or water restriction
c. Atropine
d. Dialysis
e. Saline, diuretics
f. Ethyl alcohol 50 percent
g. B_6
h. BAL (dimecaprol)
i. Penicillin
j. Naloxone (Narcan)
k. Hypotonic saline
l. Glucose
m. Nonspecific supportive therapy ± sedatives
n. Propranolol (Inderal)

8. What is the pattern of inheritance of the following diseases that cause dementia?

1. Wilson's disease
2. Huntington's chorea
3. Adrenoleukodystrophy
4. Porphyria, acute intermittent
5. Familial Alzheimer's disease

a. Sex-linked recessive
b. Autosomal recessive
c. Autosomal dominant

9. Which clinical findings are associated with bulbar or pseudobulbar palsy?

1. Depressed gag reflex
2. Reduced voluntary palate movement
3. Atrophy of tongue

a. Bulbar palsy
b. Pseudobulbar palsy
c. Both

    4. Dysphagia
    5. Increased jaw jerk
    6. Dysarthria
    7. Emotional lability
    8. Decreased jaw jerk
    9. Aphasia
    10. Dementia

10. Which diseases are associated with bulbar or pseudobulbar palsy?

1. Alzheimer's disease	a. Bulbar palsy
2. Poliomyelitis	b. Pseudobulbar palsy
3. Bilateral frontal lobe infarcts	c. Both
4. ALS	
5. Vertebrobasilar artery occlusions	
6. Encephalitis	
7. Botulism	
8. Multiple sclerosis	
9. Postanoxic encephalopathy	
10. Myasthenia gravis	

11. Which of the following conditions are reversible forms of dementia?

a. Uremia	n. Cryptococcal meningitis
b. Hepatic encephalopathy	o. SSPE
c. Postanoxic encephalopathy	p. Mononucleosis encephalitis
d. Porphyria cutanea tarda	q. Cerebral syphilis
e. African porphyria	r. Hypertensive encephalopathy
f. Acute intermittent porphyria	s. Lacunar state
g. Myxedema	t. Subdural hematomas
h. Kernicterus	u. Alzheimer's disease
i. Combined system disease	v. Pick's disease
j. Hypercalcemia	w. Creutzfeldt-Jakob disease
k. Mercury poisoning	x. Myoclonic epilepsy
l. Wernicke-Korsakoff snydrome	y. Wilson's disease
m. Pellagra	z. Parkinson's disease

12. Which commonly used medications may cause dementia?

13. What is the most common form of dementia accompanied by a peripheral neuropathy?

14. Which is the most common EG finding in patients with early Alzheimer's disease?
    a. Theta and delta activity
    b. Periodic complexes
    c. High-voltage fast activity
    d. Normal or slight slowing of the background activity

15. In which conditions is cerebral atrophy found on CT scans?

a. Alzheimer's disease	d. Normal pressure hydrocephalus
b. Down's syndrome	e. Encephalitis
c. Normal aging	f. Pseudotumor cerebri

16. With which condition is cerebral atrophy, as detected by CT, most closely associated?
    a. Alzheimer's disease
    b. Intellectual impairment
    c. Old age

17.   Positron emission tomography (PET) and other studies have demonstrated decreased cerebral glucose metabolism and decreased oxygen consumption in Alzheimer's disease. How is it known that Alzheimer's disease does not result from cellular hypoxia?

18.   From which area of the brain do the majority of cerebral cortex cholinergic fibers originate?
   a.   Hippocampus
   b.   Basal ganglia
   c.   Frontal lobe
   d.   Nucleus basalis Meynert

19–22.   Choline acetyltransferase (CAT) is the fundamental enzyme in synthesis of acetylcholine (ACh). What is the effect of the following substances on ACh activity?

19. Neostigmine	a. Increases ACh activity
20. Scopolamine	b. Decreases ACh activity
21. Organic phosphate insecticides	c. Does not change ACh activity
22. Physostigmine	

23.   What are the features of multi-infarct dementia that are *not* present in Alzheimer's disease?
   a.   Prominent physical impairments, e.g., spasticity
   b.   History of hypertension and cerebrovascular infarctions
   c.   Helpfulness of EEG in diagnosis
   d.   A CT scan showing multiple lucencies
   e.   Improvement in symptoms with antihypertensive treatment

24.   Which are frequently found features of Wernicke-Korsakoff syndrome?
   a.   CT scan that is normal or shows atrophy
   b.   Confabulation
   c.   Hemorrhage in portions of the limbic system
   d.   Full recovery after diagnosis

25.   Why do many patients with active neurosyphilis have negative blood VDRL tests?
   a.   Autoimmune diseases often cause false-negative tests.
   b.   After years, the VDRL naturally reverts to being negative.
   c.   Small doses of antibiotics, given for unrelated reasons, partially but inadequately treat syphilis and the VDRL reverts to being negative but neurosyphilis continues.
   d.   Very high antibody levels interfere with the test.

26.   Since a large proportion of patients with neurosyphilis have negative CSF VDRL tests, how should the clinician proceed?
   a.   In the appropriate clinical setting, if there is CSF pleocytosis and increased protein concentration, treatment for neurosyphilis should be given despite a negative CSF VDRL
   b.   Obtain a CSF FTA-ABS test
   c.   Do lumbar puncture on all patients with dementia
   d.   Do lumbar puncture on all patients with a positive blood VDRL

27.   Of the following, which is the most accurate blood test for syphilis?
   a.   VDRL
   b.   Microhemagglutination assay (MHA-TP)
   c.   Wasserman
   d.   Colloidal gold curve

28.   Which are characteristics of Pick's disease?
   a.   Preserved visuospatial ability
   b.   Familial tendency
   c.   Preserved parietal lobe despite otherwise generalized cerebral atrophy

d. Argentophilic intraneuronal bodies
e. Transmissibility to monkeys
f. Ready clinical identification

29. What are neurologic complications of professional boxing?
   a. Dementia pugilistica
   b. Intracranial bleeding
   c. Parkinsonism
   d. Dysarthria
   e. Spasticity and other corticospinal tract signs

30. Which forms of intellectual deterioration are associated with peripheral neuropathy?
   a. Alzheimer's disease
   b. Wernicke-Korsakoff syndrome
   c. Metachromatic leukodystrophy
   d. Uremia
   e. Nitrous oxide abuse
   f. Acute intermittent porphyria
   g. Combined system disease / (B$_{12}$ deficiency)
   h. Polyarteritis

31. Which movement disorders are associated with functionally incapacitating cognitive impairments?
   a. Choreoathetosis
   b. Lesch-Nyhan syndrome
   c. Dystonia musculorum deformans
   d. Tourette's syndrome
   e. Essential tremor
   f. Rigid form of Huntington's chorea

32. Which forms of dementia tend to develop in several members of a family?
   a. SSPE
   b. Pick's disease
   c. Alzheimer's disease
   d. Subdural hematomas

ANSWERS

1. a. Seizures, strokes, and psychosis (the three S's)
   b. Dementia, incontinence, and gait apraxia
   c. Headache, papilledema, and bilateral Babinski signs
   d. Dementia, tremor, rigidity, and Kayser-Fleischer corneal rings
   e. Dementia, chorea, and, in young adults, rigidity
   f. Dementia with psychotic appearance, acneiform skin rash, headache, and lethargy
   g. Nonspecific mental dullness and peripheral neuropathy
   h. Recurrent episodes of delirium, seizures, peripheral neuropathy, and abdominal pain with dark red urine (acute intermittent porphyria only)
   i. A confusional state with nystagmus, ocular paresis, ataxia, and peripheral neuropathy
   j. Rarely occurring, excited, confusional state
   k. Adenoma of face, seizures, and dementia, usually beginning in childhood
   l. Lethargy, confusion, and asterixis
   m. Slowly developing dementia, ataxia, and myoclonus, usually in rural boys
   n. Rapidly developing dementia, pyramidal and extrapyramidal motor findings, and myoclonus

2. a. Serum T$_4$ level
   b. Serum B$_{12}$ level
   c. Watson-Schwartz test or urine porphyrin levels

    d.   Serum heavy metal tests or finger nail analysis
    e.   Serum heavy metal tests
    f.   CSF-VDRL, if positive (see text)
    g.   EEG (periodic complexes) and CSF measles antibody
    h.   Serum electrolytes
    i.   Serum electrolytes
    j.   Bloody or xanthochromic CSF from a LP or a CT scan showing blood
    k.   CT scan
    l.   EEG (periodic complexes) and brain biopsy (spongyform encephalopathy)
    m. Serum ceruloplasmin level and slit-lamp examination
    n.   CT scan
    o.   EEG (triphasic waves) and liver function tests
    p.   Cryptococcal antigen test of the CSF

3. b, e, f, g, j, k, l, n

4. a.   Subarachnoid hemorrhage, chronic meningitis, but mostly idiopathic
    b.   CT scan and cisternography

5. No. Since senile plaques and neurofibrillary tangles are found in normal, aged brains, routine histologic examination cannot be diagnostic. If enzyme studies can be performed, a lowered acetylcholine or choline acetyltransferase level would be virtually diagnostic.

6. a. 3; b. 5; c. 4; d. 3; e. 2; f. 6;

7. 1. e; 2. e; 3. j; 4. j; 5. d; 6. a; 7. m; 8. b; 9. h; 10. m; 11. f; 12. h; 13. c; 14. m; 15. h; 16. m; 17. g; 18. m; 19. m, g; 20. n

8. 1. b; 2. c; 3. a; 4. c; 5. c

9. 1. a; 2. c; 3. a; 4. c; 5. b; 6. c; 7. b; 8. a; 9. b; 10. b

10. 1. b; 2. a; 3. b; 4. c; 5. a; 6. b; 7. a; 8. b; 9. b; 10. a

11.

a.	Yes		n.	Yes
b.	Yes		o.	No
c.	No		p.	Yes
d.	No		q.	Yes
e.	No.		r.	Yes
f.	Yes		s.	No
g.	Yes		t.	Yes
h.	No		u.	No
i.	Yes		v.	No
j.	Yes		w.	No
k.	No		x.	No
l.	Yes		y.	Yes
m.	Yes		z.	No

12. Insulin, steroids, bromides, reserpine, L-dopa, scopolamine, atropine, methyldopa (Aldomet)

13. Wernicke-Korsakoff syndrome

14. d

15. a, b, c

16. c

17. Since several studies have demonstrated that oxygen *extraction* is normal, the O_2 consumption is low because cerebral requirements are low. In addition to Alzheimer's disease, in many other conditions in which cerebral metabolism is lowered, the oxygen consumption is secondarily lowered. As a practical point, giving oxygen to Alzheimer's disease patients will not reverse the dementia.

18. d

19. a (but not in the brain)

20. b

21. a (but not in the brain)

22. a

23. a, b, d

24. a, c (the mamillary bodies are part of the limbic system)

25. b, c, d

26. a

27. b

28. a, b, c, d

29. a, b, c, d, e

30. b, c, d, e, f, g, h (see Table 5-2)

31. a (but not always), b, f

32. b, c

8

Aphasia and Related Disorders

Language impairment, *aphasia*,* differs from generalized intellectual impairment, dementia (Chapter 7), both in its circumscribed neuropsychologic characteristics and in its origin, which is usually a single, discrete cerebral lesion, such as a cerebrovascular accident (CVA) (Chapter 11). More important, unlike dementia, aphasia usually results from damage to certain areas of the *dominant hemisphere,* the cerebral hemisphere that governs language function.

Language function includes verbal language (speaking and listening), written language (reading and writing), and even sign language. In addition, the dominant hemisphere integrates language with intellect, emotion, and the sensory modalities (such as the tactile, auditory, and visual systems), and thus provides the primary avenue for conscious communication of thoughts and experience.

However, the dominant hemisphere does not necessarily govern languages that are learned as adults, including "second languages," or writing that is based on pictures (e.g., hieroglyphics) rather than letters. It also plays a minimal role in imparting that combination of inflection, rhythm, and tone that compose the *prosody* of speech. In music, too, the dominant hemisphere usually has less influence than the nondominant one, at least with regard to people who have no particular creative or interpretive musical skills. However, those people with such musical skills have been shown to process music, as language, in the dominant hemisphere.

Cerebral hemisphere dominance for language is accompanied by control of fine, rapid hand movements ("handedness") and, to a lesser degree, reception of vision and hearing. For example, right-handed people, who have left cerebral hemisphere dominance, not only prefer their right hand for writing and throwing a ball, but their right foot for kicking, right eye when peering through a telescope, and right ear for listening to words spoken in both ears (*dichotic listening*).

Autopsy and radiologic studies have shown that the superior surface of the domi-

---

*Patients with aphasia and related disorders may receive assistance from the American Speech-Language-Hearing Association, 10801 Rockville Pike, Rockville, Maryland 20852, (301) 897-5700.

nant temporal lobe has significantly greater cortex area than that of the nondominant lobe because it has more gyri and deeper sulci. This region, the *planum temporale*, contains important elements of the language pathway. Notably, according to some reports, the normal cortical asymmetry is lacking in some patients with autism and chronic schizophrenia—two conditions with prominent language abnormalities.

About 90 percent of all people are left hemisphere dominant for language and are right-handed. Of the others, many are also left hemisphere dominant but appear to be ambidextrous or even left-handed. Many people who are truly ambidextrous excel in playing certain sports and performing on musical instruments. These people may have been endowed with language and motor skill function in their right as well as left hemisphere.

In contrast, left-handed people may also have naturally occurring right hemisphere dominance or, instead, their right hemisphere may have become dominant as a consequence of congenital cerebral injury on the left (Chapter 13). Left-handed people are found in disproportionate numbers among those who excel in various skilled endeavors and, as might be expected, also among those who are mentally or physically impaired. For example, a greater than expected number of left-handed people are musicians, artists, mathematicians, and athletes.[*] However, left-handed people are also over-represented among children with dyslexia and other learning disabilities, stuttering, and general clumsiness. Likewise, this disproportionate left-handedness is also found among people with mental retardation, epilepsy, and certain major psychiatric disorders, including autism and some forms of schizophrenia. Also, left-handed persons are prone to thyroid and gastrointestinal tract immune disorders.

Although the left hemisphere is usually dominant, and this chapter will assume it always is, under certain circumstances dominance must be established with certainty. For example, when the temporal lobe must be partially resected because of intractable partial complex epilepsy (Chapter 10), only a limited resection of the dominant temporal lobe would be permissible to avoid creating aphasia. Cerebral dominance can be established with the *Wada test* in which sodium amobarbital is injected directly into each carotid artery: When the dominant hemisphere is perfused, the patient becomes briefly aphasic.

APHASIA

Functional Neuroanatomy

Impulses conveying speech, music, and uncomplicated sound travel from the ears along the acoustic (eighth cranial) nerves into the brainstem. Crossed and uncrossed brainstem tracts bring them to the primary auditory cortex, *(Hechl's) gyri,* in each temporal lobe (see Fig. 4-15). Most music and a portion of other impulses remain in

---

*Closely examining this general rule about athletes, Hemenway (see references) found that left-handed athletes tend to be more successful than right-handed ones only in those sports that are directly competitive and have active defenses, such as baseball, tennis, fencing, and boxing. In these sports, left-handed athletes have a tactical advantage, such as a left-handed batter's greater closeness to first base. In other sports, such as swimming, golf, and pole vaulting, Hemenway found little difference between right- and left-handers. Thus, he doubts that right hemisphere dominance confers an advantage for athletes.

the nondominant hemisphere. Those conveying language are transmitted to *Wernicke's* area, which is in the dominant temporal lobe, and travel in a semicircle within the *arcuate fasciculus* through the temporal and parietal lobes to *Broca's area* (Fig. 8-1). Within this pathway, words are converted into language and integrated with other psychologic information and various sensory modalities. Broca's area, which is immediately anterior to the motor centers for the right arm, face, larynx, and pharynx, serves to articulate the processed, integrated language.

Using this model, several language patterns and clinicopathologic correlations have been postulated. When people repeat aloud what they hear, impulses go to Wernicke's area, pass through the arcuate fasciculus, and arrive at Broca's area for speech production (Fig. 8-2). When people read aloud, impulses are initially received by each occipital lobe's visual cortex (see Fig. 4-1); however, those from the left visual field are received by the right occipital cortex and must travel through the posterior corpus callosum. Then impulses from the visual cortices of both occipital lobes merge and travel through the arcuate fasciculus to Broca's area (Fig. 8-3).

Thus people cannot repeat phrases if they have lesions in the left temporal, parietal, or frontal lobe. Morever, lesions that damage Broca's area are also apt to damage the adjacent motor cortex and thus cause dysarthria and right hemiparesis as well as aphasia. However, lesions that cause aphasia as a result of Wernicke's area or arcuate fasciculus damage are not associated with dysarthria or hemiparesis. Finally, lesions that damage the posterior corpus callosum interrupt the path for written information received by the left visual field as it travels from the visual cortex of the right hemisphere to the language centers of the left hemisphere.

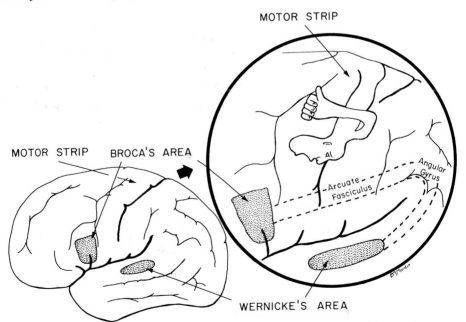

Fig. 8-1. The left cerebral hemisphere contains Wernicke's area in the temporal lobe and Broca's area in the frontal lobe. They are connected by the arcuate fasciculus. Adjacent to Broca's area is the motor area for the right hand and face.

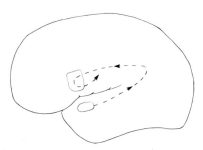

Fig. 8-2. When patients repeat aloud, language is received in Wernicke's area and transmitted through the parietal lobe by the arcuate fasciculus to Broca's area. This area innervates the adjacent cerebral cortex for the tongue, lips, larynx, and pharynx, as well as for the right face and arm.

Clinical Evaluation

In previous years, aphasia was divided according to various systems. In one of the most widely used, it was classified as *receptive* (*sensory*) or *expressive* (*motor*) on the basis of the relative impairment of verbal reception or expression; however, this nomenclature was not practical because almost all aphasic patients had mixtures of receptive and expressive impairments. The neurologic community has now adopted a division of aphasia into *nonfluent* and *fluent* based on the quality of a patient's verbal output (Table 8-1). Most cases can now be reliably classified as either nonfluent or fluent. In addition, clinicopathologic correlations have been confirmed with isotopic brain scan, computed tomography (CT), positron emission tomography (PET), and autopsy studies.

These varieties of aphasia are usually evident during conversation, history taking, or mental status examination. To detect subtle cases, reach an exact diagnosis, or demonstrate the findings, a series of verbal tests can be administered. This entire sequence might be performed with written requests and responses; however, with rare exceptions (described below), written deficits will parallel verbal deficits. The standard aphasia tests evaluate three basic language functions:

- *Comprehension,* which is tested by asking the patient to follow simple requests, such as picking up one hand.
- *Naming,* by asking the patient to say his or her own name and that of common objects, such as a pen or key.
- *Repeating,* by asking the patient to recite several short phrases, such as "The boy went to the store."

Nonfluent Aphasia

Nonfluent aphasia is characterized by a paucity of speech. Whatever speech is produced consists almost only of single words and short phrases, with preferential use

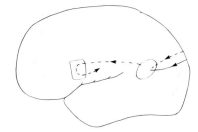

Fig. 8-3. When patients read aloud, visual impulses are received by the occipital visual cortex regions. Both send impulses to the left parietal region. Those from the left visual field, which are received in the right cortex, must first pass through the posterior corpus callosum (see Figs. 4-1 and 8-4).

Table 8-1
The Salient Features of the Motor Aphasias

Feature	Nonfluent Aphasia	Fluent Aphasia
Previous descriptions	Expressive Motor Broca's	Receptive Sensory Wernicke's
Spontaneous speech	Nonverbal	Verbal
Content	Paucity of words, mostly nouns and verbs	Complete sentences with normal syntax
Articulation	Dysarthric, slow, stuttering	Good
Errors		Paraphasic errors Nonspecific phrases Circumlocutions
Response on testing		
Comprehension	Preserved	Impaired
Repetition	Impaired	Impaired
Naming	Impaired	Impaired
Associated deficits	Hemiparesis (arm, face > leg)	Hemianopsia Hemisensory loss
Localization of lesion	Frontal lobe (in or near Broca's area)	Temporal or parietal lobe (occasionally diffuse)

of highly meaningful words, such as nouns and verbs. Speech is slow, typically at a rate of less than 50 words per minute. Moreover, articulation is poor and the cadence so irregular that the speech pattern is sometimes called "telegraphic." For example, in response to a question about food, a patient might stammer ". . . fork . . . steak . . . eat . . ."

Patients with nonfluent aphasia are neither able to say their own name or the names of common objects, nor to repeat simple phrases. However, they have relatively normal comprehension. This can be illustrated by their ability to follow verbal requests, such as "Close your eyes" or "Raise your left hand." This combination of inability to speak correctly and preserved ability to follow verbal requests was what originally caused nonfluent aphasia to be designated expressive.

Nonfluent aphasia, since it stems from a Broca's area lesion, is characteristically associated with paresis of the right arm and lower face. It is also associated with *buccofacial apraxia,* which is not merely paresis, but inability to execute normal facial, lip, and tongue movements. Aphasic patients are not able to speak distinctly partly because of buccofacial apraxia. When buccofacial apraxia is severe, it can lead to virtual mutism, so-called *aphemia.* To evaluate buccofacial apraxia, the examiner asks people to say "La . . . Pa . . . La . . . Pa . . . La . . . Pa . . . ," blow out an imagined match, or protrude their tongue in different directions. Patients will not be able to follow these abstract requests but will be able to use the same muscles reflexly, i.e., they will be able to say a few words, sing, eat, or blow out an actual match.

Nonfluent aphasia patients so often become frustrated, tearful, and distraught that emotional disturbances have been considered characteristic. While emotional disturbances with aphasia may be common, many patients, particularly those who have had several CVAs, may actually be revealing signs of either dementia, pseudobulbar palsy (Chapter 4), or both. In fact, signs of nonfluent aphasia, dementia, and pseudobulbar palsy are apt to be confused with each other and, because all can originate in frontal lobe injury, may occur together.

The lesion responsible for nonfluent aphasia and the associated hemiparesis, located in or near Broca's area, is almost always a discrete structural injury, such as a middle cerebral artery occlusion. Diffuse cerebral injuries, such as metabolic disturbances or Alzheimer's disease, are practically never the cause.

An extreme form of nonfluent aphasia is *global aphasia,* which is characterized by virtually complete loss of language function. Aside from uttering some unintelligible sounds and following an occasional gestured command, patients with global aphasia are mute and unresponsive. Their devastating language impairment is accompanied by (right) hemiplegia, a comparably severe motor deficit. Responsible lesions are so extensive that most of the left hemisphere, including both Broca's and Wernicke's areas, is injured. Internal carotid artery occlusions and penetrating head wounds are two of the most frequent causes.

Fluent Aphasia

Fluent aphasia consists of plentiful, articulate speech that contains complete, grammatically correct sentences spoken at a relatively normal rate of 100 words per minute. It is characterized by many words being used incorrectly or nonsensically. These words, which are called *paraphasic errors* or *paraphasias,* may make conversation unintelligible.

Paraphasias include real words being substituted for others, such as "clock" for "watch" (a related paraphasia). Unrelated words may be substituted, such as "glove" for "knife" (an unrelated paraphasia). Also, altered words may appear, such as "breat" for "bread" (a literal paraphasia). More striking, strings of nonsensical coinages (*neologisms*) may be used, such as "I want to fin gunt in the fark."

Besides using paraphasias, patients may speak in *circumlocutions,* as though they were trying to avoid dealing with their word-finding difficulty. They may also employ nonspecific terms, such as substituting *shirt and the thing* for *shirt and tie.* Likewise, patients tend toward tangential discussions, as though once the wrong word was chosen, they pursue the idea triggered by their error.

Nevertheless, speech prosody is true to patients' emotions, Also, most patients will still be able to produce a melody even though they may be unable to say lyrics. For example, patients can hum a tune, such as "Jingle Bells," but if they attempt to sing, their lyrics will be strewn with paraphasias.

In contrast to nonfluent aphasia, fluent aphasia is associated with minimal physical deficits (Table 8-2). Significant hemiparesis is generally lacking. Usually, right-sided hyperactive deep tendon reflexes (DTRs) and a Babinski sign are the only motor signs present. However, right-sided sensory impairment and homonymous hemianopsia may be present because of interruptions of the sensory and visual cerebral pathways.

Lesions that cause fluent aphasia are usually discrete structural ones, such as small CVAs, in the temporoparietal region. They often damage Wernicke's area or the arcuate fasciculus. However, hypotension, anoxia, or carbon monoxide poisoning may bring about a fluent aphasia by damaging a crescent of cerebral cortex above the arcuate faciculus and isolating the Wernicke–Broca axis from the rest of the cerebral cortex. More important, unlike nonfluent aphasia, fluent aphasia is sometimes caused by diffuse cerebral injury, including Alzheimer's disease.

Varieties of fluent aphasia have been described, but most descriptions are not

Table 8-2

Clinical Evaluation for Aphasia

Spontaneous speech: fluent versus nonfluent
Verbalization tests
    Comprehension (ability to follow requests)
    Naming (common objects: tie, keys, pen)
    Repetition (simple phrases, complex phrases)
Specific abnormalities
    Circumlocutions, Tangents
    Nonspecific phrases
    Paraphasic errors
        Related ("spoon" for "fork")
        Unrelated ("football" for "fork")
        Literal ("fark" for "fork")
        Neologistical ("needle" for "fork")
Reading and writing (repeat above tests)
Associated physical signs
    Corticospinal tract
        Hemiparesis (especially lower face and arm)
        Babinski sign
    Motor skills
        Buccolingual apraxia
        Limb apraxia
    Sensory system
        Loss of cortical modalities (position, stereognosis)
    Visual tracts
        Homonymous hemianopsia
        Superior quadrantanopsia (with temporal lobe lesions)

---

only complex and turn on subtle points, but their clinicopathologic correlations are unreliable because of individual variations in anatomy, language lateralization, and speech production. Nevertheless, several varieties are recognizable. One is *anomia*, which is simply an inability to name common objects. It is associated with Alzheimer's disease, in which cases it may be found along with dementia. Another variety is *transcortical aphasia*, which results from isolation of the Wernicke–Broca axis. Since the language system itself is intact but no longer able to receive input from the rest of the cerebrum, patients can repeat whatever they hear, including long phrases, but they cannot initiate meaningful conversation.

MENTAL ABNORMALITIES WITH LANGUAGE IMPAIRMENTS

Distinguishing among aphasia, dementia, and their coexistence is more than an academic exercise. A diagnosis of aphasia almost always suggests that a patient has had a discrete dominant cerebral hemisphere injury. Since a CVA or other structural lesion would be the most likely cause, the appropriate evaluation would include CT (Chapter 20). In contrast, a diagnosis of dementia suggests that the most likely cause would be Alzheimer's disease or another diffuse process, and the evaluation might include an EEG, CSF analysis, and various blood tests as well as CT.

Patients with dementia in its early stages are usually fully verbal, articulate, and able to perform well on the three standard language function tests. However, an exception is patients in whom anomia is associated with dementia. This impairment probably results from people's naming ability, which unlike their other basic language functions, is heavily dependent on memory and thus particularly vulnerable to intellectual decline. Those with severe dementia have a paucity of speech and a limited vocabulary. When these patients do speak, they tend to have *perseverations*, repetitions of thoughts and words; *echolalia,* a form of perseveration in which they parrot visitors' questions; and *palilalia,* which is repetition of their own words.

Although aphasia and dementia may be confused with each other, they can be distinguished. Patients with nonfluent aphasia usually have had the sudden onset of marked language impairment and dysarthria accompanied by right hemiparesis. Those with dementia, which takes months or more to develop, typically have no hemiparesis or dysathria, and can say their own name and those of common objects, follow simple requests, and repeat phrases.

Patients with fluent aphasia are also apt to be misdiagnosed as having dementia because they might have trouble recounting the date and place, repeating a series of numbers, and following requests. They may be identified because they usually are unable to give their own name, identify common objects, or perform well on the other standard language tests. Moreover, their language will almost always be strewn with paraphasias. Patients with dementia, in contrast, can almost always say their own name and those of common objects, follow simple requests, and repeat simple phrases. Even if patients have anomia, they seldom use paraphasias.

Sometimes patients might be found to have both aphasia and dementia. This combination might occur in cases of multi-infarct dementia or when a person with Alzheimer's disease sustains a CVA. Such cases, apart from being tragic, are notoriously difficult to diagnose because aphasia invalidates all but the most sophisticated tests.

While the distinction between both forms of aphasia and dementia may be difficult, that between fluent aphasia and *schizophrenic speech* can be even more troublesome. These two conditions are confused because of common language abnormalities that include circumlocutions, tangentialities, and neologisms. Moreover, as the thought disorder of schizophrenic patients becomes more pronounced, their language abnormalities increase in frequency and become more similar to those of fluent aphasia. Also, patients with aphasia are apt to have emotional disturbances because the abrupt onset of the inability to communicate may be as bewildering as suddenly finding themselves in a country where everyone speaks a foreign language.

Despite these similarities, many differences can be discerned. Schizophrenic speech usually develops in patients who are in their third decade and have had longstanding mental disturbances. In schizophrenic speech, neologisms and other paraphasias are usually neither frequent nor conspicuous, and the content follows the rules of grammar. Moreover, comprehension is almost always preserved.

In contrast, people who develop aphasia are usually in their sixth or seventh decade and, aside from having cardiovascular disease, are in good health. Although they may be distraught, they are often but not always aware that their problem is not comprehending spoken language and they request help. Possibly because of self-monitoring, their responses are shorter and more pointed. If a right homonymous hemianopsia or other lateralized finding can be elicited, aphasia from a cerebral lesion is indicated; however, such physical deficits unfortunately are sometimes not found because either they are subtle or the patient's excitement or inability to cooperate precludes a proper examination.

Language usage abnormalities, but not aphasia, are also a prominent aspect of *childhood autism*. Autistic children begin to speak later than normal and often remain mute until they do so. Their grammar is poor, incorrect pronouns are assigned ("pronoun reversal"), and echolalia is common. Also, they have limited prosody and generally do not use gestures meaningfully. Otherwise, their language abnormalities have only sight similarity to aphasia. In particular, autistic children do not display several of the cardinal features of aphasia: paraphasias, anomias, and comprehension impairment.

Mutism and apparent language abnormalities can also be associated with psychogenic disturbances. In these situations, the language impairment is usually transient, inconsistent, and amenable to suggestion. An amobarbital interview might be attempted, but the examiner should first request that responses be in writing. In this way, patients with psychogenic mutism will reveal intact language function.

Perhaps the most common aphasia-like psychogenic condition is word-finding difficulties attributable to psychodynamic processes. This condition is so close to aphasia that it cries out for a neurologic explanation. One example is a person's momentary inability to recall well-known names. This phenomenon, which is akin to anomia, might be the result of diffuse cerebral cortical dysfunction as in Alzheimer's disease, but in this case one with purely psychologic manifestations. Another example is the Freudian slip, such as a newscaster's reference to "Treachery Secretary Regan," which neurologists might interpret as a paraphasia.

RELATED DISORDERS: ALEXIA, AGRAPHIA, AGNOSIA, AND APRAXIA

Although aphasia is the most frequently occurring language disorder, several others are important and also referable to injury of the dominant hemisphere. *Alexia*, reading inability, and *agraphia*, writing inability, are almost always found together; however, an important exception is *alexia without agraphia*. This is a rare condition in which people cannot read but can transcribe dictation or write their thoughts, and then be unable to read their own writing.

This syndrome results from a destructive lesion encompassing the dominant (left) occipital lobe and adjacent posterior corpus callosum (Fig. 8-4). Patients are unable to see anything in their right visual field because of the left occipital cortex lesion. In addition, those left visual impulses that do reach the right occipital cortex cannot be conveyed to the language centers of the left hemisphere. Thus, patients cannot comprehend written material presented to either visual field. However, they can still write full sentences from memory, imagination, or dictation because these forms of information reach the language centers through intact pathways that can communicate with all the necessary areas. In pure cases, despite the right homonyous hemianopsia and alexia, other language and physical abilities of patients remain intact.

Agraphia may also occur in the controversial *Gerstmann's syndrome*. In this condition, which has been attributed to lesions in the *angular gyrus* of the dominant parietal lobe (Fig. 8-1), agraphia is accompanied by three other abnormalities: *acalculia* (impairment of arithmetic skills), *finger agnosia* (inability to identify fingers), and *left/right confusion*. The state of Gerstmann's syndrome as a distinct clinical entity has been questioned because patients rarely display all four components simul-

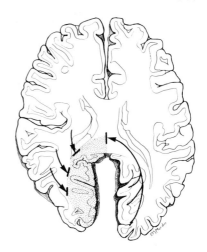

Fig. 8-4. *Alexia without agraphia* is caused by lesions that damage the left occipital lobe and the posterior corpus callosum. Visual impulses are not received by the damaged left occipital cortex. Those that do reach the right cortex cannot be transmitted across the damaged corpus callosum to the left cerebral language centers. Thus, written language is incomprehensible; however, since the language and motor centers themselves remain intact, writing is still possible.

taneously, and those who do have most components usually also have fluent aphasia. Nevertheless, the constellation of Gerstmann's signs, even if they do not constitute a syndrome, is useful in evaluating children for dyscalculia and other learning disabilities. In particular, children with dyscalculia are frequently found to have poor handwriting (agraphia), and left-right confusion accompanied by physical signs of dominant hemisphere injury, such as right-sided hyperactive DTRs or a Babinski sign (Chapter 13).

Another neuropsychologic disturbance that can be the result of dominant hemisphere injury is *agnosia*. This is a perceptual disorder in which patients cannot recognize objects despite intact sensory systems, intellectual capabilities, and language function. It should not be confused with either dementia or aphasia—other conditions in which patients might not be able to say the names of objects. An example of agnosia is if a man were shown a stop sign and, even though he could name it and describe its physical characteristics, he would be unable to explain its meaning. Another perceptual disturbance, *prosopagnosia,* is the inability to recall familiar faces or identify objects out of their usual (visual) context, such as a shirt pocket cut from a shirt. Unlike aphasia, prosopagnosia is more often the result of bilateral occipitotemporal lesions.

Color agnosia or *anomia,* a variety of agnosia, is the inability to recognize color correctly. It does not result from color blindness, dementia, or aphasia, but supposedly from damage to the dominant occipitotemporal region. Patients with color agnosia are unable to name the colors of painted cards or other colored objects; however, in striking contrast, they are able to match cards of the same color and also recite the colors of common objects, such as the sky. Because of their dominant (left) posterior cerebral damage, patients often also have a right homonymous hemianopsia and aphasia (also see *agnosia,* Chapter 12, Visual Disturbances).

Apraxia, which is the motor system's equivalent of aphasia, is the inability to execute learned actions despite normal strength, sensation, coordination, and, more important, comprehension. This impairment is thought to result from either faulty integration, or "disconnection," of motor with sensory and language centers, or possibly a failure of "motor association areas" to plan complex motor sequencing.

Typically, patients with apraxia cannot perform a particular movement at the request of the examiner, but they might still be able to do it as an automatic or unconscious action if sufficient cues (actual objects) are provided or by imitating the examiner. While several clinically useful varieties of apraxia have been described (Table 8-3), the most important ones are the two varieties of *ideomotor apraxia: buccofacial* and *limb apraxia*. Both are associated with aphasia and attributable to injury of the dominant frontal or parietal lobe (Fig. 8-5).

Buccofacial apraxia, which is associated with nonfluent aphasia, is characterized by patients' inability to move their cheeks, lips, or tongue in response to specific requests. In testing for this apraxia, people may be asked to stick out their tongue, repeat "Pa . . . Ka . . . Pa . . . Ka . . . ," pretend to use a straw, or make chewing movements. Patients will not be able to perform many of these actions purely as demonstrations, but with actual food they will eat and stick out their tongue, chew, and use a straw. Also, even though they might not be able to speak, they can often sing.

In limb apraxia, which is associated with both fluent and nonfluent aphasia, patients cannot use the limbs on either side of their body to execute simple actions. Patients are not able to salute; pretend to brush their teeth, comb their hair, or kick a ball; or move their hands in certain patterns. Characteristically, when asked to pretend to use an object, these patients will use their hand as though it were the object. However, as in the other apraxias, patients will be able to perform commands if supplied with cues or by imitating the examiner.

In *ideational apraxia*, still another form of apraxia, patients cannot perform motor activities that require several sequential steps. For example, patients cannot pretend to remove a cigarette from a pack and then light it, or pretend to fold a letter, place it into an envelope, and then affix a stamp. Although patients might complete

Table 8-3
Common Apraxias

Apraxia	Tests	Lesion's Usual Location	Associated Deficits
Constructional	Copy figure or arrange matchsticks	Nondominant parietal lobe	Left hemi-inattention
Ideational	Pretend to take a cigarette from a pack and light it, i.e., a complex sequential action	Both frontal lobes or entire cerebrum	Dementia
Ideomotor		Dominant posterior frontal or anterior parietal lobe	Aphasia
Buccofacial	Pretend to blow out a match, use a straw, or repeat syllables		
Limb	Pretend to brush teeth, unlock a door, or pick up a ball, i.e., a simple action		
Gait	Walk, start-stop-start, turn	Entire cerebrum especially, normal pressure hydrocephalus	Dementia

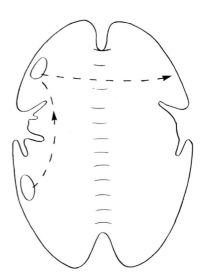

Fig. 8-5. In a schematic overview of the brain, commands for purposeful skilled movements are received by Wernicke's area in the posterior dominant (left) cerebral hemisphere. They are transmitted anteriorly to the motor regions of that hemisphere and then, through the anterior corpus callosum, to the contralateral motor strip. Interruptions of the path within the left cerebral hemisphere result in ideomotor apraxia of both arms. Lesions in the anterior corpus callosum will interrupt only those impulses destined to control the left arm and leg.

segments of these tasks, they cannot complete the entire sequence in order. Ideational apraxia is usually found to result from either diffuse cerebral disease or injuries of both frontal lobes. It is closely associated with and often a manifestation of dementia.

NONDOMINANT HEMISPHERE SYNDROMES

Hemi-inattention

While aphasia and the other disturbances discussed so far, such as agraphia and apraxia, are attributable in large measure to injuries of the dominant hemisphere, several important psychologic disturbances are attributable to nondominant hemisphere injury. The most important disorder associated with nondominant injury is *hemi-inattention (hemispatial neglect)*. It originates in injury of the nondominant parietal lobe cortex or the underlying structures, including the thalamus or reticular activating system.

Patients with right parietal lobe infarction characteristically ignore visual, tactile, and other stimuli that originate from their left side. Typically, they will not perceive objects in their left visual field despite suggestions that important things can be seen there (Fig. 8-6). Also, when both sides of their body are touched, patients neglect the left-sided stimulation (*extinction on double simultaneous stimulation (DSS)*)and report that only their right side was touched. Sometimes patients even fail to shave the left side of their face and leave their left side undressed (*dressing apraxia*).

A crucial aspect of hemi-inattention is the failure of patients to accept any associated physical deficit (*anosognosia*), which is usually a left hemiparesis. When patients do have left hemiparesis, they deny, rationalize, or employ other defense mechanisms. In the initial phase of a nondominant parietal lobe CVA, patients often refuse to accept physical therapy and hospital routine. All patients with left hemiparesis should be checked for anosognosia, especially since it can cause management problems.

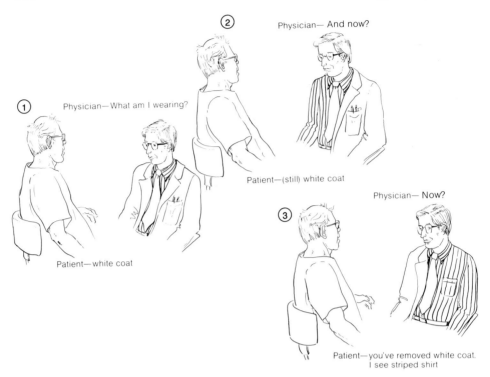

Fig. 8-6. In a classic demonstration of left *hemi-inattention*, the patient, neglecting left-sided stimulation, perceives only that the examiner is wearing whatever he sees in his own right visual field. Even if the patient's problem were simply a left homonymous hemianopsia, he still would have explored and discovered, with his intact right visual field, that the examiner was half-dressed.

Another manifestation of nondominant hemisphere injury is *constructional apraxia,* in which patients lose their ability to integrate visual information with fine motor skills (Table 8-3). In particular, *visual-spatial* perceptual impairments often prevent them from copying simple figures or arranging matchsticks in patterns (Fig. 8-7).

Aprosody

Several authors have recently described how patients with nondominant hemisphere lesions cannot appreciate emotional aspects of speech. They are said to have *aprosody.* For example, such a patient would be unable to discern the contrasting implications of the question, "Are you going to the dance?" asked first by a gleeful mother, then by a jealous friend. Not only are patients unable to discern other people's emotional tone, they themselves speak in a monotone, being unable to confer affective nuance. They are also unable to sing because, although they can repeat the lyrics to a song, they cannot convey its melody.

In many patients, aprosody is accompanied by loss of nonverbal forms of communication, or the *paralinguistic components* of speech, such as facial expression and limb gesture, that normally lend credence, emphasis, and most important, affect to

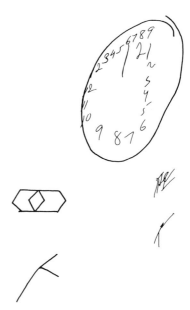

Fig. 8-7. When asked to draw a clock, a patient with _constructional apraxia_ drew an incomplete circle, repeated (perseverated) the numerals, and placed them asymmetrically. When attempting to copy the figure on the left, the patient repeated several lines, failing to draw any figure. The patient also misplaced and rotated the position of the lower figure.

the meaning of spoken words. However, this loss may also be caused by diminished physical abilities resulting from several conditions unrelated to nondominant hemisphere injuries, such as parkinsonism and depression.

Several authors have also suggested that the nondominant hemisphere is responsible not only for prosody and the other qualities already discussed, but for general affect, complex nonverbal processes, holistic cognitive approach, and impulsiveness. The dominant hemisphere, they suggest, is responsible for verbal, sequential, analytic cognitive processes, and for reflectiveness.

DISCONNECTION SYNDROMES

While many psychologic functions are governed almost entirely by either one hemisphere or the other, the multitude of human endeavors, including learning and expression of emotion, require communication between both hemispheres. Appropriate interhemispheric connections are the myelin-coated axonal (white matter) bundles, _commissures,_ of which the most conspicuous is the _corpus callosum._ Others are the massa intermedia and the anterior, posterior, and hippocampal commissures.

Injuries that damage the commissures deprive each hemisphere of some of the other's information and thus lead to a group of interesting psychologic disturbances called _disconnection syndromes._ One disturbance that has already been discussed is alexia without agraphia (Fig. 8-4). Another, the _anterior cerebral artery syndrome,_ is an injury to the corpus callosum produced by infarction of the anterior cerebral arteries. In this condition, not only are both frontal lobes damaged, but information cannot pass from the left hemisphere language centers to the appropriate right hemisphere motor center. Thus, although the patient's left arm and leg will have normal spontaneous movement, these limbs will not respond to an examiner's verbal or written requests, i.e., the patient will have unilateral (left-sided) limb apraxia (Fig. 8-5).

The corpus callosum also occasionally fails to develop in utero (*congenital absence*) and sometimes it is damaged by excessive consumption of red wine (*Marchiafava-Bignami syndrome*). Disconnection signs may be present in these cases but they are subtle and variable.

Split Brain

The most important disconnection syndrome is the "split brain," which is the result of surgical sectioning of the corpus callosum performed for control of intractable epilepsy (Chapter 10). In split brain cases, since the cerebral hemispheres are virtually isolated from each other, examiners may present certain information exclusively to one of the patient's hemispheres. For example, by showing the patient pictures, writing, and other visual information within one visual field, only the contralateral hemisphere will receive the information (Fig. 8-8). Likewise, tactile information can be presented to only one hemisphere by having a blindfolded patient touch objects with the contralateral hand. However, since auditory pathways are duplicated in the brainstem (see Fig. 4-15), sounds that are heard in only one ear are received to a certain extent by both hemispheres. A variety of striking abnormalities can be demonstrated by appropriate testing largely because visual, other sensory, and emotional data from the right hemisphere cannot be transmitted to the language centers of the left hemisphere.

In testing a patient's left cerebral hemisphere function, written words are presented to the right visual field or objects are placed in the right hand. The patient can respond correctly by speaking and by writing with his or her right hand. To written and verbal requests for particular right arm and leg movements, the patient also responds correctly; however, his or her left limbs are unable to follow the same requests because of left limb apraxia (Figs. 8-5 and 8-8).

In testing right hemisphere function, visual information is shown in the patient's left visual field. Since impulses cannot travel to the language centers, the patient cannot read, respond to written requests, or name objects. Nevertheless, the patient is able to use the left hand to copy complex figures. He or she is also able to perform well on tests of mathematical ability, facial recognition, and perception of emotion.

Sophisticated testing has shown that not only can each hemisphere experience emotion, but also each hemisphere might simultaneously experience a different, sometimes conflicting, emotion. For example, a picture that evokes humor can be shown in one visual field and one that evokes sadness in the other. In this case, tests of each hemisphere will reveal a different emotion.

In addition, each hemisphere also has been shown to reason independently by nonverbal, if not verbal, processes and to learn properly presented facts, sequences, and ideas. However, some information obtained by one hemisphere cannot be shared with the other. In particular, since patients cannot describe information that is presented to the right hemisphere, many of their experiences do not reach conscious expression or cannot be verbalized.

Split brain studies have suggested that in normal persons the two hemispheres of the brain might have independent knowledge, thought processes, and emotions. Also, they indicate that emotions in the right hemisphere may be less accessible to verbal description. Moreover, although the functions of the cerebral hemisphere may complement each other, they might occasionally conflict.

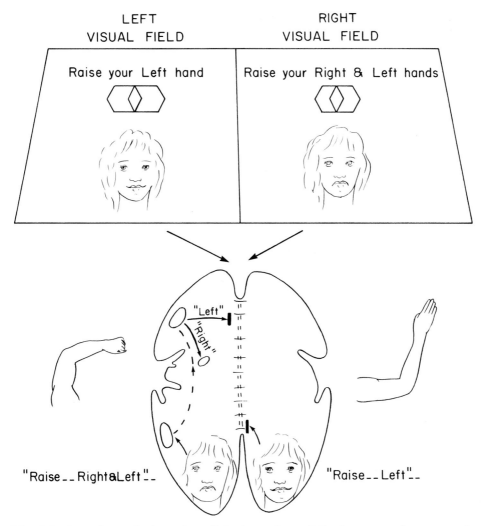

Fig. 8-8. In patients who have the split brain syndrome following a commissurotomy, the right hemisphere may receive written requests and "see" pictures shown in the left visual field. This hemisphere is unable to "read" the message but it can guide the left hand to copy pictures. The left hemisphere can read requests shown in the right visual field and, with the right hand, follow them; however, since the language areas cannot send information through the corpus callosum, the left hand does not follow the commands. Only pictures and faces shown to the left hemisphere can be described by the patient; however, in nonverbal ways, the right as well as the left hemisphere can initiate a response.

REFERENCES

Bear DM: Hemispheric specialization and the neurology of emotion. Arch Neurol 40:195, 1983

Benson DF: Aphasia, Alexia, and Agraphia. New York, Churchill Livingstone, 1979

Bryden MP, Ley RG: Right-hemisphere involvement in the perception and expression of emotion in normal humans. In Heilman KH, Satz P (eds): Neuropsychology of Human Emotion. New York, The Guilford Press, 1983

Critchley M, Henson RA (eds): Music and the Brain: Studies in the Neurology of Music. London, William Heinemann Medical Books Ltd, 1977

Damasio AR, Damasio H: The anatomic basis of pure alexia. Neurology 33:1573, 1983

Damasio AR, Damasio H, Hoesen GWV: Prosopagnosia: Anatomic basis and behavior mechanisms. Neurology 32:331, 1982

Darley FL: Aphasia. Philadelphia, W.B. Saunders, 1982

Faber R, Abrams R, Taylor MA, et al: Comparison of schizophrenic patients with formal thought disorder and neurologically impaired patients with aphasia. Am J Psychiatry 140:1348, 1983

Ferro JM, Martins IP, Tavora L: Neglect in children. Ann Neurol 15:281, 1984

Gazzaniga MS, Risse GL, Springer SP, et al: Psychologic and neurologic consequences of partial and complete cerebral commissurotomy. Neurology 25:10, 1975

Gerson SN, Benson DF, Frazier SH: Diagnosis: Schizophrenia versus posterior aphasia. Am J Psychiatry 134:966, 1977

Geschwind N: Specializations of the human brain. In Flanagan D (ed): The Brain: A Scientific American Book. San Francisco, W. H. Freeman Co, 1979.

Hemenway D: Bimanual dexterity in baseball players. N Engl J Med 309:1587, 1983

Heilman KM, Valenstein E (eds): Clinical Neuropsychology. New York, Oxford University Press, 1979

Hier DB, Mondlock J, Caplan LR: Behavioral abnormalities after right hemisphere stroke. Neurology 33:337, 1983

Homan RW, Criswell E, Wada JA, et al: Hemispheric contributions to manual communication (signing and finger-spelling). Neurology 32:1020, 1982

Mazziotta JC, Phelps ME, Carson RE, et al: Tomographic mapping of human cerebral metabolism: Auditory stimulation. Neurology 32:921, 1982

Ross ED, Harney JH, Utamsing C, et al: How the brain integrates affective and propositional language into a unified behavior function. Arch Neurol 38:745, 1981

Straub RL, Black FW: The Mental Status Examination in Neurology, 2nd Ed. Philadelphia, F. A. Davis Co, 1985

Weinstein EA, Friedland RP (eds): Advances in Neurology: Hemi-Inattention and Hemisphere Specialization. New York, Raven Press, 1977

Weintraub S, Mesulam MM, Kramer L: Disturbance in prosody: A right-hemisphere contribution to language. Arch Neurol 38:742, 1981

QUESTIONS

1–5. Formulate the following cases:

Case 1

A 68-year-old man suddenly develops right hemiparesis. He only utters "Oh, Oh!" when stimulated. He makes no response to questions or requests. His right lower face is paretic, and both the right arm and leg are flaccid and immobile. He is inattentive to objects in his right visual field.

Case 2

A 70-year-old man has been unable to speak fully or use his right arm since suffering a cerebrovascular accident (CVA) the previous year. He can only say "weak, arm," "go away," and "give . . . supper me" with slurring. On request, he can raise his left arm, protrude his tongue, and close his eyes. He can name several objects, but he cannot repeat phrases. His right arm is paretic, but he can walk.

Case3

Over a period of 6 weeks, a previously healthy 64-year-old woman has developed headaches, progressively severe difficulty finding words, and apparent confusion. She speaks continuously and incoherently: "Go to the warb," "I can't hear," "My heat hurts." She is unable to follow commands, name objects, or repeat phrases. On examination, there is pronation of the outstretched right arm, a right Babinski sign, and papilledema. Visual fields cannot be tested.

Case 4

A 34-year-old man with mitral stenosis has the sudden onset of language difficulty after a transient left-sided headache. While fully articulate and able to follow requests and repeat phrases, he has difficulty in naming objects. For example, when a pen, pin, and penny are held up in succession, he frequently uses the name of one for the other and repeats the name of the preceding object; however, he can point to the "money," "sharp object," and "writing instrument" when these objects are placed in front of him. No abnormal physical signs are detected on neurological examination.

Case 5

A 54-year-old man complains of several months of difficulty in thinking and being unable to remember the word he desires. Although his voice quivers, he is fully conversant and articulate. He is able to write the correct responses to questions; however, his answers are slow and poorly written. He is able to name six objects, follow double requests, and repeat complex phrases. On further testing, he has difficulty recalling six digits, three objects after three minutes, and both recent and past events. Judgment seems intact. The remainder of the neurologic examination is normal.

6–10. Match the lesions that are pictured schematically with those expected in cases 1–5.

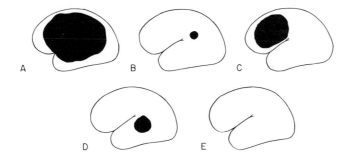

11–26. Match the lesion with the expected associated finding(s).

11. Paresis of one recurrent laryngeal nerve	a. Dysarthria,including hoarseness
	b. Dysphagia
12. Pseudobulbar palsy	c. Dementia
13. Bulbar palsy	d. Dyscalculia
14. Dominant hemisphere temporal lobe lesion	e. Fluent aphasia
	f. Constructional apraxia
15. Lateral medullary syndrome	g. Dyslexia
16. Laryngitis	h. Deafness
17. Dominant hemisphere angular gyrus lesion	i. Mutism
	j. Left-right disorientation
18. Dominant hemisphere parietal lobe lesion	k. Finger agnosia
	l. Hyperactivity
19. Nondominant hemisphere parietal lobe lesion	m. Sixth cranial nerve palsy
	n. Alexia
20. Bilateral frontal lobe tumor	o. Ataxia

21. Bilateral anterior cerebral   p.   Dressing apraxia
    artery infarction   q.   Anosognosia
22. Streptomycin toxicity   r.   Hemi-inattention
23. Alcohol intoxication   s.   Left limb apraxia
24. Periaqueductal hemorrhagic
    necrosis (Wernicke's encephalopathy)
25. Dilantin toxicity
26. Infarction of left posterior
    cerebral artery

27–33. An 8-year-old boy has difficulty learning how to read in the fourth grade. At times he is also a behavior problem in school. Which of the following conditions might be the cause of his difficulties?

27. Mental retardation
28. Congenital cerebral injury
29. Dyslexia
30. Visual impairment
31. Auditory impairment
32. Psychiatric disturbances
33. Unsupportive home environment

34. A 70-year-old man complains of the sudden inability to read. While he can write his name and many sentences that are dictated to him, he cannot read aloud or copy written material. His speech is fluent and contains no paraphasic errors. On further examination, it is found that he can see objects only in his left visual field. What is this man's difficulty and where is the responsible lesions(s)?

35. A 68-year-old man has a car accident in which he drifted into oncoming traffic. When questioned by police, he was unaware of a weak left arm. On examination by a physician, the patient was shown to have a left homonymous hemianopsia, a mild left hemiparesis (which the patient denied) and failure to recognize his weak left arm. What intellectual processes are apparent?

36. A 60-year-old woman with longstanding depression has agitation, a language disturbance, and dysarthria. She was initially misdiagnosed as having an exacerbation of her psychiatric disorder. However, subsequently she was recognized as suffering from an aphasia that was characterized by a paucity of words and impaired ability to express herself. She was also shown to have a mild right hemiparesis. A CT scan indicated an occlusion of the left middle cerebral artery. In planning her rehabilitation management, which additional associated findings should be sought?

    a. Constructional apraxia   d. Left homonymous hemianopsia
    b. Gait apraxia   e. Buccofacial apraxia
    c. Limb apraxia   f. Ideational apraxia

37. Patients with nondominant hemisphere lesions are reported to have loss of the normal inflections of speech and diminished associated facial and limb gestures. What are the technical terms used to describe these findings?

38. A man, who has undergone a corpus callosum commissurotomy for intractable seizures, is shown a typewritten request to raise both arms. What will be his response when the request is shown in his left visual field? In the right visual field?

39–44. With which other conditions are the various forms of apraxia associated?

39. Gait   a. Aphasia
40. Constructional   b. Hemi-inattention
41. Ideational   c. Dementia

42.	Limb	d.	Dysarthria
43.	Buccofacial	e.	Incontinence
44.	Ideomotor	f.	Left homonymous hemianopsia
		g.	Right homonymous hemianopsia
		h.	Aprosody

ANSWERS

1–5.
Case 1. This is a case of complete loss of language function, *global aphasia*, with right hemiplegia and homonymous hemianopsia. The cause is probably an occlusion of the left internal carotid artery creating a large infarction of the left hemisphere.

Case 2. Since he can manage only a few phrases or words in a telegraphic pattern, he has *nonfluent aphasia*, which is typically accompanied by right hemiparesis in which the arm is more paretic than the leg. The lesion encompasses Broca's area and the adjacent cortical motor region. It was probably caused by an occlusion of the left middle cerebral artery.

Case 3. The patient has *fluent aphasia* characterized by a normal quantity of speech beset by paraphasic errors and only subtle right-sided corticospinal tract abnormalities. There is probably a lesion in the left parietal or posterior temporal lobe. The headaches and papilledema, given her age, previous good health, and the course of the illness, suggest that it is a mass lesion, such as a glioblastoma multiforme (Chapter 19).

Case 4. This is a case of anomic aphasia, which is a variety of *fluent aphasia* where language impairment is restricted to the improper identification of objects, i.e., a naming impairment. While its origin may be Alzheimer's disease, since this patient has mitral stenosis and the illness began suddenly with a headache, it was probably caused by a small embolic CVA (Chapter 11).

Case 5. The patient does not have any sign of aphasia. His difficulty with memory might be either early dementia or psychogenic inattention. Further evaluation that might be performed could include neuropsychological studies or laboratory tests that might reveal an origin or dementia, such as an EEG and a CT scan.

  6. *Case* 1, drawing a
  7. *Case* 2, drawing c
  8. *Case* 3, drawing d
  9. *Case* 4, drawing b or d
  10. *Case* 5, drawing e
  11. a
  12. a, b, c
  13. a, b
  14. e
  15. a, b, o
  16. a
  17. d, j, k (Gerstmann's syndrome)
  18. d, e, g, j, k
  19. f, g, p, q, r
  20. c, possibly also a, b, and i
  21. s and possibly c and i
  22. h, o
  23. a, d, o

24.   c, m, o

25.   o

26.   n

27–33.   All Yes

34.   He clearly has alexia, as demonstrated by his inability to read, and also a right homonymous hemianopsia. He does not have agraphia because he can transcribe dictation and write words from memory. Nor does he have aphasia. Thus, he has the syndrome of alexia without agraphia. This syndrome is caused by a lesion in the left occipital lobe and posterior corpus callosum. The left occipital lesion would explain the failure of visual information to pass from the intact right visual cortex through the corpus callosum to the left (dominant) hemisphere for integration (Fig. 8-4). Since memory and auditory circuits, as well as the corticospinal system, are intact, he can write words that he hears or remembers. Such lesions are usually caused by infarctions of the left posterior cerebral artery or by infiltrating brain tumors, such as a glioblastoma multiforme.

35.   He probably had the accident because a left homonymous hemianopsia prevented him from seeing oncoming traffic. More important, he has anosognosia (failure to recognize one's illness). As in this man, these perceptual distortions characteristically are found in patients with parietal lobe lesions.

36.   c, e. Limb and buccofacial apraxias are associated with dominant hemisphere lesions. Their identification is important because these impediments are potentially major obstacles in speech and physical therapies.

37.   Aprosody and loss of paralinguistic components of speech.

38.   When the request is shown in his left visual field, he will raise neither arm because the written information will not reach the left hemisphere language centers. When the request is shown in his right visual field, the information will reach the language centers and he will raise his right hand; however, the command to move his left hand may not reach the right hemisphere's motor center (see Fig. 8-8).

39.   c, e

40.   b, f, h

41.   c

42.   a, g

43.   a, d, g

44.   a, g

9

Headaches

Headaches are common conditions that can be barometers of emotional stress, chronic and recurrently incapacitating illnesses, or symptoms of serious disease. Their clinical importance lies also in their sometimes being accompanied by unusual symptoms, such as visual hallucinations, and the contributing role, which is usually exaggerated, of psychologic factors.

Several varieties of headache that are usually cited as chronic have distinctive patterns, are associated with unusual symptoms, and are affected by psychologic factors. These are *muscle contraction* (or *tension*) headaches, *migraines,** *cluster* headaches, *postconcussive* headaches, and *trigeminal neuralgia* (tic douloureux). Diagnosis in most cases is based not on physical or laboratory findings, which are usually normal, but on the patient's description of the headache and of its response to particular medicines.

On the other hand, acutely occurring or steadily progressive but otherwise non-specific headaches may be manifestations of an underlying disease that can lead to permanent neurologic injury or death. These diseases are *temporal arteritis, intracranial mass lesions, pseudotumor cerebri, meningitis,* or *subarachnoid hemorrhage.* Although the patient's description of the headache is not particularly helpful, abnormalities in the neurologic examination and laboratory tests usually permit an accurate and possibly life-saving diagnosis to be made.

MUSCLE CONTRACTION (TENSION) HEADACHES

Despite recently acquired evidence that implicates cranial vascular dysfunction, tension headaches are still generally attributed to achy contraction (tension) of the frontal, nuchal (neck), and other scalp and face muscles (Fig. 9-1). They typically

---

*Patients who have migraines may receive assistance from The National Migraine Foundation, 5252 North Western Avenue, Chicago, Illinois 60625, (312) 878-7715.

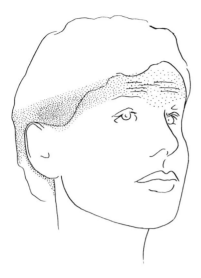

Fig. 9-1. Patients with muscle contraction (tension) headaches usually complain of a band-like squeezing, symmetric pressure at their neck, temples, or forehead.

develop in the afternoon and may be produced by physical fatigue, cervical spondylosis, or excessive light or noise, as well as by emotional stress (Table 9-1). They are found almost exclusively in adults, more frequently in women than in men, and, probably because of psychologic rather than genetic reasons, in successive family members.

Therapy

Ideally a clear-cut psychologic or physical origin should be demonstrated; however, the relief of a headache with simple measures not only indicates the headache's

Table 9-1
Important Items in a Headache History

What is its nature?
  Severity: mild, moderate, severe
  Type: throbbing,* aching, sharp
  Location: unilateral (hemicranial),* bilateral, frontal, periorbital*
  Precipitants: stress, relief of stress,* menses,* missing meals,* too little or too much sleep,*
    glare,* alcohol,* chocolate,* medications (vasodilators, birth control)*
  Relief: rest, sleep,* alcohol, coffee, vasoconstrictors*
What symptoms are associated with the headache?
  Aura:* visual, personality change
  Autonomic dysfunction:* nausea, vomiting, polyuria
  Photophobia (light),* hyperacusis (noise)*
What are its temporal characteristics?
  Were they present in childhood?*
  What is their duration?
  Do they begin in the morning?*
  Do they occur during sleep?*
  Are they most frequent on weekends?*
  Are they associated with menses?*
  Do they occur in clusters?
Is there a history of car-sickness as a child?*
Is there a parent or sibling with similar headaches?*

  *Symptoms that indicate migraines.

benign origin but provides the cure. Several successful therapies have been empirically established. Although practice may differ, certain steps are usually followed by neurologists:

- *Step 1.* In *abortive* therapy, simple analgesics should be taken at the very start of a headache (or any pain) to prevent its full development. Thus, medicine should be left in the car, kept at work, and placed in pocketbooks and taken at the first inkling of a headache. Patients should first try common analgesics, such as aspirin, acetaminophen (e.g., Tylenol), or combinations of caffeine with aspirin (e.g., APC or Excedrin) (Table 9-2). Nonnarcotic prescription medications, such as Fiorinal, may elicit a better response, but this is mostly because of a physician's implicit endorsement.
- *Step 2.* Preventive, or *prophylactic,* therapy should be given if abortive therapy is ineffective or requires excessive medicine. Minor tranquilizers (e.g., diazepam) or combinations of sedative and vasoactive medicines (e.g., Bellergal-S) are often helpful if taken daily. Especially effective are amitriptyline (Elavil) and other antidepressants in small doses administered mostly at night, even in patients who are not overtly depressed (see Chapter 14, Pain).
- *Step 3.* Insight-oriented psychotherapy and classic psychoanalysis directed toward headaches have not been significantly beneficial. Whether such modalities help the headache patient by providing insight or reduction in anxiety is a different but also unanswered question. An alternate nonpharmacologic approach has been biofeedback training or conditioning (which costs about $500 in 1985). Studies have shown that this is effective in reducing headaches and decreasing medicine intake for about six months in about 50 percent of carefully selected patients. Biofeedback results are similar whether monitoring is of an electroencephalogram (EEG), electromyogram (EMG), skin temperature, blood pressure, or pulse.

MIGRAINES

According to a theory that has been strongly challenged but not replaced, migraines result from brief constriction of cerebral arteries, usually in the carotid artery system (see Fig. 11-1), followed by prolonged, flaccid dilation during which unsuppressed pulsations stretch the arterioles. The pulsatile distention, it is also suggested, may release bradykinin-like substances that give rise to the headache.

Migraine and its varieties are thought by many investigators to be a genetic illness that is expressed through serotonin metabolism abnormalities. Studies have shown that plasma serotonin falls during the attack of migraine; that serotonin antagonists, such as methysergide (Sansert), prevent migraines; and that reserpine, which reduces serotonin, induces them. However, hormone fluctuations and actions of a myriad of other substances have also been implicated.

In the *classic variety* of migraine, which affects only about 20 percent of patients, the headache is preceded by an *aura*, which can be almost any symptom of brain dysfunction but which is almost always the same visual hallucination (Table 9-3). This usually involves a partial graying of the visual field (*scotoma*), flashing zig-zag lines (*scintillating scotomata*) (Fig. 9-2), tubular vision, or aberration of the appearance of objects (*metamorphosia*). Although olfactory hallucinations may be a migraine aura, they are more likely to be a manifestation of a partial complex seizure (Chapter 10). Cyclic abdominal pain in children may be an aura.

Table 9-2

Medications for Headache*

Medicine	Composition
APC	Aspirin
	Phenacetin
	Caffeine
Bellergal-S	Phenobarbital
	Ergotamine
	Belladonna
Bufferin	Aspirin
	Aluminum glycinate
	Magnesium carbonate
Cafergot†	Ergotamine
	Caffeine
Cafergot P-B†	Ergotamine
	Caffeine
	Belladonna
	Pentobarbital
Elavil	Amitriptyline
Excedrin	Aspirin
	Acetaminophen
	Salicylamide
	Caffeine
Fiorinal	Butalbital
	Caffeine
	Aspirin
Inderal‡	Propranolol
Lithium	Lithium
Midrin	Isometheptene
	Dichloraphenazone
	Acetaminophen
Steroids	Prednisone
	Dexamethasone
Sansert‡	Methysergide
Valium	Diazepam
Wigraine	Ergotamine
	Caffeine

*Consult package insert for indications, dosage, contraindications, precautions, and side-effects.

†Available in both suppository and tablet form.

‡Prophylactic use.

Table 9-3

Causes of Visual Hallucinations*

Delirium tremens (DTs)
Drug intoxication
    Illicit: LSD and other hallucinogens
    Medicinal: L-dopa, scopolamine, and others
Migraines, classic variety
Narcolepsy (Hypnopompic and hypnogogic hallucinations)
    (Chapter 17)
Sudden blindness, e.g., Anton's syndrome (Chapter 12)
Seizures (Chapter 10)
    Elementary (visual)
    Complex partial

*Commonly cited neurologic conditions.

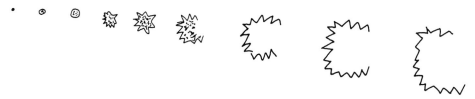

Fig. 9-2. Patients, particularly children, may provide valuable diagnostic information if they are asked to draw what they "see" during a headache. A patient describing the aura (a scintillating scotoma) that she sees before her (classic) migraine states, "In the early stages, the area within the lights is somewhat shaded. Later, as the figure widens, you can sort of peer right through the area. Eventually, it gets so wide that it disappears." Typically, this scotoma has an angulated margin, which is brightly lit, and an opaque interior that began as a star and expanded into a crescent.

In the *common variety,* which affects about 75 to 80 percent of migraine patients, there is no preceding aura. The headache is characteristically 4 to 24 hours in duration, throbbing, and dull, and initially felt on one side of the head (hemicranially) and behind or around the eye (retro- or periorbitally) (Fig. 9-3). Although typically hemicranial initially, in about 50 percent of patients the headaches move to the opposite side or becomes generalized. Accompanying symptoms, including nausea, vomiting, photophobia, hyperacusis (sensitivity to noise), and polyuria, may be as troublesome as the headache itself and often lead to prostration.

In some cases, migraines are accompanied by mood changes and other alterations in the mental state (Table 9-4). Patients may become depressed and withdrawn and seek dark and quiet places to escape from people as well as from light and noise. If unable to find solitude, they may become distraught. At the beginning of a headache, patients occasionally become feverishly active and work excessively. During this time, they also drink large quantities of water and crave food or sweets, particularly chocolate. Children may seem to be confused and also often become overly active. When children can rest, they may be so unable or unwilling to respond that they are said to be in a "stupor." After a migraine clears, especially if it ends with sleep, patients sometimes feel euphoric.

Classic and common migraines, like tension headaches, are more common in women than in men and tend to affect more than one family member. However, migraines occur in children and adolescents as well as adults, and they begin in the

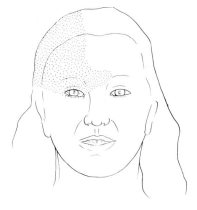

Fig. 9-3. Patients with migraines have throbbing, hemicranial headaches that, in about 50 percent of cases, either move to the other side of the head or become generalized.

Table 9-4

Causes of Altered Mental State*

Drugs
  Illicit
  Medicinal
Metabolic aberrations, e.g., hypoglycemia
Migraines
Seizures (Chapter 10)
  Absence
  Partial complex
Sleep attacks, e.g., narcolepsy, sleep apnea naps (Chapter 17)
Transient global amnesia (Chapter 11)
Transient ischemic attacks (TIAs) (Chapter 11)

*Commonly cited, transient, recurrent neurologic conditions.

early morning rather than the afternoon. In women, migraines often first start at menarche, recur premenstrually, and may be aggravated by birth control pills. In men and women, migraines may occur during REM sleep (Chapter 17), sometimes exclusively (*nocturnal migraines*).

Another important characteristic of migraines is that they can be precipitated by certain physical factors, such as skipping meals (hypoglycemia), excessive sleep, menses, alcohol,* and stress. The role of stress is particularly interesting. In addition to stress precipitating migraines, as it probably does tension headaches, in many patients *relief* of stress is associated with migraine. For example, a woman who may have a difficult job might awaken Saturday or Sunday mornings with migraines. Likewise, at the start of a vacation, especially after examinations, students often develop migraines. However, contrary to popular beliefs, migraines affect people in all socioeconomic groups and all personality types. Obsessive persons, although possibly more disturbed by having migraines, may be no more susceptible.

Other Migraine Varieties

Migraines that occur in children, *childhood migraines,* are similar to classic and common varieties except that more boys than girls are affected, visual auras occur more often, nausea and vomiting are even more troublesome, and children are more liable to develop hyperactivity, confusion, and stupor.

In *basilar migraines,* mental changes, which include confusion and unresponsiveness, and headaches are accompanied by symptoms that reflect cerebellum and brainstem dysfunction, such as ataxia, vertigo, and diplopia. This variety of migraine, which particularly affects children, is believed to arise from changes in the vertebrobasilar rather than the carotid artery system (see Fig. 11-2).

Hemiplegic migraines, which may occur in both children and adults, are characterized by hemiparesis, hemiparesthesia, and sometimes aphasia preceding or accompanying otherwise typical hemicranial migraine headaches. Sometimes the hemiparesis may even develop without an associated headache. In evaluating a patient

---

*The alcoholic "drinks" that are most likely to precipitate a migraine are red wine and brandy, and the least likely, vodka and white wine. Alcoholic drinks can also provoke cluster headaches. However, they ameliorate tension headaches.

with transient hemiparesis, the physician must consider the possibility of hemiplegic migraines, along with transient ischemic attacks (TIAs), postictal (Todd's) hemiparesis, and psychogenic disorders. Hemiplegic migraine deficits occasionally become permanent, just as though a patient had experienced a cerebrovascular accident (CVA). This condition, a *complicated migraine,* is virtually the same as a stroke. Thus, women with migraines who are over 35 years of age should not take oral contraceptives because of their association with a slightly increased incidence of stroke.

Migraine-Like Conditions

Many people who eat certain foods, take particular medications, or "insult" their body in other ways, develop headaches that mimic migraines. Similarly, these substances can precipitate a typical migraine in susceptible persons. The best known examples of foods precipitating headaches are the *Chinese restaurant syndrome,* which is caused by monosodium glutamate (MSG), and the *hot dog headache,* which is caused by the nitrites found in processed meats. Another is the *ice cream headache,* caused by any very cold food overstimulating receptors in the pharynx. Despite many claims, few people actually develop headaches after eating foods that contain tyramine, such as ripened cheese, or those that contain phenylethylamine, particularly chocolate.

An interesting headache condition that occurs frequently is the *caffeine-withdrawal headache*. It develops in people who have a steady coffee intake but fail to drink their morning cup(s). This headache, which is often accompanied by anxiety, can be relieved with medications containing caffeine as well as with black coffee. These headaches pose a dilemma for heavy coffee drinkers, in whom excessive caffeine leads to irritability, palpitations, and gastric burning but foregoing or missing coffee leads to rebound headaches and anxiety.

Antianginal medicines, such as nitroglycerin or isosorbide (Isordil), which contain nitrites or act directly on cerebrovascular tone, may cause headaches. Elderly patients in whom atherosclerosis leads to cerebrovascular insufficiency and poor arteriole muscle tone are particularly vulnerable. Curiously, whereas some calcium channel blockers, such as nifedipine (Procardia), precipitate headaches, others, such as verapamil (Calan), may be useful in prophylaxis. Oral contraceptives not only induce or exaggerate headaches, but as already mentioned, their use may be complicated by CVAs.

Migraine-like headaches often occur after strenuous physical activity. Even during sexual intercourse or masturbation, a migraine-like headache, *coital cephalgia,* may develop. Nevertheless, physicians should be cautious in concluding that a severe headache occurring during athletic or sexual activity results from a benign, migrainous vascular change. Instead, such a headache may have resulted from an intracerebral or subarachnoid hemorrhage caused by rupture of a cerebral aneurysm.

Therapy of Migraines

In migraine treatment, several specific steps are usually followed by neurologists:

- *Step 1.* Using a "headache diary," in which patients note the days of headaches and physically and emotionally significant events, physicians and patients might identify the precipitating factors of a migraine. If these factors cannot be avoided, at least they can be anticipated.

- *Step 2.* Abortive medicines, which must be taken immediately, usually consist of vasoactive agents, sometimes in combination with analgesics or sedatives. Medicines beneficial in tension headaches, such as Fiorinal, are often effective in common migraines. If analgesics are ineffective, medicines that consist predominantly of powerful vasoconstrictors, such as Cafergot or Wigraine, may be given to interrupt the vascular changes that lead to the headache. Patients who develop migraines at night may try taking medicine at bedtime. If oral medications are unsatisfactory, suppositories should be tried because they are usually better absorbed, more rapidly effective, and less likely to cause nausea. Sublingual tablets, another alternative, are more socially acceptable but less effective. After taking medicines, patients should remain at rest in a darkened room and, if possible, sleep. If nausea or vomiting are prominent, antiemetic suppositories, which generally contain phenothiazines, should also be used.
- *Step 3.* Prophylactic therapy is usually suggested if headaches occur more than two or four times a month or if abortive medicines are taken excessively. Prophylactic therapy not only reduces headache frequency and intensity, it reduces patients' need for all medicines and allays their fear. Propranolol (Inderal), a beta-adrenergic blocker, is widely used for migraine prophylaxis as well as for treatment of angina and essential tremor (Chapter 18). It changes sympathetic tone and counters anxiety. Methysergide (Sansert), which is a congener of LSD that interferes with serotonin metabolism, is another highly effective prophylactic medicine; however, it may induce mood changes and, if taken for more than 6 months, retroperitoneal fibrosis. Antidepressants are also effective in migraine prophylaxis. They may be useful not only because they reduce or alter REM sleep, during which many migraine headaches develop, but also because they frequently act as analgesics (Chapter 14).
- *Step 4.* Neither insight-oriented psychotherapy nor classic psychoanalysis has been shown in adequately controlled studies to be an effective migraine treatment. Biofeedback and relaxation therapy has helped small numbers of patients but only for a limited time. All such therapies are less effective in migraines than tension headaches.

TENSION-MIGRAINE COMBINATION

Descriptions of tension headaches and migraines imply that these conditions are entirely different and readily diagnosed (Table 9-5). However, this distinction may be artificial, and these two headaches may represent only the ends of a spectrum of a single headache disorder. In practice, many patients have a combination of tension headaches and migraines that seems to blend, vary, and recur. This combination is so common that it is virtually a migraine variety.

Whether these headaches are actually separate illnesses or not, physicians should determine what portion of their patients' headaches are migraines. If headaches are unilateral, throbbing, present in the morning, accompanied by nausea, precipitated by menses, or evoked by the other known migraine precipitants, the diagnosis of migraine is appropriate. Physicians should not expect patients to have an aura or even

Table 9-5

Comparison of Muscle Contraction
(Tension) and Common Migraine Headaches

	Tension	Migraine
Age at onset	Middle-age	Childhood, adolescence
Location of headache	Symmetric	Hemicranial*
Nature of headache	Dull	Throbbing*
Associated symptoms	None	Nausea, hyperacusis, photophobia
Time of onset	Afternoon	Early or late morning†
Effect of alcohol	Reduces headache	Worsens headache

*In approximately one half of patients.
†May develop during REM sleep and be present on awakening.

a severe, incapacitating headache before diagnosing migraine. Appropriate therapy remains the prescription of medications, such as propranolol, that are more effective for migraines than for tension headaches. Overall, therapy for combination headaches will be more successful if physicians concentrate on the diagnosis and treatment of the migraine component.

CLUSTER HEADACHES

Cluster headaches are probably caused by a form of cerebrovascular imbalance different from that responsible for migraines. They have no family tendency, affect men more than women and usually begin between age 20 and 40 years. In fact, they are the only form of chronic headache to develop more frequently in men than women.

These headaches are called "cluster" because they occur in groups of one to three daily that last from several weeks to a few months. Clusters occur most often in the spring, and cluster-free intervals range from 3 months to several years.

The headache itself, which usually lasts one-half to three hours, is located periorbitally. It is nonthrobbing and very painful, with pain seeming to bore from the eye straight backwards into the head. Characteristic accompaniments are ipsilateral eye tearing, conjunctival congestion, nasal stuffiness, and a partial Horner's syndrome (Fig. 9-4). Headaches may occur randomly throughout the day, but they may be precipitated by alcoholic drinks and they have an especially strong tendency to develop during REM sleep. Unlike migraines, cluster headaches are not preceded by an aura or accompanied by nausea. They are not associated with mental changes but the pain is often so severe that patients say that they want to kill themselves.

Treatment with abortive medicines is usually ineffective for a cluster headache because of its abrupt onset and relatively short duration. However, oxygen inhalation at 10 to 12 L/min may provide relief. Even prophylactic treatment with methysergide, propranolol, and amitriptyline may be unsatisfactory. One prophylactic preparation that has proved notably effective is lithium, given because cluster headaches were known to be cyclic and developed in middle-aged persons. Alternatively, steroids, such as prednisone and dexamethasone, are helpful for several weeks. Psychotherapy and biofeedback, however, provide no benefit.

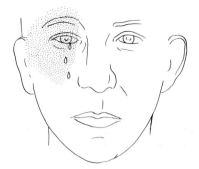

Fig. 9-4. Patients with cluster headaches usually have unilateral periorbital pain accompanied by ipsilateral tearing and nasal discharge, along with ptosis and miosis (a partial Horner's syndrome).

POSTCONCUSSIVE (POSTTRAUMATIC) SYNDROME

After *minor* head trauma, usually as a result of motor vehicle accidents, people with a continual, generalized, dull headache that is accompanied by nonspecific impairments, which typically includes easy fatigability, "dizziness" (lightheadedness), insomnia, and mental difficulties, are said to have postconcussive syndrome. The symptoms, which often prevent patients from working, are unexpectedly severe and prolonged, lasting several months to years. In contrast, soldiers, football players, children, and many others who sustain comparable or more severe head injuries rarely develop the postconcussive syndrome. When postconcussive symptoms last longer than 6 months, especially if litigation is unsettled, psychogenic factors including outright malingering may be predominant.

The neurologic etiology, to the extent that it does exist, is not established. However, microscopic lacerations of meningeal, cerebrovascular, or cerebral structures and shearing of cerebral matter have been postulated. In addition, if occipital headache is present, that aspect of the syndrome might originate from wrenching of cervical muscles, ligaments, and nerve roots ("whiplash" injury).

Although medical symptoms often include memory impairment, inattentiveness, and depression, routine neuropsychologic tests rarely confirm cognitive deficits. Only sophisticated tests can establish the existence of these complaints and not be subverted by patients' mimicking disabilities.

Another factor to consider besides factitious impairments is the patient's premorbid intellectual and personality state. Highly intelligent and strongly motivated people may not appear to have deficits. On the other hand, young adults who have a history of learning disabilities or attention deficit disorders are likely to develop serious incapacity when they sustain traumatic injury and psychologic shock from a motor vehicle accident.

Despite unequivocal evidence of cognitive, personality, and physical impairments, in most cases CT scans and EEGs are normal. However, brainstem auditory evoked responses (Chapter 15) have been reported to be abnormal, indicating the syndrome may have an anatomic basis in brainstem dysfunction.

The most successful therapies have been those directed toward muscle contraction. Effective medicines are mild analgesics, muscle relaxants, and amitriptyline. Physical therapy, including cervical traction, may provide relief whether or not whiplash injury has occurred. Psychotherapy may be useful if patients have developed posttraumatic anxiety or the injury has precipitated depression. Also, to eliminate at least one incentive for prolonged disability, litigation should be settled as quickly as possible. In some cases, however, incapacity has continued after settlements were reached.

TRIGEMINAL NEURALGIA (TIC DOULOUREUX)

Trigeminal neuralgia consists of brief, 20-second to 30-second jabs of excruciatingly sharp pain extending along one of the three divisions of the trigeminal nerve. The division most often affected is V_2 (see Fig. 4-11). Pain can occur spontaneously or be elicited by touching certain areas called *trigger zones,* or by certain facial movements, such as those made while eating or brushing teeth. Episodes of pain may occur a dozen times daily; however, it may recede for many months.

Trigeminal neuralgia affects women twice as often as men and develops relatively late in life, typically between the ages of 50 and 60 years. A lifelong, recurring condition, it is one of the most important causes of headache in the elderly (Table 9-6).

The condition has been shown to originate, in most cases, from compression by an aberrant cerebral blood vessel of the trigeminal nerve root as it emerges from the brainstem. Another but less frequent cause, accounting for most cases in young adults, is multiple sclerosis. Whatever the cause, treatment is usually begun with carbamazepine (Tegretol). In the majority of patients, in whom an aberrant vessel is probably responsible for the neuralgia, the most effective procedure is a craniotomy to place a barrier between any vessel compressing the trigeminal nerve and the nerve itself.

ACUTELY OCCURRING OR PROGRESSIVELY SEVERE HEADACHES

Temporal Arteritis

Temporal arteritis is a disease of unknown etiology in which the temporal and other cranial arteries become inflamed. Since histologic examination of affected arteries reveals giant cells, the condition is properly called *giant cell arteritis.*

Patients are almost always older than 55 years. They usually have a dull, continual headache in one or both temples that may radiate towards the jaw ("jaw claudication"). In advanced cases, patients' temporal arteries are reddened and tender.

Table 9-6

Headaches in the Elderly*

Brain tumors: glioblastoma, metastasis
Cerebrovascular insufficiency
Cervical spondylosis
Migraines, especially medication-induced
Subdural hematomas
Temporal arteritis
Trigeminal neuralgia (tic douloureux)

*Commonly cited chronic neurologic conditions.

Temporal arteritis is also characterized by signs of systemic illness, such as malaise, low grade fever, and weight loss.

Since untreated arterial inflammation will lead to occlusion, serious complications develop in cases when diagnosis is delayed. Most important, ophthalmic artery occlusion will cause blindness and cerebral artery occlusion will result in cerebral infarctions. A temporal artery biopsy is the definitive test, but it is often unnecessary, hazardous, or impractical. In over 90 percent of cases, an erythrocyte sedimentation rate (ESR) elevated above 40 mm provides an easily obtainable adequate confirmation. Timely treatment with steroids will quickly relieve the headaches and prevent complications.

Intracranial Mass Lesions

Patients with brain tumors and subdural hematomas often have headaches as their first or most bothersome symptom (Chapter 19). These headaches also are usually dull and either unilateral or generalized. They are worse if intracranial pressure is raised, as when people cough, or in the early morning, when REM sleep occurs. Although brain tumor headaches may awaken patients, usually it is migraines and cluster headaches (which also develop in REM sleep) that most frequently occur at night.

When mass lesions cause headache, they also usually produce other signs either of increased intracranial pressure, such as papilledema, or of cerebral impairment, such as seizures. But no matter how unlikely is a brain tumor, neurologists order computerized tomography (CT) in almost all patients with unexplained progressive headaches, and an ESR in those over 55 years of age.

Chronic Meningitis

Chronic meningitis, most often from *Cryptococcus,* may cause continual, dull headaches and be accompanied by signs of systemic illness and dementia. These effects can be corrected if the illness is diagnosed early enough (Chapter 7). Patients who have impaired immune systems, including the elderly, those taking steroids, and those with AIDS, are susceptible. A CT scan, which must be performed before a lumbar puncture, may show communicating hydrocephalus. The lumbar puncture will yield cerebrospinal fluid (CSF) that has a lymphocytic pleocytosis, low glucose concentration, and possibly positive test results for antigens, such as *Cryptococcus.* Since fungi and tuberculosis organisms may take weeks to culture (Chapter 20), the diagnosis must be based on the preliminary CSF results.

Pseudotumor Cerebri

Pseudotumor cerebri (benign intracranial hypertension) is virtually restricted to young obese women who have menstrual irregularities. It gives rise to papilledema and a dull, generalized headache. Pseudotumor appears to be caused by fluid accumulation within the brain interstitium that raises CSF pressure, often to levels over 400 mm H_2O. If untreated, pseudotumor will lead to blindness from optic atrophy (Chapter 12). Treatment usually consists of diuretics, weight loss through dieting, repeated lumbar punctures, and sometimes steroids. In refractory cases, CSF shunting procedures are required.

Bacterial Meningitis and Subarachnoid Hemorrhage

In young adults, two life-threatening, headache-producing illnesses are bacterial meningitis and subarachnoid hemorrhage. Bacterial meningitis is usually caused by *Meningococcus* or *Pneumococcus*. It often spreads in epidemic fashion among young adults in confined areas, such as dormitories or military training camps, causing a rapidly developing, severe headache that is accompanied by photophobia, malaise, fever, and nuchal rigidity. At the slightest indication of these symptoms, the CSF must be examined and treatment started with penicillin or another antibiotic.

Viral infections that cause headaches may involve the brain, causing *encephalitis,* or the meninges, causing *viral meningitis*. These conditions, which are usually much more benign than bacterial infections, are diagnosed with CSF analysis, CT, and EEG. However, one particular virus, Herpes simplex, is noteworthy as the most frequent cause of nonepidemic, serious encephalitis. Herpes virus damages the inferior surface of the frontal and temporal lobes. Thus, in addition to having fever, somnolence, and delirium, patients have partial complex seizures and memory impairment. Some patients who have sustained bilateral temporal lobe damage have developed a human variety of the Klüver-Bucy syndrome (Chapter 16), which usually affects only monkeys subjected to removal of both temporal lobes.

The other important acutely occurring headache is caused by *subarachnoid hemorrhage* from a ruptured *berry aneurysm*. In this condition, patients usually suddenly develop an extraordinarily severe headache, prostration, and nuchal rigidity—symptoms similar to those in bacterial meningitis. Subarachnoid hemorrhage often occurs during exertion, straining at stool, and sexual intercourse. However, mild or otherwise atypical subarachnoid hemorrhages ("leaks") are not as dramatic and are often disregarded or confused with common migraines, tension headaches, or a "head cold." The correct diagnosis of subarachnoid hemorrhage may be made from evidence of blood on CT scans or the CSF being bloody or xanthochromic (yellow from blood breakdown).

SUMMARY

In evaluating patients with tension headaches, migraines, and other chronic, recurrent headaches, the diagnosis rests on the history and, to a certain extent, on the patient's own response to medicines. Psychologic factors play some role in these headaches but cannot be readily altered.

Patients with either acutely occurring or progressively severe headaches are apt to have life-threatening illnesses. A careful neurologic examination is in order and usually so is a CT scan to diagnose a brain tumor, subdural hematoma, or other mass lesion. Those who might have pseudotumor cerebri, meningitis, or subarachnoid hemorrhage usually should have a lumbar puncture. Patients older than 55 years with an unexplained, chronic headache should have an ESR as an emergency procedure.

REFERENCES

Abramowicz M (ed): Drugs for migraine. The Medical Letter 26:95, 1984

Bell NW, Abramowitz SI, Folkins CH: Biofeedback, brief psychotherapy and tension headaches. Headache 23:162, 1983

Bergtsson BA, Malmuall BE: Giant cell arteritis. Acta Med Scand 658(suppl):1, 1982

Blanchard EB, Andrasik F, Arena JG, et al: Nonpharmacologic treatment of chronic headache: Prediction of outcome. Neurology 33:1596, 1983

Cohen MJ, McArthur DL, Rickles WH: Comparison of four biofeedback treatments for migraine headache: Physiologic and headache variables. Psychosomatics 42:463, 1980

Dalessio DJ (ed): Wolff's Headache and Other Head Pain. New York, Oxford University Press, 1980

Dikmen S, Reitan RM, Temkin NR: Neuropsychological recovery in head injury. Arch Neurol 40:333, 1983

Lance JW: Headaches related to sexual activity. J Neurol Neurosurg Psychiatry 39:1226, 1976

Lance JW: Headache. Ann Neurol 10:1, 1981

Lance JW: Mechanism and Management of Headache, 4th ed. London, Butterworths, 1982

Lauritzen M, Olsen TS, Lassen NA: Regulation of regional cerebral blood flow during and between migraine attacks. Ann Neurol 14:569, 1983

Martin MJ: Muscle-contraction (tension) headache. Psychosomatics 24:319, 1983

Noseworthy JH, Miller J, Murry T, et al: Auditory brainstem responses in postconcussion syndrome. Arch Neurol 38:275, 1981

Raskin NH: Migraine. Psychosomatics 23:897, 1982

Richards W: The fortification illusions of migraines. Sci Am 224:89, 1971

Rothner AD: Headaches in children. Headache 19:156, 1979

Rowe MJ, Carlson C: Brainstem auditory evoked potentials in postconcussion dizziness. Arch Neurol 37:679, 1980

Sacks OW: Migraine: Understanding a Common Disorder. Berkeley, University of California Press, 1985

Saper JR: Headache Disorders: Current Concepts and Treatment Strategies. Boston, John Wright, 1983

Sternbach RA, Dalessio DJ, Kunzel M, et al: MMPI patterns in common headaches disorders. Headache 20:311, 1980

QUESTIONS

1–4. A 17-year-old Marine recruit has developed a moderately severe, generalized headache, lethargy, and nuchal rigidity.

    1. What disease must be considered first?

    2. What diagnostic procedure must be performed first?

    3. What would the typical result be?

    4. What is the therapy?

5–9. A 45-year-old man has had moderate bitemporal headaches, then the gradual onset of stupor over a 5-day period. He has episodes of unusual, repetitive behavior, complaints of unusual smells, and photophobia. On examination he has fever, delerium, mild nuchal rigidity, and bilateral long tract findings.

    5. What might the episodic behavioral disturbances indicate?

    6. What do the delerium and long tract findings suggest?

    7. What is the most common cause of sporadic (nonepidemic) encephalitis?

    8. What areas of the brain are particularly susceptible?

    9. What are the major sequelae of this infection?

    10. A young hypertensive housewife suddenly develops severe right retro-orbital pain, prostration, and a right third cranial nerve palsy. What is the most likely cause?

    11. A middle-aged hypertensive man has the sudden onset of the worst headache of his life while watching television. Although he has nausea and vomiting, he is able to speak coherently. What are the likely possible causes?

12. An elderly, depressed man has a moderately severe generalized headache and decreased attention span but no "hard" findings. What entities should be given special consideration?

13. What medicines are known to cause headaches?

14–25. Match the disease with the characteristic symptoms.

14.	Tic douloureux	a.	Severe ocular pain, "red eye," decreased vision
15.	Bell's palsy		
16.	Pseudotumor cerebri	b.	Papilledema, generalized headache, and menstrual irregularity
17.	Basilar migraine		
18.	Subarachnoid hemorrhage		
19.	Temporal arteritis	c.	Mastoid pain followed by facial palsy
20.	Angle-closure glaucoma		
21.	Subdural hematoma	d.	Lancinating pain in the jaw
22.	Postconcussive headache	e.	Moderate headache, focal seizures, fever
23.	Childhood cerebellar tumor		
24.	Viral meningitis	f.	Mild headache and hemiparesis
25.	Hemiplegic migraine	g.	Chronic pain, depressed sensorium
		h.	Temporal pain, blindness, high sedimentation rate
		i.	Prolonged dull headaches, inattention, and insomnia
		j.	Generalized headache, nuchal rigidity
		k.	Horner's syndrome
		l.	Headache, nausea, vomiting, and ataxia

26. What features of a headache suggest that it is a migraine?

27. What are common precipitants of migraine headaches?

28. How do migraine headaches in children differ from those in adults?

29. In what neurologic disorders are visual hallucinations experienced?

30–33. At what ages do the following headaches usually occur (more than one age period may be appropriate)?

30.	Migraine, classical	a.	Childhood
31.	Migraine, common	b.	Adolescence
32.	Cluster	c.	Middle age
33.	Temporal arteritis	d.	Older age

34–37. Which of these headaches are relieved by sleep?

34. Classical migraine

35. Common migraine

36. Cluster

37. Temporal arteritis

38–44. Which of these headaches awaken a patient from sleep?

38. Classical migraine

39. Common migraine

40. Brain tumor

41. Subdural hematoma

42. Tension
43. Cluster headaches
44. Conversion reaction
45. In what stage of sleep do migraine and cluster headaches begin?
46. What laboratory tests are associated with migraine headaches?
47. A group of many severe periorbital headaches occurs every winter when the patient goes to Miami. This is typical of what kind of headache?
48. What are the diseases or conditions that cost industry the largest number of people-hours?

49–51. Which of the following headaches follow family patterns?
49. Migraine headaches
50. Cluster headaches
51. Tension headaches

52–56. Which medicines are useful for the following headaches?

52. Tension headaches
53. Infrequently occurring classical migraine
54. Frequent, severe common migraine
55. Cluster headaches
56. Occasionally occurring mild migraine

a. Methysergide (Sansert)
b. Propranolol (Inderal)
c. Cafergot
d. Aspirin compounds
e. Aspirin, phenacetin, caffeine, and barbiturate compounds
f. Lithium

57–60. What are the prominent adverse effects of the following medications?
57. Methysergide (Sansert)
58. Propranolol (Inderal)
59. Cafergot
60. Aspirin

61. Which headache variety is cyclic or periodic, develops in middle-aged persons, and responds to lithium treatment?

62. Which tests are likely to be abnormal in patients with postconcussive syndrome?
   a. CT scan
   b. Lumbar puncture
   c. EEG
   d. Brainstem auditory-evoked responses

63. Which procedures may alleviate postconcussive headache?
   a. Neck muscle massage
   b. Use of antidepressant medications
   c. Concluding all litigation
   d. Use of major tranquilizers

64. Which headache variety occurs more often in men than women?
   a. Classic migraine
   b. Common migraine
   c. Pseudotumor cerebri
   d. Trigeminal neuralgia
   e. Tension headaches
   f. Cluster headaches

65. Which therapies are appropriate for pseudotumor cerebri headaches?
   a. Repeated lumbar punctures
   b. Antidepressants
   c. Diuretics
   d. Steroids
   e. Muscle massage
   f. Biofeedback

66–73. Match the headache with its most likely cause:

66. Tic douloureux
67. Hot-dog headache

a. Giant cell inflammation of extra- and intracranial arteries

68. Coital cephalgia
69. Pseudotumor cerebri
70. Temporal arteritis
71. Chinese restaurant syndrome
72. Nocturnal migraine
73. Antianginal medication-induced headaches

b. Autonomic nervous system dysfunction
c. Vascular compression of the trigeminal nerve
d. Nitrites
e. Monosodium glutamate
f. Intracerebral fluid retention
g. Nightmares
h. REM sleep
i. NREM sleep
j. Night terrors
k. Cerebral as well as coronary artery dilation

74. Why might tricyclic antidepressant (TCA) medications be helpful in migraine headaches in people without overt depression?
  a. TCA may improve sleep patterns
  b. TCA may increase the concentration of serotonin, which is analgesic
  c. TCA are analgesic themselves
  d. TCA are endorphins
  e. Such patients may have occult depression

75. Why is rectal or parenteral administration preferable to oral administration of vasoconstrictors, such as ergotamine, for migraines?

76. Which of the following are reasonable criteria for changing from abortive to prophylactic migraine therapy?
  a. More than four migraines monthly
  b. Tinnitus from aspirin-containing medications
  c. Ergotism
  d. Habitual narcotic use
  e. Once monthly classic migraines

77. Which conditions are apt to occur in several family members, although not necessarily on a genetic basis?
  a. Temporal arteritis
  b. Tuberous sclerosis
  c. Multiple sclerosis
  d. Migraines
  e. Absence (petit mal) seizures
  f. Cluster headaches
  g. Pick's disease
  h. Tension headaches

78. During which periods are women's migraines exacerbated?
  a. Premenstrually
  b. When depressed
  c. In the first trimester of pregnancy
  d. When nursing
  e. Menopause
  f. When taking oral contraceptives
  g. At menarche
  h. During middle age

79. Which observations suggest that serotonin metabolism abnormalities are causally related to the development of migraines?
  a. Propranolol (Inderal) is a good prophylactic medication
  b. Dexamethasone suppression tests are abnormal in migraine patients
  c. Platelet serotonin concentrations fall before migraines
  d. Reserpine, which depletes serotonin, precipitates migraines
  e. Methysergide (Sansert), which interferes with serotonin, prevents migraines

80. A 35-year-old man, who suffers several migraine attacks a year, developed a uniquely severe headache during sexual intercourse. Two evenings later, such a headache recurred during masturbation. What advice should be given to the patient?

ANSWERS

1. Acute bacterial meningitis, particularly meningococcal, is a common, often fatal disease in military recruits, school children, and other young people brought to confined areas.

2. The possibility of bacterial meningitis merits immediate investigation with a lumbar puncture for cerebrospinal fluid (CSF) analysis.

3. With bacterial meningitis, the CSF reveals a low glucose concentration (0–40 mg/100 mL), high protein concentration (greater than 100 mg/100 mL), and a polymorphonuclear pleocytosis (over 100/mL).

4. Although alternatives have been suggested, penicillin, 20,000,000 U/day intravenously, remains the standard treatment.

5. He may be having partial complex seizures originating in the uncus of the temporal lobe, i.e., "uncinate fits."

6. He probably has cerebral as well as meningeal involvement.

7. Herpes simplex encephalitis is the most common, nonepidemic encephalitis.

8. Herpes simplex encephalitis has a predilection for the temporal lobes, which include the uncus and portions of the limbic system.

9. Temporal lobe encephalitis may cause not only partial complex seizures but, because of the limbic system involvement, profound memory impairment and in rare cases a form of the Klüver-Bucy syndrome (Chapter 16).

10. While there are many causes of severe retro-orbital pain, a third nerve palsy indicates that a posterior communicating artery aneurysm has ruptured and caused a subarachnoid hemorrhage.

11. Any newly occurring or unique headache is potentially serious. In view of the hypertension, such a headache suggests a cerebral or subarachnoid hemorrhage. Migraine or cluster headaches, which may appear in middle-age, might be the correct diagnosis; however, they should be considered only when headaches have become a chronic illness (often requiring months of observation) and potentially fatal conditions have been excluded.

12. While elderly people are subject to most forms of headaches, they are prone to develop a variety of conditions (Table 9-6) that probably reflect a depressed immune system, atherosclerotic and fragile cerebral vessels, or iatrogenic disturbances. Also, they may be more prone than younger people to have headache as a symptom of depression.

13. Nitroglycerin, long-acting vasodilators (e.g., Isordil), and some other antianginal medications cause headaches. Reserpine causes a dull frontal pain and nasal stuffiness. The monoamine oxidase (MAO) inhibitors cause hypertensive headaches if foods containing tyramine are eaten. Birth control pills precipitate or exacerbate migrainous headaches.

14. d	**20.** a
15. c	**21.** f, g, i, or l
16. b	**22.** i
17. l	**23.** l
18. j	**24.** j
19. h	**25.** f

26. Typically, a migraine is unilateral (in 50 percent), pulsating, and accompanied by autonomic nervous system dysfunction, e.g., nausea, vomiting, fatigue, and diaphoresis. Classic migraines, which are relatively infrequent (20 percent of migraine sufferers have the classic variety), will be preceded by auras, which are most often visual scotoma.

27. Menses, glare, alcohol, too much sleep, missing meals (hypoglycemia), and relief of stress may precipitate migraines.

28. While patients of all ages may have visual auras and autonomic dysfunction, these symptoms may be the primary or exclusive manifestation of migraines in children. Children are also more prone to develop the basilar artery migraine variant. Behavioral disturbances, such as agitation or withdrawal, are often more pronounced in children.

29. Migraines, seizures originating in the temporal or occipital lobes, drugs, narcolepsy, and alcohol withdrawal (DTs) all may precipitate visual hallucinations.

30.	a, b, c	**44.**	No
31.	a, b, c	**45.**	REM
32.	c	**46.**	Low plasma serotonin
33.	d	**47.**	A cluster headache
34.	Yes	**48.**	Low back pain and headache
35.	Yes	**49.**	Yes
36.	No	**50.**	No
37.	No	**51.**	Yes
38.	Yes	**52.**	d or e
39.	Yes	**53.**	c
39.	Yes	**54.**	a or b
40.	Yes	**55.**	f, sometimes a or b
41.	Yes	**56.**	d or e
42.	No	**57.**	Retroperitoneal fibrosis
43.	Yes	**58.**	Bradycardia, asthma, cardiac failure

59. Nausea and vomiting in acute stage; vascular spasm, claudication, and muscle cramps with prolonged use, i.e. *ergotism*

60. Painful gastric distress, gastroduodenal bleeding, and easy bruisability

61. Cluster headaches were initially treated with lithium because of their similarity to manic-depressive illness.

62. c and d, but neither positive nor negative results have definite diagnostic value.

63.	a, b, c	**69.**	f
64.	f	**70.**	a
65.	a, c, d	**71.**	e
66.	c	**72.**	h
67.	d	**73.**	k
68.	b	**74.**	a, b, c, e

75. Parental or rectal vasoconstrictor medication administration produces effective blood levels much faster than oral administration. Early treatment is essential because once vasodilation is established, migraines are relatively refractory to vasoconstriction treatments. In addition, when a patient has a migraine, gastric atony prevents absorption of orally administered medications.

76. a, b, c, d

77. b, c, d, e, g, h. Tension headaches may occur in families, but this incidence is presumably not on a genetic basis.

78. a, c, e, f, g

79. c, d, e

80. While the patient might have merely developed a coital migraine, the development of a uniquely severe headache in any patient, especially when it occurs during vigorous activity, requires further evaluation. In particular, a subarachnoid or intracerebral hemorrhage must be considered. A CT scan or lumbar puncture, depending upon the circumstances, is usually performed because the possibility of a potentially fatal subarachnoid hemorrhage should always be borne in mind when confronted with a patient who describes having the "worse headache" of his or her life.

10

Seizures

Major seizure varieties, such as partial complex, are characterized by specific clinical features and electroencephalographic (EEG) patterns. They are associated with distinctive etiologies, age at the onset of the seizures, and appropriate therapies. The tendency to have recurrent seizures, *epilepsy,** is an important neurologic condition that affects about 6 of every 1,000 people.

A psychiatrist should know as much about seizures as any other neurologic condition. Seizures can mimic psychiatric disturbances, have prominent cognitive and affective components, and be precipitated by psychotropic medicines. Moreover, patients with epilepsy often develop mental aberrations. The most specific laboratory test for seizures, the EEG, is also important for diagnosis of metabolic encephalopathy (an important form of "delirium") and certain dementias but is not useful for many other neurologic conditions.

This chapter, after discussing the nature and uses of EEG, reviews the clinical features of major seizure varieties, EEG diagnosis, and appropriate therapies. Emphasizing mental changes brought about by seizures and their therapy, it includes discussions of related neurologic, psychologic, and medication-induced disorders.

EEG

Normal and Abnormal

The routine EEG records cerebral electrical activity detected by "surface" or "scalp" electrodes (Fig. 10-1).† Four frequency bands of cerebral activity, called by Greek letters, tend to occur over certain parts of the cerebrum and under particular conditions (Table 10-1).

---

*Patients with epilepsy may receive assistance from the Epilepsy Foundation of America, 4351 Garden City Drive, Landover, Maryland 20785, (301) 459-3700.

†The cost of a routine EEG in 1985 is approximately $150.

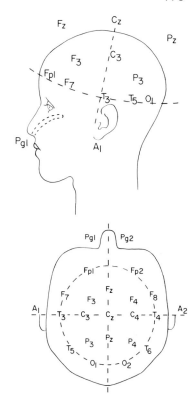

Fig. 10-1. In the standard array of scalp electrodes, most are named for the underlying brain and odd-numbered ones are on the left and even-numbered on the right. The P_g electrodes are from the nasopharyngeal leads; the C electrodes, the center of the skull; and the A electrodes, the ears.

In normal persons, the dominant, or *background* EEG activity is in the *alpha* range of 8 to 13 cycles-per-second, or Hertz (Hz), and occurs over the occipital region (Fig. 10-2). Alpha activity is prominent when people are relaxed with their eyes closed, but it disappears if they open their eyes, concentrate, or become anxious. Thus, it accurately monitors freedom from anxiety and is useful in biofeedback, "alpha training," and other behavior modification techniques. Alpha activity is also lost when people fall asleep or take any medicine that affects mental function, and it slows in the elderly and in almost every neurologic illness.

Beta activity, frequencies faster than 13 Hz, usually has lower voltage and overlies the frontal lobes. While present in normal persons, its relative proportion is increased when people are concentrating, anxious, or using minor tranquilizers.

Theta (4 to 7 Hz) and *delta* (1 to 3 Hz) frequencies are usually absent in healthy, alert adults, but are normally seen in children, in all people as they fall into deep sleep

Table 10-1
Common EEG Rhythms

Activity	Hz (cycles/sec)	Usual Location
Alpha	8–13	Posterior
Beta	>13	Anterior
Theta	4–7	Generalized*
Delta	1–3	Generalized*

*May be focal.

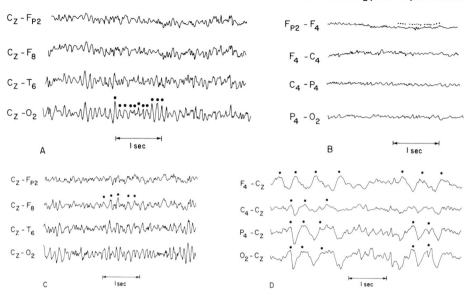

Fig. 10-2. (A) *Alpha* activity is the regular 11-Hz activity overlying the occipital lobe. (B) *Beta* activity is the low voltage, irregular 17-Hz activity overlying the frontal lobe. (C) *Theta* activity is the 5-Hz activity overlying the right frontal lobe. (D) *Delta* activity is the high voltage 2- to 3-Hz activity present over the entire hemisphere.

(Chapter 17), and in many people with relatively trivial disturbances, such as migraine headaches. When present diffusely over the entire brain, slow activity may indicate a degenerative condition or metabolic derangement. When found over a particular area or in *phase reversal* (Fig. 10-3), it may indicate a cerebral lesion, but its absence does not exclude one. Overall, since minimal provocation creates EEG slowing, it is nonspecific.

Whatever their frequency, unusually pointed waves, "sharp waves" or "spikes," indicate a cerebral lesion or a predisposition to epilepsy. When in phase reversal, they indicate an irritative focus that is likely to produce a seizure. However, the finding of sharp waves or spikes does not prove that a patient suffers from a seizure disorder, but that he or she has the possibility of having one.

Uses

SEIZURES

The greatest usefulness of the EEG is in diagnosing and categorizing seizures. During a seizure (*ictus*), *paroxysmal* EEG activity may arise from either normal or abnormal background activity. Paroxysms usually consist of bursts of spikes, slow waves, or complexes of both.

Ideally, an EEG would be done during the ictus, but seizures rarely occur during routine recordings. When they do, EEGs may be obscured by muscle movement artifact. The EEGs obtained immediately after the seizure, in the *postictal period*, generally show only slow, low voltage activity, called "postictal depression." Fortu-

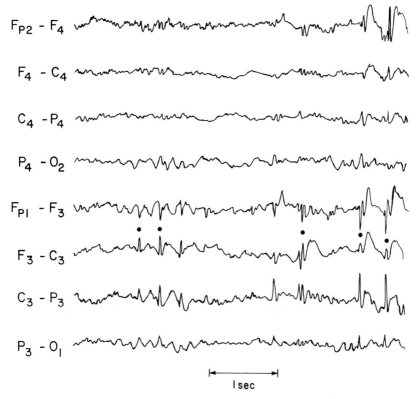

Fig. 10-3. On at least five occasions (marked by dots), sharp waves and spikes, in *phase reversal,* appear to point toward each other. They originate from the F_3 electrode, which is over the left frontal lobe. A finding of such isolated, phase-reversed sharp waves is associated with seizures; however, without further clinical or EEG evidence, it is insufficient for diagnostic purposes.

nately, EEGs obtained between seizures, in the *interictal period,* contain specific abnormalities that suffice for definitive diagnosis in up to 80 percent of cases. However, since about 20 percent of epilepsy patients have essentially normal routine EEGs, normal interictal EEGs do not exclude a diagnosis of seizures.

Several maneuvers are used to evoke diagnostic EEG abnormalities in suspected epileptics. For example, patients are asked to hyperventilate for about three minutes or look directly into a stroboscopic light during the EEG. If these maneuvers do not yield diagnostic information and a strong suspicion of seizures persists, an EEG is performed after sleep deprivation. In about one third of epileptic patients, this EEG reveals abnormalities that were not apparent on routine studies.

In some cases, specially placed electrodes will reveal abnormalities undetectable by scalp electrodes. For example, nasopharyngeal or sphenoidal electrodes can detect discharges from the inferior-medial (mesial) surface of the temporal lobe (Fig. 10-4). Also, electrodes experimentally placed in the subdural space or within the cerebral cortex have revealed an epileptic focus.

A recently introduced technique, *telemetry,* consists of simultaneous videotape recording and correlating a patient's EEG and behavior for several hours, overnight,

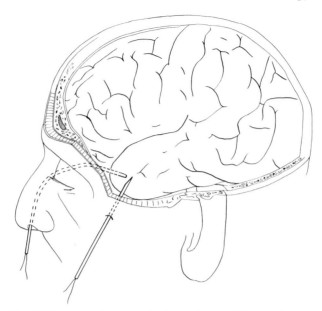

Fig. 10-4. *Nasopharyngeal electrodes,* which are inserted through the nostrils, reach to the posterior pharynx. There, separated by the thin sphenoid bone, they are adjacent to the mesial surface of the temporal lobe. (Refer to Figs. 20-1 and 20-13 to see the distance between the mesial surface of the temporal lobe and the scalp, and also the relationship of the temporal lobe to the sphenoid bone). *Sphenoidal* electrodes are inserted through the skin to reach the lateral, external surface of the sphenoid wing. There they are near the inferior surface of the temporal lobe.

or, in difficult cases, several days.* Telemetry is especially valuable in diagnosing partial complex seizures and disorders that mimic seizures, such as "hysteric" seizures or pseudoseizures (see below).

TOXIC-METABOLIC ENCEPHALOPATHY

Another use of the EEG is in detecting the ingestion of barbiturates and other drugs, hepatic or renal failure, encephalitis, or other conditions leading to mental impairment or depressed sensorium. During the initial phases, when patients are merely withdrawn or agitated and do not yet manifest cognitive impairment, the EEG may lose its alpha activity and develop generalized theta and delta activity.

In hepatic or uremic encephalopathy, there are often repetitive *triphasic waves* (Fig. 10-5). In hepatic failure, this pattern is characteristic and may appear before the bilirubin is raised. While other EEG changes found in encephalopathy can be confused with those induced by medications, sleepiness, or congenital injuries, a normal EEG virtually rules out a toxic-metabolic encephalopathy.

---

*The cost of telemetry for several hours in 1985 is approximately $600.

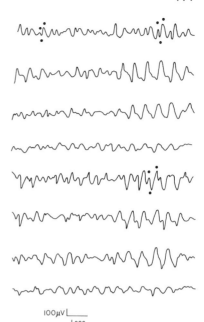

Fig. 10-5. This EEG obtained from a patient with hepatic encephalopathy reveals typical *triphasic waves,* which can be seen in the first and fifth channel. There is also lack of organized background activity.

100μV

1 sec

DEMENTIA

In early Alzheimer's disease, the alpha background characteristically slows from about 12 Hz down to 8 Hz. While this is still normal, virtually all patients with moderately advanced Alzheimer's disease have slow-wave activity. Unfortunately, patients with multi-infarct dementia have similar abnormalities, preventing EEG differentiation between these two conditions (Chapters 7 and 11).

In contrast, the EEG is much more helpful in diagnosing subacute sclerosing panencephalitis (SSPE) and Creutzfeldt-Jakob disease (Chapter 7). In these conditions, dementia is accompanied by myoclonic jerks and an EEG showing *periodic complexes* (Fig. 10-6).

The EEG is also useful in diagnosing the *locked-in syndrome,* in which people sustain pontine or medullary infarctions (Chapters 2 and 11) that prevent them from speaking or moving their trunk or limbs. However, since the cerebrum and upper brainstem are normal, they have normal cerebral activity despite their physical impairment and therefore a normal EEG.

Patients with the locked-in syndrome must be differentiated from ones in a *persistent vegetative state,* which typically follows cardiac arrest or drug overdose. These patients have marked cerebral cortex injury, but preserved brainstem function, and profound dementia accompanying inability to speak or move. As would be expected from extensive cerebral cortex damage, their EEGs are markedly abnormal.

The EEG is also useful in distinguishing pseudodementia from dementia (Chapter 7). Whereas in pseudodementia the EEG is normal or shows only slightly slowed background activity, in advanced dementia from almost any cause it shows theta and delta activity. Nevertheless, in the many patients who have mixed depression and mild dementia, the EEG is of little help.

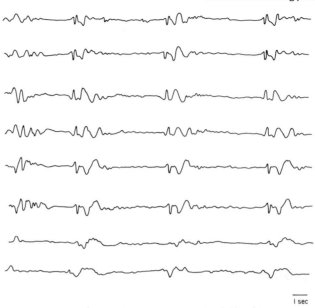

I sec

Fig. 10-6. *Periodic complexes* are seen in all channels as four fairly regular bursts of electrical activity followed by minimal activity, so-called "burst-supression." Periodic complexes are associated with myoclonic jerks, and together they are cardinal features of two dementing illnesses, subacute sclerosing panencephalitis (SSPE), which occurs in children, and Creutzfeldt–Jakob disease, which occurs in the elderly (Chapter 7).

STRUCTURAL LESIONS

The EEG is not a good test for detecting or excluding structural lesions such as brain tumors, abscesses, cerebrovascular accidents (CVAs), or subdural hematomas. It might be normal in many of these conditions; when abnormal, it cannot distinguish between them. Computed tomography (CT) is more reliable and cost-effective (Chapter 20).

PSYCHIATRIC DISTURBANCES

Aside from drug abuse, toxic-metabolic encephalopathy, and some causes of dementia, the EEG is virtually useless for diagnosing psychiatric illness. First, approximately 15 percent of "normal" people have nonspecific EEG changes, such as an occasional spike or slow wave. Also, there is no consensus on how many patients with psychosis have EEG abnormalities or what they are. Further compounding the difficulty is the fact that both adults and children with either mental retardation or minimal brain dysfunction often have mild, nonspecific abnormalities similar to those attributable to age or state of awareness.

In addition, psychotropic medications can induce prominent EEG alterations that can persist for up to two months after their withdrawal. Phenothiazines, butyrophenones, tricyclic antidepressants, and lithium may cause background slowing, theta and delta activity, and occasional nonfocal sharp waves. Phenothiazines tend to produce these abnormalities in the frontal and temporal lobes. Diazepam

(Valium), barbiturates, and some other minor tranquilizer-sedatives typically induce beta activity.

Moreover, these medications do more than merely cause EEG artifacts. Many increase patients' tendency to have seizures. Those with anticonvulsant properties such as diazepam and barbiturates, provoke seizures and sleep disorders when withdrawn abruptly.

Changes in the EEG also follow electroconvulsive therapy (ECT). During and immediately after ECT, EEG changes resemble those of a generalized tonic-clonic seizure. With increasing numbers of treatments, ECT induces more persistent slow-wave activity, lasting up to three months over the frontal lobes or the entire cerebrum.

Slowing of the EEG induced by ECT is generally associated with memory impairment but also with a more effective treatment of endogenous depression. When ECT is unilateral, EEG slowing is less pronounced and is usually seen much more over the treated side.

VARIETIES OF SEIZURES

Most seizures and varieties of epilepsy are classified either as *partial,* with either elementary (simple) or complex symptoms, or as *generalized,* usually *absences* or *tonic-clonic* (Table 10-2). Partial seizures originate from paroxysmal electrical discharges in a "focus," a limited region of the cerebral cortex which is usually injured by a structural lesion. Partial seizures with motor symptoms have their focus in the contralateral frontal lobe; those with sensory symptoms, in the parietal lobe; those with visual symptoms, in the occipital or temporal lobe, and those with auditory symptoms, in the temporal lobe.

During and between partial seizures, the EEG typically shows abnormalities in channels overlying the particular focus. Since neither the entire cortex nor deep structures are involved when seizures begin, or often throughout their entire course, consciousness is always preserved.

Although partial seizures usually last between several seconds and several minutes, occasionally they continue for hours or days, while the discharge remains confined to its original focus. In such cases, called *epilepsy partialis continua* or *focal status epilepticus,* symptoms persist and interfere with normal activity. Sometimes discharges become more extensive and, enlarging in a slow, brushfire-like manner, involve adjacent cortical areas and create additional symptoms. They can also spread over the entire cortex or shoot through the corpus callosum to the other cerebral

Table 10-2
An Abridged Version of the International
Classification of Epilepsies

Partial (or focal) epilepsies
   Partial seizures with elementary symptomatology
   Partial seizures with complex symptomatology
Generalized epilepsies
   Primary generalized epilepsies
     Absences (petit mal)
     Tonic-clonic (grand mal)

hemisphere. Once the entire cerebral cortex is engulfed in this manner (*secondary generalization*), patients lose consciousness and develop bilateral motor activity and EEG abnormalities in all channels.

In contrast to partial seizures, discharges in generalized seizures arise from the thalamus or other subcortical structures and immediately spread upward to the entire cerebral cortex. Also, generalized seizures are usually caused by a genetic disorder or metabolic aberration. Moreover, they are characterized by unconsciousness and generalized EEG abnormalities, although not necessarily by gross motor activity. Like other seizures, generalized seizures can persist, in which cases they are called *generalized status epilepticus*.

PARTIAL SEIZURES

Partial Elementary Seizures

Partial seizures are said to have *elementary* symptoms when their clinical manifestation is only a particular movement, a single sensation, or a simple phenomenon. However, if there is impaired consciousness, with or without psychologic abnormalities or coordinated motor activity, seizures are said to have *complex* symptoms.

Seizures with elementary *motor* symptoms, formerly called "focal motor seizures," usually consist of rhythmic jerking (clonic movement) of an area that may be as limited as one finger or as extensive as an entire side of the body (Fig. 10-7). These

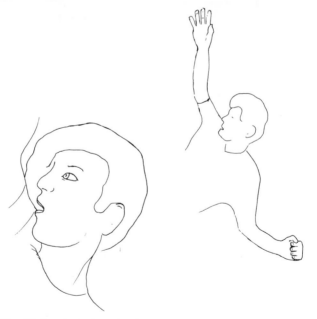

Fig. 10-7. A patient having a partial seizure with motor symptoms has his head, neck, and eyes deviated toward the right, his right arm extended, and his left flexed. This position, an adversive seizure, suggests that the seizure originated in the left frontal lobe.

seizures can develop into focal status epilepticus or undergo secondary generalization. Sometimes, in a "jacksonian march," a seizure discharge spreads along the motor cortex, and movements that began in a finger extend to the entire arm and then the face.

After any partial motor seizure, affected muscles may be weakened. A postictal monoparesis or (Todd's) hemiparesis may last as long as 24 hours. Thus, the differential diagnosis of transient hemiparesis includes transient ischemic attacks (TIAs), hemiplegic migraines, psychologic aberrations, and Todd's hemiparesis.

Seizures with elementary *sensory* symptoms usually consist of tingling or burning paresthesias in regions of the body that have extensive cortical representation, such as the face. Rarely, sensory loss, a "negative symptom," might be the sole manifestation of such a seizure.

Partial elementary seizures with "special sensory" symptoms, such as auditory, visual, or olfactory ones, can also occur. Although such seizures create vivid, realistic sensations, they are almost always recognized by patients as being hallucinations.

Auditory symptoms are usually repetitive noises, musical notes, or single words that have no meaning. Visual symptoms usually consist of bright lines, spots, stars, or splotches of color that move slowly across the visual field or, like scenes in a kaleidoscope, rotate around the center of vision. However, more elaborate visual phenomena and visual phenomena combined with auditory or emotional symptoms are "complex" symptoms that must be differentiated from other visual hallucinations (Table 9-3 and Chapter 12).

Olfactory symptoms usually consist of vaguely recognizable smells. The most frequent one is "burning rubber." Since these olfactory hallucinations usually result from discharges in the *uncus* of the temporal lobe, partial seizures with olfactory symptoms are often called *uncinate seizures* or *uncinate fits.* If discharges spread to involve larger areas of the temporal lobe, typical partial complex seizures ensue.

EEG, ETIOLOGY, AND TREATMENT

During partial elementary seizures, EEGs may show spikes, slow waves, or spike-wave complexes overlying the seizure focus. For example, during a seizure with motor symptoms, such EEG abnormalities may be prominent in channels recording frontal lobe activity (Fig. 10-8). In addition, during the interictal period, the EEG may continue to reveal occasional spikes in these channels.

Although partial seizures can develop at any age, they usually begin in late childhood or adolescence. They can be caused by various cerebral lesions, but depending upon the patient's health and age at the onset of the seizure, particular lesions may be suspected. When children develop partial seizures, the common causes are congenital cerebral injuries and neonatal meningitis. Also, children with congenital conditions, such as tuberous sclerosis, almost always develop partial seizures (Chapter 13). Thus, these children often have mental retardation and "cerebral palsy" as well as seizures.

Another cause of partial seizures in childhood is rolandic (centrotemporal) epilepsy. These seizures usually consist of facial movements and speech arrest. Unlike most other forms of partial epilepsy, centrotemporal epilepsy is not associated with underlying structural lesions, but is inherited (in an autosomal dominant pattern) and remits by puberty.

For young adults, the most common causes of partial elementary seizures are

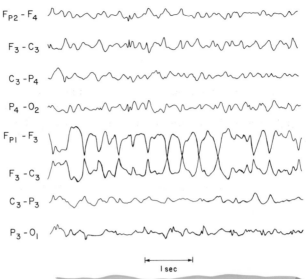

$F_{P2}-F_4$

F_3-C_3

C_3-P_4

P_4-O_2

$F_{PI}-F_3$

F_3-C_3

C_3-P_3

P_3-O_1

I sec

Fig. 10-8. This EEG obtained during a partial seizure with motor symptoms contains a paroxysm of 4-Hz sharp wave activity with phase reversals referable to the F_3 electrode. Since this electrode overlies the left frontal region, the seizure probably consists of right face or arm motor activity and, in 50 percent of cases, a deviation of the head and eyes to the right.

head trauma, arteriovenous malformations (AVMs), and previously asymptomatic congenital injuries. In addition, patients with severe mental disturbances, particularly autism, are apt to develop seizures. For people 40 to 60 years old, primary or metastatic brain tumors are the single most common cause. However, people who are older are more likely to develop seizures from CVAs than tumors.

Treatment of uncomplicated partial seizure cases begins with removal of an underlying lesion provided neurosurgery will not endanger vital centers. Standard anticonvulsants, given alone or in combination, are carbamazepine (Tegretol), phenytoin (Dilantin), or phenobarbital. Unfortunately, their use may be complicated by cerebellar atrophy; allergic skin reactions, including the Stevens-Johnson syndrome; hepatitis; or hematologic abnormalities. Also, even at therapeutic blood concentrations, anticonvulsants can induce cognitive impairment and changes in affect. In all varieties of epilepsy, the clinical response of patients and the anticonvulsant concentrations in their blood must be monitored to balance seizure control benefits against anticonvulsant side effects.

Partial Complex Seizures

Partial complex seizures, which usually begin between a patient's late childhood and early 30s are the single most frequent seizure variety, affecting about 65 percent of epilepsy patients. This high frequency is reflected in clinical studies and is especially important to be aware of when analyzing studies of psychiatric disorders in epilepsy patients.

Many old studies of epilepsy patients were likely to be misleading because they did not acknowledge the preponderance of patients who had partial complex seizures, relied upon patients' descriptions of nonspecific sensations, and did not require EEG correlation. Current studies, which use telemetry, have defined ictal and postictal seizure manifestations and separated them from nonseizure disturbances.

Nevertheless, many unsettled issues continue to revolve around partial complex seizures. A major one is the genuineness of the broad range of purported ictal symptoms, including violence. Another is the relationship between partial complex epilepsy and interictal mental abnormalities, such as personality disorders, psychosis, and cognitive impairment.

Before describing partial complex seizures any further, a preliminary note on nomenclature must be inserted. These disorders have been known in the past under two less cumbersome titles: *psychomotor seizures* and *temporal lobe seizures*. However, the first term is properly applied only to a rare variety of partial complex seizures with exclusively behavioral abnormalities. The latter term is no longer used because these seizures originate in the frontal and other lobes rather than the temporal lobe in about 10 percent of cases, this term often belies the location of the focus. Moreover, it is inconsistent with the current classification of seizures, which relies upon symptoms rather than anatomic origin.

About 10 percent of patients who have seizures begin with a premonitory sensation, an *aura,* which is actually an elementary partial seizure. With or without the aura, during the seizure patients are typically inattentive, uncommunicative, and have impaired consciousness.

The most important physical characteristic of partial complex seizures are *automatisms,* which are simple, repetitive, and purposeless movements. They are present in over 80 percent of these seizures, found more frequently than psychologic aberrations, and never occur without accompanying loss of awareness. Although automatisms can be found in absence seizures (see below), they are much more frequent in partial complex seizures, where they almost always involve both the face and hands. They usually consist of swallowing, kissing, lipsmacking, and other facial motions, or fumbling, scratching, rubbing the abdomen, and other hand movements (Fig. 10-9).

Patients may stand, walk, or develop the same postures as seen in adversive seizures (Fig. 10-7). In about 25 percent of cases, patients may utter brief phrases or mutter unintelligibly. Occasionally, they lose their body tone and collapse (*temporal lobe syncope*).

Rarely, special sensory phenomena, which are more elaborate than in partial

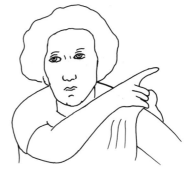

Fig. 10-9. During partial complex seizures, patients are typically dazed. They perform rudimentary, purposeless actions, such as this woman's pulling on her clothing. Repetitive, simple body movements, *automatisms,* such as lip smacking, are present in 80 percent of cases.

elementary seizures, can occur. Patients may have complex visual hallucinations that include macropsia and micropsia (where objects appear, respectively, larger or smaller than reality), or auditory ones that consist of meaningless, repetitive sounds or words. Visual hallucinations supposedly originate more frequently in the right cerebral hemisphere, but auditory sensations are equally likely to originate in either hemisphere. However, since seizure patients often have congenital cerebral injuries and tend to be left-handed, one cannot assume that their left cerebral hemisphere is dominant (Chapter 8).

Many symptoms that might indicate seizures cannot be accepted in isolation. For example, the various "experiential phenomena," such as *déjà vu, jamais vu,* dreamlike states, mind–body dissociations, and floating feelings, are rarely associated with paroxysmal EEG abnormalities. They are too nonspecific and they have been so romanticized that they have virtually no diagnostic value when described by a well-read patient.

Another frequent disturbance with a dubious association with partial complex seizures is the *rising epigastric sensation.* This is a feeling of swelling in the abdomen that, as if progressing upwards within the body, turns into tightness in the throat and a feeling of suffocation. Although this symptom is sometimes an aura, it has a striking similarity to a common psychogenic disturbance, *globus hystericus,* in which people also feel occlusion of the throat and an inability to breathe.

About 90 percent of partial complex seizures, whatever their ictal manifestions, sooner or later undergo secondary generalization. Thus, a guideline for differentiating them from a recurring psychogenic event is that at least every 1 to 2 years partial complex seizures explode into generalized seizures.

In contrast, a decidedly uncommon event, despite its frequent occurrence in popular literature, is *partial complex status epilepticus.* Only about two dozen cases have been described in neurologic journals, and many were not documented with telemetry. When this condition occurs, patients have confusion, sometimes accompanied by aphasia, automatisms, and other purposeless motor activity, lasting for $1\frac{1}{2}$ to 24 hours (Ballenger). Confusion is so pronounced that patients are incapable of thought and complicated activity, much less homicidal rampages. However, the attack may be severe enough to merit its description *ictal psychosis.*

ICTAL SEX AND VIOLENCE

Sexually related symptoms and actions are occasionally attributed to partial complex seizures. However, in many people, seizure-like symptoms that occur during sexual activity are probably the result of anxiety or hyperventilation. Although epileptic patients commonly fumble with buttons or tug at their clothing, and thus may seem to partially undress, true exhibitionism is extraordinarily rare.

Nevertheless, rudimentary sexual activities, such as masturbation, scratching of the perineum, and pelvic thrusting, do occur. For example, in one study, 4 of 61 patients with refractory partial complex seizures had such activity; however, it was not accompanied by more complex sexual behavior (Spencer). Only several times has sexual intercourse or orgasm as a seizure symptom been reported in the neurologic literature. When sexual behavior results from a seizure, its focus is found most often in the frontal or temporal lobe and in the right more than the left hemisphere.

The extent of *ictal violence,* violence as a manifestation of seizures, has been controversial. However, by excluding experiential phenomena as being equivalent to a partial complex seizure and relying on telemetry, several observations have been made (Delgado-Escueta). Such violence occurs in less than 0.1 percent of seizures. When violence does occur, it is not accompanied by a major affective state, such as rage, and it is fragmented, unsustained, and neither directed nor destructive, i.e., it is not "aggressive." For example, it usually consists only of brief, random shoving, pushing, or kicking or of verbal abuse, such as screaming; however, it does not consist of sequential activities or interactions required with people or mechanical devices, such as cars or guns. In addition, seizures with violent manifestations, like other seizures, are not provoked by social factors, such as threats.

On the other hand, some authors have attributed aggressive violence to seizures (Pincus). Also, fifteen times between 1889 and 1981, seizures have been used as a defense for the purpose of legal appeals in cases of murder, homicide, manslaughter, or disorderly conduct.

INTERICTAL MENTAL ABNORMALITIES

Previous studies had found that patients who seemed to have seizures originating in the temporal lobe (*temporal lobe epilepsy*) had distinctive personality trait abnormalities (Bear). They described patients as being hyposexual, humorless, circumstantial, and overly concerned with general philosophic questions, such as the order of the universe. In addition, they were noted to have *hypergraphia,* a tendency to write excessively and compulsively. However, recent studies, often based on telemetry, have refuted many of these contentions, finding no distinctive personality traits in patients with partial complex seizure epilepsy (Guerrant, Mungas, Stevens).

Previous studies also suggested that different emotional and intellectual abnormalities depended upon whether the seizure focus was in the right or left temporal lobe. Supposedly, right-sided foci predisposed a patient to anger, sadness, and elation, and left-sided ones to ruminative and intellectual tendencies. However, recent evidence indicates there is no difference in personality traits when foci are in different temporal lobes, or even other brain areas (Rodin). Furthermore, no difference in personality traits is apparent among patients with different varieties of epilepsy.

In several old but frequently cited studies, 10 percent of temporal lobe epilepsy patients were found to have "schizophrenic-like" or "schizophreniform" psychosis; and, conversely, psychotic epilepsy patients were found to have temporal lobe epilepsy much more than either generalized epilepsy or nonneurologic illness (Slater, Flor-Henry). This interictal psychosis, as acute schizophrenia, was characterized by hallucinations, thought disorders, paranoid ideation, and illusions and responded to conventional antipsychotic medications. The psychosis began on the average at age 30 years and was most often present when epilepsy had begun between ages 5 and 10 years. Therefore, it became evident more than 10 years after the onset of epilepsy. Male epilepsy patients who were left-handed and had a left-sided seizure focus were supposedly more susceptible. Although most studies reported that the psychosis was more likely to occur if seizures were poorly controlled, some reported it was precipitated by anticonvulsant suppression of seizures and a "forced normalization" of the EEG.

However, in these studies, many patients who were diagnosed as having temporal lobe epilepsy had only experiential symptoms or occasional EEG temporal lobe spikes—criteria that by themselves would not now be considered diagnostic. Also, the high incidence of temporal lobe epilepsy among psychotic patients may be only a reflection of the large proportion (65 percent) of all epilepsy patients who have partial complex seizures. Moreover, in addition to the usual uncertainty about whether the left hemisphere of epileptic patients is actually dominant, newer studies have questioned the alleged preponderance of left-sided foci in patients with partial complex seizures and psychosis. The newer studies have found, too, that emotional and cognitive difficulties in epileptic children with unilateral temporal lobe epilepsy do not differ significantly in magnitude depending on whether the right or left lobe contains the focus.

Despite controversy regarding many interictal mental abnormalities, there has been general agreement that patients with partial complex and other seizures, except for absences, are liable to suffer from mental retardation or progressive intellectual (cognitive) deterioration. Investigators discovered that when epilepsy began in early childhood, 10 to 25 percent of patients had mental retardation. One typical study found that about 50 percent of partial complex seizure patients and 25 percent of generalized tonic-clonic seizure patients developed inattentiveness, impaired memory, and slowed speech (Guerrant).

These cognitive and other mental changes, in addition to seizures, have been ascribed to perinatal anoxia, prematurity, and other congenital brain injuries (Chapter 13). Thereafter, seizures themselves may cause head trauma, cerebral anoxia, and massive electrical discharges, which are all likely to cause further, cumulative damage. Another cause of progressive cognitive impairment is anticonvulsants. Even at therapeutic concentrations, almost all can lead to impaired concentration.

Moreover, anticonvulsant intoxication is the factor most often responsible for development of acute confusion in epileptics. Less common causes are partial complex or absence status epilepticus, head trauma, or the residue of seizures, i.e., postictal confusion.

Another established interictal trait of epilepsy patients is a high incidence of crime. For example, among incarcerated men, the incidence of epilepsy is at least four times as great as in the general population; however, crimes of adult epileptic prisoners are no more violent than those of nonepileptic ones (Whitman). The consensus among investigators is that the origin of the criminiality is not epilepsy, but that seizures, head trauma, and other brain injuries lead to poor impulse control, lower socioeconomic status, and other conditions that predispose persons to crime.

Depression is also supposedly commonplace, especially in patients who have developed epilepsy in middle age or later. The incidence of suicide is four to five times greater in epilepsy patients and even greater in men and those who have partial complex seizures. In committing suicide, patients frequently overdose with anticonvulsants, especially phenobarbital.

Tricyclic and tetracyclic antidepressants, while permitted, must be given cautiously since they lower the seizure threshold. Of these medications, maprotiline (Ludiomil) may be the most epileptogenic in depressed patients. Individual psychotherapy, group therapy, and self-help groups, but not psychoanalysis, have helped most seizure patients with, or even without, depression.

Another of the psychiatric aspects of epilepsy is recurrent seizures that are refractory to routine management. Two common causes are noncompliance with anticonvulsant regimens and pseudoseizures. Therefore, when epilepsy management is complicated by inexplicably refractory seizures, valuable diagnostic tests are frequent determinations of anticonvulsant levels in the blood and telemetry.

EEG

During a partial complex seizure, the EEG will typically show paroxysms of spikes, slow waves, or other abnormalities in channels overlying the temporal or frontotemporal region. Even though the seizure focus may be unilateral, EEG abnormalities are found bilaterally in almost all cases because of the presence of additional foci or projections from a single focus.

In the interictal period, the routine EEG reveals spikes or spike and slow-wave complexes over the temporal lobes in about 40 percent of known cases. With an appropriate history, such EEG abnormalities are specific enough to corroborate the diagnosis.

Also, about 90 percent of persons with anterior temporal spikes on the EEG will have partial complex seizures. Nevertheless, spikes without seizure symptoms should not by themselves be considered diagnostic for seizures.

If nasopharyngeal leads and sleep recordings are used, EEG abnormalities will be found in as many as 80 percent of cases (Fig. 10-10). After that test, if cases remain a diagnostic problem, especially where episodic behavioral abnormalities are believed to result from seizures, telemetry must be used as the definitive test. In short, the EEG diagnosis of partial complex seizures should be approached with a routine EEG, which has a 40 percent yield; an EEG with nasopharyngeal leads during sleep, for an 80 percent yield; and then telemetry, with virtually a 100 percent yield.

Since partial elementary and partial complex seizures usually originate from structural lesions, CT scans are routinely performed (Chapter 20). They are also performed in most cases of tonic-clonic seizures because clinical and EEG data may not be able to distinguish between genetically induced primary generalized seizures and partial seizures that have undergone secondary generalization. Cases in which CT scans might be avoided are those of drug- or alcohol-withdrawal seizures and absences (see below).

In partial seizures, a CT scan may reveal a structural lesion or temporal lobe atrophy, even where the neurologic examination is normal. It will also reveal many tumors, tuberous sclerosis nodules, large infarctions, and AVMs. However, it will not show mesial temporal sclerosis, neonatal injuries, or cryptic temporal lobe vascular malformations.

Positron emission tomography (PET) has been used to study cerebral metabolism during seizures and interictal periods. In partial complex seizures, the affected tempo-

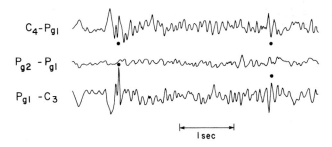

Fig. 10-10. An interictal EEG with nasopharyngeal electrodes (P_{g1} and P_{g2}) shows phase-reversed spikes that routine scalp electrodes may not detect.

ral lobe typically is hypermetabolic during the ictus and hypometabolic interictally. Curiously, the metabolic alterations are unrelated to the clinical and EEG manifestations of these seizures.

ETIOLOGY

Lesions that cause partial complex seizures include those that cause partial elementary seizures, but also temporal lobe AVMs, hamartomas, astrocytomas, and mesial temporal sclerosis. This last condition, which is probably the most common cause of partial complex seizures, is thought to lead to sclerosis of the "Sommers" sector of the hypocampus and temporal lobe atrophy. In addition to temporal lobe lesions, in about 10 percent of cases the seizure originates in a structural lesion outside of the temporal lobe.

Partial complex and elementary seizures are almost never precipitated by alcohol- or drug-withdrawal, emotional factors, or external social factors, such as threats. However, like other seizures, they may be precipitated by menses, intercurrent illness, and malabsorption of anticonvulsants.

TREATMENT

Treatment of partial complex seizures usually begins with the same anticonvulsants used in treatment of partial elementary seizures. Also, mysoline (Primidone) is sometimes helpful. More often, combinations of two or three anticonvulsants are required. In using multiple anticonvulsants, it is necessary to follow blood concentrations especially closely to avoid frequent seizures or mental impairments and other signs of anticonvulsant intoxication. When seizures tend to occur premenstrually, acetazolamide (Diamox) is given.

Patients sometimes are advised to undergo a temporal lobectomy for intractable partial complex seizures. Suitable candidates must have a unilateral, single temporal lobe seizure lesion identifiable on clinical, EEG, and radiographic testing. Wada tests (Chapter 8) are performed to avoid postoperative aphasia and the Klüver-Bucy syndrome (Chapters 12 and 16). In properly selected cases, temporal lobectomy reportedly results in a more than 75 percent reduction in seizure frequency. In addition, about 50 percent of patients have a postoperative reduction in rage attacks, aggressive behavior, and psychotic disturbances (Falconer).

Patients with multiple seizure foci causing seizures that undergo secondary generalization may benefit from a commissurotomy, a sectioning of the corpus callosum (Chapter 8). This procedure interrupts the spread of discharges between cerebral hemispheres. Despite the extent of the surgery, postoperative deficits are so subtle that special neuropsychologic tests are required to demonstrate the major consequence of commissurotomy, the split-brain syndrome (see Fig. 8-8).

GENERALIZED SEIZURES

Generalized seizures are characterized by an immediate loss of consciousness accompanied by symmetric, synchronous, paroxysmal EEG discharges. These seizures are usually the result of either an autosomal dominant genetic disorder, a physiologic disturbance, or a metabolic aberration, including drug and alcohol withdrawal. Unlike partial seizures, generalized seizures lack an aura, lateralized motor or sensory disturbances, and focal EEG abnormalities. Also, they practically never result from brain tumors, cerebral infarctions, or other cerebral cortex injuries. Most generalized seizures are of either the absence (*petit mal*) or tonic-clonic (*grand mal*) variety.

Absences

Absence seizures usually begin between ages 4 and 10 years. Unlike other major seizure varieties, they usually disappear in early adulthood. However, in about 40 percent of patients, tonic-clonic seizures develop at some time.

Absences, which may occur many times daily, are 1-second to 10-second lapses in attention accompanied in almost all cases by automatisms, subtle clonic limb movements, and blinking (Fig. 10-11). Notably, the blinking occurs rhythmically at 3 Hz, the frequency of the associated EEG abnormality. Although children do not have retrograde amnesia and they maintain muscle tone and bladder control, their mental and physical activity is interrupted. After the ictus, as though it had never occurred, there is no confusion, agitation, or sleepiness.

Children with unrecognized absences may be misdiagnosed as being inattentive or mentally retarded. More important, they may be misdiagnosed as having partial complex seizures, even though the two conditions can be differentiated (Table 10-3). The distinction is especially important when, on rare occasions, *absence status epilepticus* leads to apathy and psychomotor retardation for several hours. This condition usually develops only in children and young adults with a history of absences who have suddenly discontinued their anticonvulsants.

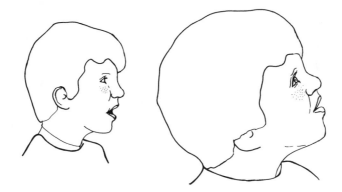

Fig. 10-11. During a typical absence, this 8-year-old boy has brief, 1- to 3-second staring spells during which he becomes glassy-eyed and mute. Typically he rolls his eyes upwards and blinks at 3 Hz. Although he loses consciousness, he maintains bodily tone and does not become incontinent. Absence seizures and the accompanying EEG abnormality (see Fig. 10-12) may be demonstrated by having the child count numbers slowly while hyperventilating. Seizures occur when the counting slows or pauses. At the end of the seizure, the child will resume counting at the appropriate number, which indicates that there is no retrograde amnesia.

Table 10-3

Comparison of Partial Complex and Absence Seizures

Feature	Partial Complex	Absence
Aura	Often	Never
Consciousness	Impaired	Lost at onset
Movements	Usually simple and repetitive but may involve some activity	Blinking, and facial and finger automatisms
Postictal behavior	Amnesia, confusion, and tendency to sleep	No abnormality, but amnesia for ictus
Frequency without treatment	1 to 2 per week	Several daily
Duration	2 to 3 minutes	1 to 10 seconds
EEG	Spikes and polyspike and waves, usually over both temporal regions	Generalized 3-Hz spike-and-wave complexes
Anticonvulsants	Carbamazepine, phenytoin, phenobarbital, primidone	Ethosuximide, valproic acid, clonazepam

EEG, ETIOLOGY, AND TREATMENT

During an absence, the EEG shows synchronous 3-Hz spike and slow-wave complexes in all channels (Fig. 10-12). However, in the interictal period, occasional asymptomatic bursts of 3 Hz spike-and-slow-wave complexes lasting 1 to 1.5 seconds may be observed. In patients with absences, either hyperventilation or photic stimulation can precipitate the characteristic clinical and EEG abnormalities.

A patient's relatives also often have absences or 3 Hz spike-and-slow-wave complexes that can be precipitated by hyperventilation. This finding supports the hypothesis that absences are inherited in an autosomal dominant pattern. In contrast to tonic-clonic seizures, absences are not associated with drug withdrawal, metabolic aberrations, or structural lesions. Therefore, CT scans and other tests are usually not performed.

Absences are treated with ethosuximide (Zarontin), valproic acid (Depakene or Depakote), or occasionally clonazepam (Clonopin). Most children readily respond to one or another of these anticonvulsants. After adolescence, anticonvulsants generally can be withdrawn slowly without precipitating recurrence of absences.

Tonic-Clonic Seizures

Tonic-clonic seizures, unlike absences, begin at any age after infancy, persist into adult life, and cause massive motor activity and profound postictal residua. Although patients may have a prodrome of malaise or mood change, tonic-clonic seizures are usually unheralded, explosive events. In the initial tonic phase, patients lose consciousness, their eyes roll upward, and their neck, trunk, and limbs extend backwards

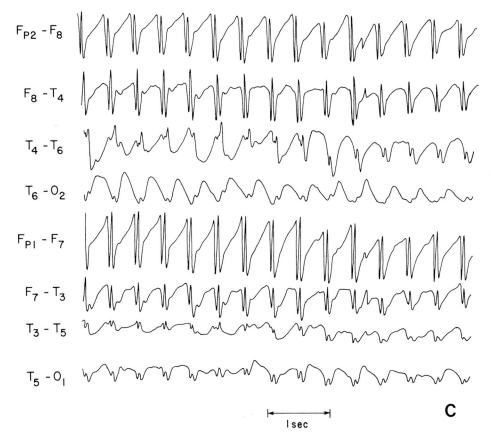

$F_{P2} - F_8$

$F_8 - T_4$

$T_4 - T_6$

$T_6 - O_2$

$F_{PI} - F_7$

$F_7 - T_3$

$T_3 - T_5$

$T_5 - O_I$

I sec

C

Fig. 10-12. During an absence, the EEG characteristically shows regular, symmetric, and synchronous 3-Hz spike-and-wave complexes. The discharge arises from and returns to a normal EEG background.

as if to form an arch. Subsequently, they have a dramatic clonic phase in which their limbs, neck, and trunk are wracked by violent jerks (Fig. 10-13).

A potential diagnostic problem is that during the tonic-clonic phases, the seizure appears similar to a partial seizure that has undergone secondary generalization. Often only a detailed history, a trained observer, or an EEG can resolve the problem.

In the postictal period, which has great diagnostic importance, patients are usually confused, disoriented, and amnesic, both for the seizure period and, in a "retrograde" pattern, the events preceding it. They may be irrational, agitated, and combative. Postictal behavioral disturbances, which can last for several hours, can be so striking as to be misdiagnosed as a functional "postictal psychosis." Such postictal disturbances must also be distinguished from partial complex status epilepticus, anticonvulsant intoxication, and a seizure-induced brain injury, such as a subdural hematoma.

EEG, ETIOLOGY, AND TREATMENT

During the tonic phase, if the superimposed muscle artifact can be eliminated by administering muscle relaxants, the EEG shows repetitive, increasingly greater spikes occurring at about 10 Hz in all channels. In the clonic phase, the spikes,

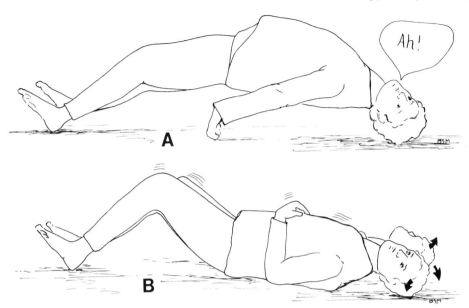

Fig. 10-13. (A) This patient in the tonic phase of a tonic-clonic seizure arches his torso and extends his arms and legs. He assumes this position because of the relatively greater strength of the extensor muscles over the flexor muscles. Simultaneous diaphragm, chest wall, and laryngeal muscle contractions force air through a tightened larynx and cause the shrill, epileptic cry. During this phase, patients often bite their tongue and involuntarily force urine out of their bladder. (B) In the clonic phase, the patient's head, neck, and legs have symmetric and forceful contractions for about 10 to 20 seconds. Saliva, which becomes aerated and often blood-tinged from tongue lacerations, appears as a froth at the mouth. The pupils dilate and the patient sweats profusely. Finally, muscular contractions become progressively less frequent and weaker. The seizure usually ends with a sigh, followed by stertorous breathing. In the immediate postictal period, patients are unresponsive.

which become less frequent but greater in amplitude, are interrupted by slow waves (Fig. 10-14).

Afterwards, the EEG shows postictal depression. The postictal EEG is often the only one available, but it can confirm the diagnosis. In contrast, following a pseudoseizure, the EEG is relatively normal.

Interictally, 20 to 30 percent of patients with tonic-clonic seizures have asymptomatic, brief bursts of spikes, polyspikes, and slow waves. Seizures and accompanying EEG abnormalities may be precipitated by photic stimulation or hyperventilation.

Many tonic-clonic seizures are the result of an autosomal dominant trait expressed between the ages of 5 and 30 years. In many of these cases, patients have a history of childhood absences.

Sleep deprivation can precipitate these seizures. For example, medical house officers, after having been on duty all night, have had tonic-clonic seizures early the following morning. In addition, stage I and stage II NREM sleep precipitate tonic-clonic seizures in epileptic patients (Chapter 17). Many epileptic patients have these seizures predominantly or exclusively while asleep, and some have seizures almost only on awakening.

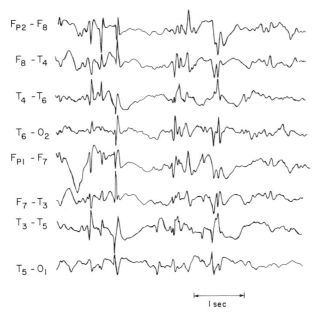

$F_{P2} - F_8$

$F_8 - T_4$

$T_4 - T_6$

$T_6 - O_2$

$F_{P1} - F_7$

$F_7 - T_3$

$T_3 - T_5$

$T_5 - O_1$

|← 1 sec →|

Fig. 10-14. During a tonic-clonic seizure, the EEG would ideally show paroxysms of spikes, polyspikes, and occasional slow waves in all channels; however, unless a muscle relaxant is administered, muscle artifact obscures this pattern. The interictal background EEG activity usually contains multiple bursts of generalized spikes. In contrast to occasional temporal lobe spikes, this is a pattern upon which a diagnosis of epilepsy can be verified.

Alcohol in itself does not precipitate seizures. However, binge drinkers often develop hypoglycemia or sleep deprivation that, in turn, triggers seizures. More important, abrupt withdrawal from chronic, excessive alcohol consumption produces "alcohol-withdrawal seizures," which usually occur the day after alcohol abstinence. Although the clinical and EEG manifestations of these seizures are similar to those in genetically determined seizures, the interictal EEG is normal.

Similarly, abrupt withdrawal from medicines with sedative effects, including diazepam (Valium), long- or especially short-acting barbiturates, and anticonvulsants, can precipitate seizures. In contrast to alcohol-withdrawal seizures, drug-withdrawal seizures do not develop until several days after abstinence, and once they begin, they often evolve into status epilepticus. Curiously, as mentioned previously, alcohol or drug withdrawal does not precipitate partial seizures.

Phenothiazines and other neuroleptics can also precipitate seizures, usually of the tonic-clonic variety, even in a person who has never had one previously. Tricyclic and tetracyclic antidepressants, monoamine oxidase inhibitors, and lithium can also precipitate seizures. In contrast, doxepin reportedly reduces the incidence of seizures.

A small but noteworthy group of children and some adults have absences or tonic-clonic seizures in response to particular sensory stimulation. In this condition, called *reflex epilepsy,* flickering lights, television pictures that have lost their vertical stability, video games, or certain patterns of letters, words, or figures can trigger seizures in susceptible persons. Even certain sounds, such as musical passages, may also cause seizures.

Treatment of tonic-clonic seizures usually includes the use of the anticonvulsants valproic acid, phenytoin, carbamazepine, and phenobarbital. One or more of them are usually given for at least 6 months, except in cases of a single seizure or ones where a precipitating factor, such as sleep deprivation or abrupt alcohol or drug withdrawal can be identified and avoided.

Any coexisting psychiatric illness must also be treated. Improvement in psychiatric illness, especially depression, is often associated with improvement in epilepsy. For patients with no history of seizures, prophylactic use of anticonvulsants is not indicated. For epileptic patients requiring phenothiazines, other neuroleptics, or antidepressants, the anticonvulsant dosage should be raised only if a seizure occurs. If a nonepileptic patient receiving a neuroleptic develops a seizure, a cerebral lesion, such as a brain tumor, must be excluded before attributing the seizure to the medication.

DISORDERS THAT MIMIC SEIZURES

Pseudoseizures

Episodes mimicking seizures are called hysteric seizures or pseudoseizures. They are more prevalent in women, children, and adolescents. Patients with pseudoseizures, like those with psychogenic hemiparesis and other psychogenic deficits, have a high incidence of character disorders, affective illness, and major psychopathology (Chapter 3).

Pseudoseizures often occur together with seizures in the same patients. In some patients, pseudoseizures are responsible for apparently intractable seizures. Therefore, although patients may seem to have only pseudoseizures, a finding of pseudoseizures should prompt an investigation for seizures, as well as psychiatric evaluation.

Unlike tonic-clonic seizures, pseudoseizures mimicking generalized seizures usually begin slowly, gradually developing flailing, alternating limb movements that may or may not be accompanied by trunk and pelvic movements. As fatigue ensues, the movements decline in intensity and regularity. Notably, they usually have no tonic phase and there is neither incontinence, tongue-biting, nor other bodily injury. Despite the apparent generalized nature of the pseudoseizure, consciousness is preserved and subsequent confusion and retrograde amnesia are absent.

If an EEG were obtained during a pseudoseizure and muscle artifact were eliminated, it would be normal. One performed afterwards, which is more feasible, would not show postictal depression. Also, the serum prolactin concentration is elevated after a seizure but not after a pseudoseizure.

Pseudoseizures mimicking partial seizures are more subtle and difficult to diagnose. Patients who mimic partial elementary seizures may have unilateral limb movement; visual aberrations or other subjective phenomena; or nonspecific sensations, such as dizziness or epigastric sensations. Although these might be symptoms of seizures, successive pseudoseizures in individual patients have more varying manifestations than genuine partial seizures, last longer than the usual limit of several minutes, and are not accompanied by dulling of the sensorium. Also, very few patients can convincingly mimic automatisms or progression to a generalized seizure. Nevertheless, telemetry is sometimes required to make an accurate and reliable diagnosis.

Episodic Dyscontrol Syndrome

The episodic dyscontrol syndrome, which is roughly equivalent to "rage attacks," consists of violent outbursts for which the patient typically claims amnesia. In contrast to violent partial complex seizures, episodic dyscontrol outbursts are purposeful, aggressive, and accompanied by a highly charged affect. Violence is barbarically destructive and consists of screaming, punching, wrestling, and throwing glasses or bottles. Also, these attacks can be provoked by threats and various other external circumstances and especially by alcohol consumption.

Episodic dyscontrol attacks are commonplace in patients with diffuse cerebral damage, especially from congenital cerebral injury or head trauma. Thus, they are apt to occur in people with neurologic impediments, borderline intelligence, or seizures. Coexistence of episodic dyscontrol syndrome and seizures probably is responsible for some reports of aggression in epileptic patients. Suggested treatments for episodic dyscontrol syndrome, in addition to excluding alcoholic beverages, have included anticonvulsants. However, none have been consistently effective.

Cerebrovascular Disturbances

Transient ischemic attacks (TIAs) resemble partial seizures in that both may involve momentarily impaired consciousness and lateralized physical deficits (Chapter 11). However, TIAs usually have a slower onset, rarely cause loss of consciousness, and tend to begin only when the patient is standing upright. Also, they are not associated with the development of new mental or physical activity.

Patients with migraine headaches may have episodes of confusion and personality change followed by a tendency to sleep (Chapter 9). They also may have hemiparesis for several hours and abnormal EEGs. In fact, the incidence of seizures in migraine patients is greater than in the general population. Correct diagnosis, which is occasionally difficult, rests on the patient's history and response to medications.

More closely resembling a partial complex seizure is transient global amnesia, in which patients suffer several hours of disorientation, memory impairment, and EEG abnormalities (Chapter 11). This condition, which is probably caused by vascular insufficiency of the temporal lobes, may be diagnosed, although with some difficulty, by attention to clinical and EEG abnormalities.

Sleep Disorders

Some apparent seizure patients are actually having sleep attacks (narcolepsy), which may be associated with momentary loss of body tone (cataplexy) (Chapter 17). Unlike seizures, however, narcolepsy has no aura, motor activity, incontinence, or postictal symptoms. Moreover, during narcolepsy, instead of the EEG showing paroxysmal activity, it displays normal rapid eye movement (REM) activity.

Metabolic Aberrations

Finally, although many medicines produce transient mental alterations resembling those found in seizures, they practically never induce movements or stereotyped thoughts. As a general rule, a first step should be to eliminate all unnecessary medications for patients with episodic mental aberrations.

Of the other metabolic disturbances, hypoglycemia is probably the most important. It may result not only from injected insulin, but from excessive alcohol consumption and supposedly from prediabetic states. However, the severity and frequency of symptomatic hypoglycemia is probably overestimated.

REFERENCES

Abramowicz M (ed) Drugs for epilepsy. The Medical Letter 25:81, 1983

Ballenger CE, King DW, Gallagher BB: Partial complex status epilepticus. Neurology 33:1545, 1983

Bear DM, Fedio P: Quantitative analysis of interictal behavior in temporal lobe epilepsy. Arch Neurol 34:454, 1977

Camfield PR, Gates R, Ronen G, et al: Comparison of cognitive ability, personality profile, and school success in epileptic children with pure right versus left temporal lobe EEG foci. Ann Neurol 15:122, 1984

Delgado-Escueta AV, Bacsal FE, Treiman DM: Complex partial seizures on closed-circuit television and EEG: A study of 691 attacks in 79 patients. Ann Neurol 11:292, 1982

Delgado-Escueta AV, Mattson RH, King L, et al: The nature of aggression during epileptic seizures. N Engl J Med 305:711, 1981

Elliot FA: The episodic dyscontrol syndrome and aggression. Neurol Clin 2:113, 1984

Engel J, Kuhl DE, Phelps ME: Local cerebral metabolism during partial seizures. Neurology 33:400, 1983

Falconer MA: Reversibility by temporal lobe resection of the behavioral abnormalities of temporal lobe epilepsy. N Engl J Med 289:451, 1973

Finlayson RE, Lucas AR: Pseudoepileptic seizures in children and adolescents. Mayo Clin Proc 54:83, 1979

Flor-Henry P: Psychosis and temporal lobe epilepsy. Epilepsia 10:363, 1969

Geoffroy G, Lassonde M, Delisle F, et al: Corpus callosotomy for control of intractable epilepsy in children. Neurology 33:891, 1983

Glista GG, Frank HG, Tracy FW: Video games and seizures. Arch Neurol 40:588, 1983

Guerrant J, Anderson WW, Fischer A, et al: Personality in Epilepsy. Springfield, Ill, Charles C Thomas, 1962

Hawton K, Fagg J, Marsack P: Association between epilepsy and attempted suicide. J Neurol Neurosurg Psychiatry 43:168, 1980

Jabbari B, Bryan GE, Marsh EE, et al: Incidence of seizures with tricyclic and tetracyclic antidepressants. Arch Neurol 42:480, 1985

Lewis DO, Pincus JH, Shanok, SS, et al: Psychomotor epilepsy and violence in a group of incarcerated adolescent boys. Am J Psychiatry 139:882, 1982

Loiseau P, Pestre M, Dartigues JF: Long-term prognosis in two forms of childhood epilepsy: Typical absence seizures and epilepsy with rolandic (centrotemporal) EEG foci. Ann Neurol 13:642, 1983

Matthews WS, Barabas G: Suicide and epilepsy. Psychosomatics 22:515, 1981

Mayeux R, Brandt J, Rosen J, et al: Interictal memory and language impairment in temporal lobe epilepsy. Neurology 30:120, 1980

Mungas D: Interictal behavior abnormality in temporal lobe epilepsy: A specific syndrome or nonspecific psychopathology? Arch Gen Psychiatry 39:108, 1982

Pincus JH: Can violence be a manifestation of epilepsy? Neurology 30:304, 1980

Ramani V, Gumnit RJ: Intensive monitoring of interictal psychosis in epilepsy. Ann Neurol 11:613, 1982

Robertson MM, Trimble MR: Depressive illness in patients with epilepsy. Epilepsia 24:109, 1983

Rodin E, Schmaltz S: The Bear-Fedio personality inventory and temporal lobe epilepsy. Neurology 34:591, 1984

Sherwin I, Peron-Magnan P, Bancaud J, et al: Prevalence of psychosis in epilepsy as a function of the laterality of the epileptogenic lesion. Arch Neurol 39:621, 1982

Slater E, Beard AW: The schizophrenic-like psychosis of epilepsy. Br J Psychiatry 95:109, 1963

Solomon GE, Kutt H, Plum F: Clinical Management of Seizures, 2nd ed. Philadelphia, W.B. Saunders, 1983

Spencer SS, Spencer DD, Williamson PD, et al: Sexual automatisms in complex partial seizures. Neurology 33:527, 1983

Stewart RS, Lovitt R, Steward RM: Are hysterical seizures more than hysteria? A research diagnostic criteria, DSM-III, and psychometric analysis. Am J Psychiatry 139:926, 1982

Stevens JR: Psychosis and epilepsy. Ann Neurol 14:347, 1983

Stevens JR, Hermann BP: Temporal lobe epilepsy, psychopathology, and violence: The state of the evidence. Neurology 31:1127, 1981

Staudemire A, Nelson A, Haupt JL: Interictal schizophrenia-like psychoses in temporal lobe epilepsy. Psychosomatics 24:331, 1983

Stromgren LS, Juul-Jensen P: EEG in unilateral and bilateral electroconvulsive therapy. Acta Psychiatr Scand 51:340, 1975

Theodore WH, Porter RJ, Penry JK: Complex partial seizures: Clinical characteristics and differential diagnosis. Neurology 33:1115, 1983

Whitman S, Coleman TE, Patmon C, et al: Epilepsy in prison: Elevated prevalence and no relationship to violence. Neurology 34:775, 1984

QUESTIONS

1–4. Match the EEG with the interpretation (see pages 198–199).

1. Fig. EEG-A
2. Fig. EEG-B
3. Fig. EEG-C
4. Fig. EEG-D

   a. Spike and polyspike and wave
   b. 3-Hz spike and wave
   c. Normal
   d. Temporal spike focus

5–8. Match the EEG with the associated seizures.

5. Interictal temporal lobe spikes
6. Generalized 3-Hz spike and wave
7. Generalized spike and polyspike and wave
8. Occipital spike and wave

   a. Tonic-clonic (grand mal)
   b. Partial elementary
   c. Partial complex
   d. Absence (petit mal)

9–16. Match the EEG pattern with its most likely cause.

9. Delta activity, phase reversal over left occiput
10. Bifrontal beta activity
11. Alpha activity

   a. Normal relaxation
   b. Hepatic encephalopathy
   c. Use of sedatives or hypnotics
   d. Brain tumor

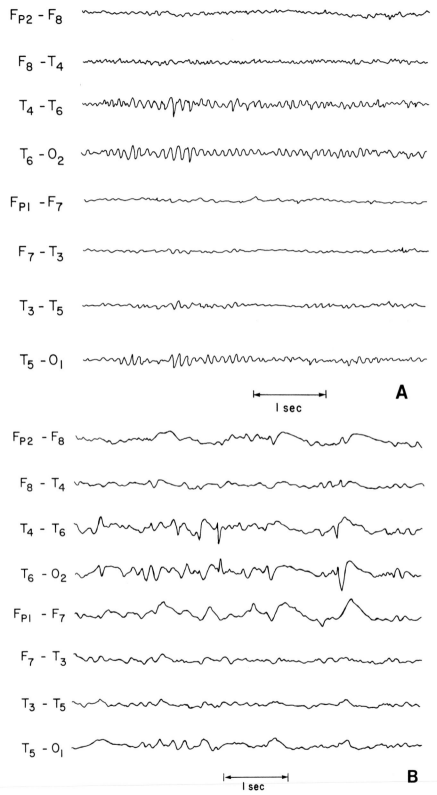

Fig. 10-EEG-A and **Fig. 10-EEG-B** (see Questions 1–4).

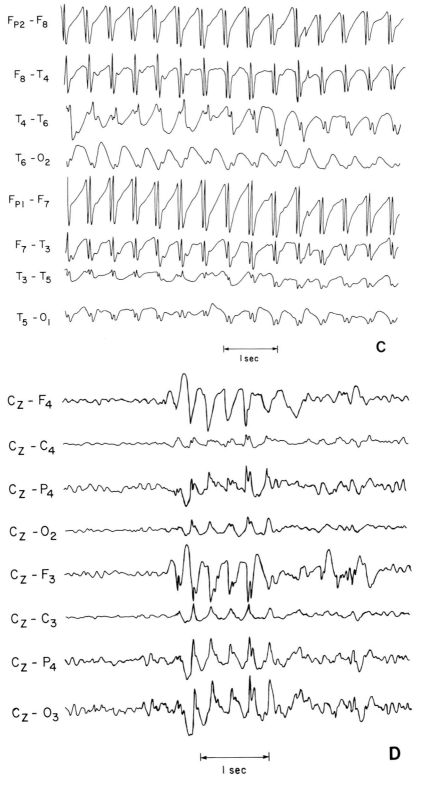

Fig. 10-EEG-C and **Fig. 10-EEG-D** (see Questions 1–4).

199

12. Triphasic waves   e.   Cerebral death
13. Rapid extraocular movement artifact   f.   REM sleep; dreaming
14. Periodic complexes   g.   Major tranquilizers
15. Generalized delta activity   h.   Psychoses
16. Electrocerebral silence   i.   Creutzfeldt-Jakob disease

17. In which conditions will an EEG be useful in making a specific diagnosis?
    a. Cerebral tumor   g. Hysteric seizures
    b. Hepatic encephalopathy   h. Manic-depressive illness
    c. Neurosis   i. Cerebellar tumor
    d. Herpes simplex encephalitis   j. SSPE.
    e. Cerebral abscess   k. Psychoses
    f. Creutzfeldt-Jakob disease   l. Status epilepticus

18–20. Match the evocative technique with the seizure(s) it might induce.

18. Hyperventilation   a.   Hysteric seizures
19. Photic stimulation   b.   Tonic-clonic (grand mal)
20. Sleep deprivation   c.   Absence (petit mal)
                                             d.   Partial complex

21–24. Identify the following statements as true or false.

21. Use of the EEG in the diagnosis of psychologic disturbances is complicated by drug-induced EEG changes.

22. Diazepam (Valium), meprobamate (Miltown), and barbiturates induce rapid (beta) EEG activity.

23. Tricyclic antidepressants and phenothiazines may induce nonfocal sharp wave EEG activity.

24. The major tranquilizers, antidepressants, and lithium may cause slowing of EEG background activity.

25. Which of the following seizure-induced symptoms or signs suggest that a cerebral lesion, such as a scar or tumor, may be the cause of the seizure?
    a. Clonic movements of the left hand only
    b. Absence
    c. Jacksonian march
    d. Uncinate seizure alone or before a partial complex seizure
    e. Postictal psychosis
    f. Psychomotor phenomena
    g. Induction following hyperventilation
    h. Thrashing movements of extremities with pelvic thrusts
    i. Incontinence
    j. Retrograde amnesia

26–33. Match the visual disturbance with the probable cause.

26. A red blotch of color in the left   a. Amaurosis fugax
    homonymous field followed by clonic   b. Partial complex seizure of temporal
    movements of the left arm and leg, then   lobe origin
    the entire body   c. Partial elementary seizure of
                                                  occipital lobe origin
27. Loss of central vision in both eyes   d. Petit mal seizure
    followed by throbbing, unilateral   e. Hysteria
    headache   f. Tension headache
                                              g. Classical migraine headache
28. Fortification scotomata   h. Delirium tremens

29. Visualization of the American flag,
    accompanied by hearing drum beats

30. Seeing and smelling garbage
31. A kaleidoscopic movement of bright lights in the right visual field
32. A "shade of gray" covering one eye for three minutes
33. Tremor, sweating, tachycardia, and seeing rodents

i. Partial elementary seizures of occipital origin with secondary generalization

34–43. The patient's age when partial (elementary or complex) seizures begin often suggests the cause. Match the cause with the age when it is likely to cause such a seizure.

34. Head injury
35. Congenital cerebral malformation
36. Arteriovenous malformation
37. Glioblastoma
38. Metastatic brain tumor
39. Sinusitis-induced cerebral abscess
40. Cerebrovascular accident
41. Conversion reaction
42. Mesial temporal sclerosis
43. Perinatal cerebral hypoxia

a. Childhood, e.g., three to eight years
b. Adolescence, e.g., 13–21 years
c. Middle age, e.g., 45–65 years

44–48. Match the seizure disorder with the drug(s) of choice and alternatives.

44. Tonic-clonic (grand mal)
45. Partial elementary motor
46. Absences (petit mal)
47. Partial seizure with secondary generalization
48. Complex partial

a. Phenytoin (Dilantin)
b. Carbamazepine (Tegretol)
c. Phenobarbital
d. Primidone (Mysoline)
e. Valproic acid (Depakene)
f. Ethosuximide (Zarontin)

49. A 30-year-old woman, who developed partial complex seizures with psychomotor symptomatology 3 years ago, has developed lethargy and confusion. Which causes of the current difficulties should be considered?
   a. Expansion of a temporal lobe tumor
   b. Development of a subdural hematoma from head trauma
   c. Partial complex status epilepticus
   d. Anticonvulsant intoxication
   e. Development of a systemic disorder, such as renal failure

50. Which of the following physical signs may indicate anticonvulsant intoxication?
   a. Hemiparesis
   b. Ataxia of gait
   c. Nystagmus
   d. Aphasia
   e. Dysarthria
   f. Lethargy or stupor
   g. Dysmetria on heel–shin testing
   h. Tremor on finger–nose testing
   i. Papilledema

51–53. Which anticonvulsant is associated with the particular adverse reaction(s)?

51. Phenytoin (Dilantin)
52. Carbamazepine (Tegretol)
53. Phenobarbital

a. Liver damage
b. Hirsutism
c. Cerebellar damage
d. Lethargy at therapeutic levels
e. Gum swelling

54. Narcolepsy is usually associated with which of the following disorders?
   a. Generalized seizures

     b. Manic-depressive illness
     c. Cataplexy
     d. Fugue states

55. A patient's head and eyes deviate to the left and the left arm extends immediately before a generalized tonic-clonic seizure develops. Where did the seizure originate?
     a. Cerebellum
     b. Right cerebral hemisphere
     c. Diencephalon
     d. Left cerebral hemisphere

56. What is the frequency with which a child's eyelids blink during an absence?
     a. 8–12/sec
     b. 3/sec
     c. Highly variable
     d. None of the above

57. Which of the following seizures may be followed by a postictal psychosis?
     a. Tonic-clonic (generalized)
     b. Absence (petit mal)
     c. Partial elementary
     d. Partial complex
     e. Partial complex with secondary generalization

58. Which seizure(s) does (do) *not* follow head trauma?
     a. Absence (petit mal)
     b. Partial complex, psychomotor variety
     c. Partial motor with Jacksonian march
     d. Tonic-clonic (generalized)
     e. Partial motor with secondary generalization

59. The interictal EEG may be of diagnostic importance in which of the following seizure disorders?
     a. Partial complex
     b. Partial elementary
     c. Tonic-clonic (generalized)
     d. Hysteric
     e. Absence (petit mal)

60. The EEG:
     a. May have abnormalities in 15 percent of clinically asymptomatic people.
     b. May be abnormal in psychologically disturbed people because of use of psychotropic medications.
     c. Usually has a background activity in the alpha (8–13 Hz) range.
     d. Will be specifically diagnostic in minimal brain dysfunction.
     e. Will be specifically diagnostic in Gilles de la Tourette's syndrome.

61. Partial complex seizures (e.g., psychomotor seizures), compared with absences (petit mal seizures), are:
     a. Longer in duration.
     b. More apt to begin in childhood.
     c. Likely to have an aura and postictal confusion.
     d. Accompanied by automatisms.
     e. Likely to disappear in young adult life.

ANSWERS

1. c	**15.** g	**29.** b
2. d	**16.** e	**30.** b
3. b	**17.** b, d, f, g, j, l	**31.** c
4. a	**18.** a, c	**32.** a
5. c	**19.** b, c	**33.** h
6. d	**20.** d	**34.** a, b, c
7. a	**21.** True	**35.** a
8. b	**22.** True	**36.** a, b
9. d	**23.** True	**37.** c
10. c	**24.** True	**38.** c
11. a	**25.** a, c, d, f	**39.** b
12. b	**26.** i	**40.** c
13. f	**27.** g	**41.** b
14. i	**28.** g	**42.** a, b

43. a

44. Drugs of choice a or b, alternatively c or e

45. Drugs of choice a or b, alternatively c

46. Drugs of choice e or f

47. Drugs of choice a or b, alternatively c

48. Drugs of choice a, b, and c or d

49. All such causes must be considered; however, in the vast majority of such cases, the cause is anticonvulsant intoxication (d)

50. b, c, e, f, g, h	**54.** c	**58.** a, d
51. b, c, e	**55.** b	**59.** a, b, c, d, e
52. a	**56.** b	**60.** a, b, c
53. d	**57.** a, d, e	**61.** a, c

11

Cerebrovascular Diseases

Cerebrovascular disease is so common that physicians might consider it in the differential diagnosis of most neurologic illnesses in adults. Unfortunately, many physicians have an unjustified pessimism toward patients with cerebrovascular disease and see them as stereotypes, epitomized by the aphorism, "A stroke is a stroke is a stroke."

Taking the opposite viewpoint, this chapter will review the recent developments in the diagnosis, prevention, and treatment of certain cerebrovascular disease while emphasizing their different physical and psychologic manifestations. This chapter will discuss only *transient ischemic attacks (TIAs)* and *cerebrovascular accidents (CVAs)* because these conditions are responsible for well over 95 percent of all cases of cerebrovascular disease, and they are the ones that virtually all physicians might encounter.

TRANSIENT ISCHEMIC ATTACKS (TIAs)

Transient ischemic attacks are brief interruptions in the blood supply to parts of the brain during which some neurologic function is temporarily lost. Full capacity is usually restored within 3 to 30 minutes, although rarely not until 12 hours. Most TIAs probably originate from platelet emboli that form within atherosclerotic extracranial arteries and then travel through the cerebral circulation. The importance of TIAs lies not only in the episodes of neurologic dysfunction, but also in their indicating underlying atherosclerotic cerebrovascular disease. Indeed, without treatment, about 25 percent of people with TIAs will develop a permanent neurologic deficit within one year.

Carotid Artery TIAs

The origin of most carotid artery TIAs is thought to be platelet emboli that originate in atherosclerotic plaques at the bifurcation of the common carotid artery.

Platelet emboli probably develop on the internal surface of narrowed (stenotic) and ulcerated plaques and travel upwards into the internal carotid artery.

Each internal carotid artery provides blood directly to the majority of the ipsilateral cerebral hemisphere and, by collateral circulation, to a portion of the contralateral hemisphere. Notably, the carotid artery also supplies the ipsilateral eye through its first branch, the ophthalmic artery (Fig. 11-1).

Therefore, TIAs of the carotid artery will often obscure vision in one eye for several minutes: People with this condition, *amaurosis fugax,* typically describe a "blanket of gray" coming down slowly in front of one eye (Table 11-1).

Symptoms of carotid artery TIAs from hemispheric ischemia are periods of (contralateral) hemiparesis, hemisensory loss, paresthesias, and hemianopsia. Of course, dominant hemisphere TIAs cause aphasia.

Under certain circumstances, confusion and personality changes may develop. When a patient with Alzheimer's disease, for example, has a carotid artery TIA, ischemia may convert a mild, compensated intellectual impairment into a marked confusional state. Likewise, when one carotid artery is markedly stenotic or occluded and the blood supply to both cerebral hemispheres is derived from the one other patent artery through the circle of Willis, ischemia of that artery will lead to generalized cerebral ischemia and mental impairment.

Several nonneurologic findings may indicate carotid artery atherosclerosis. Using a stethoscope, a physician might hear a murmur, or *bruit,* over the carotid artery bifurcation. Such a sound, suggesting an arterial stenosis or at least roughening, is important if it is heard over the artery from which TIAs are thought to originate.

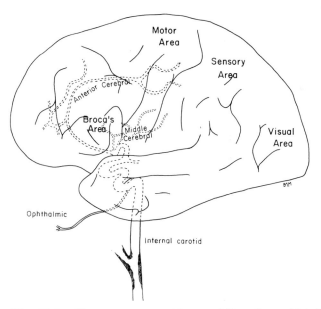

Fig. 11-1. The common carotid artery bifurcation, which is in the neck, forms the external and internal carotid arteries. Within the cranial cavity the internal carotid artery gives rise to the ophthalmic and then the anterior and middle cerebral arteries. Atheromatous plaques at the common carotid artery bifurcation are the source of most platelet emboli.

Table 11-1
Carotid Artery TIAs

Symptoms
   Ipsilateral amaurosis fugax
     Contralateral hemiparesis, hemianopsia, and/or hemisensory loss
     Aphasia
Associated findings
   Carotid bruit
   Retinal artery emboli
Noninvasive tests
   Ultrasonography
   Digital intravenous arteriography (DIVA)
Invasive tests
   Arteriography
Therapy
   Medical: platelet inhibitors, e.g., aspirin
   Surgical: carotid endarterectomy, extracranial-intracranial arterial
     bypass

Another indication is a retinal artery embolus (Hollenhorst plaque), which is supposedly atheromatous material from the ipsilateral carotid artery.

LABORATORY TESTS

In most cases where there is brief motor and sensory loss, the diagnosis of a carotid artery TIA may be made reliably on the basis of the clinical evaluation; however, several unrelated conditions might also cause transient paresthesias, motor or sensory loss, confusion, or even monocular visual loss. Commonly cited alternatives to TIAs are impaired cerebral blood flow from cardiac arrhythmias; a sensory seizure; postictal (Todd's) hemiparesis (Chapter 10); migraine attacks (Chapter 9); metabolic derangements, such as hypoglycemia; and psychogenic disturbances (Chapter 3).

Since TIAs are considered precursors of strokes or may be confused with other conditions, many neurologists recommend a series of tests to confirm the diagnosis and search for atherosclerotic lesions at the carotid bifurcation. A routine evaluation includes an electrocardiogram (ECG) and sometimes a 24-hour study of the cardiac rhythm (a Holter monitor). An EEG might be performed if there is a possibility that the patient is having seizures. A CT scan is almost always performed to exclude CVAs (see below) and cerebral mass lesions. On the other hand, lumbar punctures and skull x-ray films are not usually indicated.

Recently, several noninvasive techniques have been introduced to visualize carotid artery stenosis. For example, ultrasound imaging and digital intravenous arteriography (DIVA) are informative and carry little risk and no necessity for hospitalization. However, the definitive test remains cerebral arteriography. It requires injection of radiopaque dye through a catheter into the carotid arteries and thus exposes the patient to the risk of a cerebrovascular accident.

THERAPY

Nonsurgical (medical) therapy is effective and preferred in many patients. Neurologists generally prescribe aspirin (one to three tablets a day) because it is the most readily available platelet inhibitor. Newer medicines, e.g., sulfinpyrazone (Anturane) and dipyridamole (Persantine), which are also antiplatelet medications, may be indicated in people who are unable to tolerate the side-effects of aspirin.

The standard surgery indicated for many cases of carotid artery bifurcation stenosis is *carotid endarterectomy*, in which the vessel is briefly opened for the removal of an atheromatous plaque. Even in experienced hands, however, it entails at least a 2 percent risk of cerebrovascular accident, myocardial infarction, or death. For patients with stenosis of the intracranial portion of the carotid artery, in an experimental *extracranial-intracranial arterial bypass*, a surgeon anastomoses a scalp artery to a superficial cerebral artery through a small hole in the skull.

Basilar Artery TIAs

The two vertebral arteries join to form the basilar artery. This group of vessels, which is usually called the *vertebrobasilar system* or, more often, simply the *basilar artery*, supplies the brainstem, cerebellum, and the inferomedial portion of the temporal lobes (Fig. 11-2).

The mechanism of basilar artery TIAs is probably similar to that for carotid artery TIAs, except that atherosclerotic plaques that give rise to basilar artery TIAs are found at the origin of the vertebral arteries (in the chest) and at their junction (at the undersurface of the brain). Since these locations are inaccessible to surgeons, endarterectomy cannot be performed.

Symptoms and signs of basilar artery TIAs are distinctly different from those of carotid artery TIAs (Table 11-2). Patients with basilar artery TIAs typically have vertigo that might be accompanied by nausea and tinnitus. Sometimes patients will have tingling around the mouth (circumoral paresthesias), dysarthria, nystagmus, or ataxia—all because of ischemia of the brainstem. On rare occasions, when all flow

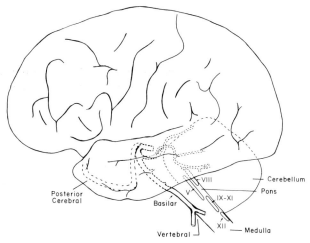

Fig. 11-2. The two vertebral arteries join to form the basilar artery. This vertebrobasilar complex supplies the brainstem, cerebellum, and the inferomedial portions of the temporal lobes. Atheromatous plaques form at the junction of the vertebral arteries.

Table 11-2

Vertebrobasilar Artery TIAs

Symptoms
    Vertigo, vomiting, tinnitus
    Circumoral paresthesias
    Dysarthria, dysphagia
    Transient global amnesia
    Drop attacks
Associated findings
    Nystagmus
    Ataxia
Noninvasive tests
    Digital intravenous arteriography (DIVA)
Invasive tests
    Arteriography
Therapy
    Medical: aspirin
    Surgical: none

through the basilar artery is interrupted and the entire brainstem becomes ischemic, a patient will have a *drop attack,* which is a brief loss of consciousness and body tone.

During a basilar artery TIA, patients are usually incapacitated because of the vertigo. Vertigo is such an important symptom that it should not be confused with other terms. It is the sensation of either revolving in space or feeling one's surroundings revolve. No substitutes should be accepted by the thoughtful physician. "Dizziness," which is frequently used, is without value because it may mean lightheadedness, giddiness, anxiety, confusion, or imbalance, as well as true vertigo.

LABORATORY TESTS

The noninvasive procedures, ultrasonography and DIVA, are not as applicable to the vertebrobasilar system as to the carotid system. While arteriography would demonstrate stenotic areas, this procedure is not performed because vertebrobasilar stenoses are not surgically accessible.

THERAPY

Medical therapy for basilar artery TIAs follows the same guidelines as that for carotid artery disease. Intracranial-extracranial arterial bypass procedures are experimental.

Transient Global Amnesia

A noteworthy but rare phenomenon associated with basilar artery TIAs is *transient global amnesia.* This condition, which sometimes occurs during sexual intercourse or other exertion in older people, probably results from ischemia of the posterior cerebral arteries. These vessels are terminal branches of the basilar artery and supply the temporal lobes (Fig. 11-2). Since the temporal lobes contain portions of the limbic system, ischemic attacks result in temporary memory impairment and personality change.

While in a state of transient global amnesia, a patient will have disorientation, amnesia, and apathy. Transient global amnesia mimics partial complex seizures, migraine attacks, metabolic derangements, and various psychologic aberrations. An EEG during an attack would be helpful in making a diagnosis of transient global amnesia.

CEREBROVASCULAR ACCIDENTS (CVAs)

In contrast to the brief neurologic deficits in TIAs, cerebrovascular accidents (CVAs), or "strokes," cause permanent physical and psychologic deficits.* In CVAs, the cerebral blood supply is irreversibly interrupted because of arterial thromboses, emboli, or hemorrhages. Portions of the brain are permanently damaged.

Risk factors for CVAs have been elucidated. The incidence of CVAs rises in almost exponential fashion after the age of 65 years, although about 20 percent of CVA victims are under the age of 65 years. An even greater risk factor than age, and one that is avoidable, is hypertension. Whether it is systolic, diastolic, or systolic-diastolic, hypertension leads to CVAs in middle-aged as well as older adults. Also, it is probably the cause of *multi-infarct dementia* (see below). Antihypertensive medications reduce the incidence of CVAs and other complications of hypertension; however, these medications themselves may cause some problems (see below).

Atherosclerosis, another risk factor, is related to age and hypertension. Even allowing for those factors, it causes myocardial infarctions, peripheral vascular disease, and TIAs, as well as CVAs. In contrast, cholesterol-rich diets, lack of exercise, and obesity, allowing for their effect on hypertension, increase the risk of CVAs only slightly.

Cardiac valvular disease, myocardial infarctions, atrial fibrillation, and probably mitral valve prolapse are risk factors because in each of these conditions, thromboses tend to form on the endocardial surface and embolize to the brain or elsewhere. Finally, oral contraceptives have been implicated as a risk factor, but they pose much less of a threat than these other factors. Their adverse influence may be confined to women who smoke or have migraine headaches. Curiously, some risk factors for coronary artery disease, such as smoking, obesity, diabetes, and increased lipids, carry little if any risk for CVAs.

Thromboses and Emboli

In thrombotic or embolic CVAs, the area of the brain that the artery supplies becomes *infarcted* and the surrounding region becomes *edematous*. Some clinical recovery seems to occur because the edema resolves; however, the infarction itself is a permanent scar which can be epileptogenic (Chapter 10).

The majority of CVAs are caused by either a thrombosis that propagates within an atherosclerotic cerebral artery or an embolus that originates within a carotid artery, i.e., an "arterial-arterial embolus." Other causes of CVAs are cardiac emboli (especially with atrial fibrillation), sickle cell disease, drug abuse, vasculitis, and blood

---

*Patients with CVAs may receive assistance from the Stroke Clubs of America, 805 12th Street, Galveston, Texas, 77550.

dyscrasias. In short, the causes of CVAs are abnormalities of the cerebral vessels, heart, or blood.

Thrombotic CVAs strike rapidly and painlessly. A disproportionate number occur suddenly during sleep, although many develop in a stuttering fashion over several days. The worst deficit in cerebral infarction occurs during the third to tenth days, when edema is most severe.

Since each of the major cerebral arteries supplies a particular area of the brain, a characteristic neurologic deficit is associated with each artery (Table 11-3). The *middle* cerebral artery infarction (Fig. 20-8), which is the most common, is associated with contralateral hemiparesis, hemisensory loss, homonymous hemianopsia and, with dominate hemisphere lesions, aphasia. Hemi-inattention and related neuropsychologic deficits may be present when the lesion is in the nondominant hemisphere. With an *anterior* cerebral artery infarction, the contralateral leg will be paretic, but if both anterior cerebral arteries are infarcted, the patient may also have pseudobulbar palsy and mental changes from bifrontal lobe damage. With a *posterior* cerebral artery infarction, contralateral homonymous hemianopsia will be detected.

Infarctions in the distribution of the basilar artery cause brainstem or cerebellar injuries. Sometimes a single, small discrete area is injured, resulting in paresis of one cranial nerve and the contralateral side of the body (Chapter 4) or in the MLF syndrome (Chapters 12 and 15). In contrast to cerebral hemisphere infarctions, *small* brainstem infarctions are unaccompanied by impairment of language or intellectual function. *Large* brainstem infarctions usually cause coma.

If desirable, for academic reasons perhaps, precise localization of brainstem infarctions is sometimes possible. With lesions of the midbrain, the ipsilateral oculomotor nerve and contralateral side of the body will typically be paretic (see Fig. 4-8). With pontine lesions, the ipsilateral abducens nerve and contralateral side of the body may be paretic (see Fig. 4-10). Finally, with lateral medullary infarctions (Wallenberg's syndrome), there is ipsilateral limb ataxia, palatal paresis, Horner's syndrome, and alternating hypalgesia (see Fig. 2-10).

Table 11-3

Cerebrovascular Accidents (CVAs) Manifestations

Carotid artery
Anterior cerebral
Contralateral lower extremity paresis
Middle cerebral
Contralateral hemiparesis, hemianopsia, and hemisensory loss
Aphasia
Hemi-inattention
Posterior cerebral
Contralateral homonymous hemianopsia
Vertebrobasilar system
Basilar artery
Total occlusion: coma or locked-in syndrome
Occlusion of branch: cranial nerve palsy with contralateral hemiparesis, internuclear ophthalmoplegia
Vertebral artery
Lateral medullary (Wallenberg's) syndrome

Hemorrhages

Hemorrhagic cerebrovascular disease, the most ominous condition, occurs when blood from a ruptured cerebral artery sprays a jet of blood directly into the brain. Hematomas often develop in the cerebral hemisphere, pons, or cerebellum. Brain damage is usually extensive and often fatal.

While thromboses begin in a slow or intermittent fashion and are painless, most hemorrhages are abrupt in onset and accompanied by headaches, nausea, and vomiting. In many cases, patients quickly lapse into stupor with profound neurologic deficits.

Most patients cannot be helped. However, two forms of hemorrhage should be identified because surgical remedies are available for these conditions. Patients with *cerebellar hemorrhages* have an occipital headache, gait ataxia, dysarthria, and lethargy. Evacuation of a cerebellar hematoma is feasible and will be lifesaving.

Subarachnoid hemorrhages are usually the result of rupture of arterial aneurysms (balloon-like dilations). Patients typically have sudden onset of an extraordinarily severe headache and nuchal rigidity; however, they may have no neurologic deficits. Neurosurgeons can occlude most ruptured aneurysms.

The symptoms of a subarachnoid hemorrhage are occasionally confused with those of a migraine headache. In subarachnoid hemorrhage, the headache is unique and severely painful. Examination will reveal nuchal rigidity. A CT scan of the head will usually reveal blood at the base of the brain. Lumbar puncture will yield bloody CSF in cases of recent onset and xanthochromic CSF in those more than several days old (Chapter 20).

CEREBROVASCULAR ACCIDENTS AND PSYCHOLOGIC ABNORMALITIES

Although atherosclerosis causes TIAs and CVAs, atherosclerosis itself does not cause intellectual, emotional, or other psychologic abnormalities. In other words, "hardening of the arteries" does not cause dementia.

Once a CVA has developed, however, psychologic abnormalities can be a prominent feature. Specific psychologic abnormalities caused by CVAs are associated with certain physical deficits. For example, dominant hemisphere CVAs that cause aphasia or Gerstmann's syndrome are associated with right-sided hemiparesis, reflex abnormalities, and homonymous hemianopsia. Likewise, nondominant parietal lobe CVAs that cause hemi-inattention, anosognosia, and constructional apraxia are associated with left-sided sensory and visual abnormalities (Chapter 8).

Deficits can, in a sense, be additive. Dementia has been found when many small CVAs have damaged a total quantity of brain, estimated to be 50 to 150 cc, irrespective of the location of the injuries. In such cases, physical impairments, such as hemiparesis, are prominent and patients are disabled if not bedridden. Also, when hemiparesis or other unilateral deficits are present in demented patients, the cause of the dementia is more likely to be CVAs than Alzheimer's disease.

Multi-infarct dementia accounts for 8 to 40 percent of all cases of dementia. This condition is similar to *etat lacunaire* in which hypertensive cerebrovascular disease causes multiple small cerebral scars (lacunes) measuring 0.5 to 1.5 cm in diameter. With successive infarctions, patients have a stepwise decrease in intellectual function and progressive physical impairments, such as paresis, clumsiness, rigidity, and reflex abnormalities. They often have partial recovery after each "mini-infarction."

Multi-infarct dementia differs from Alzheimer's disease in that it has an abrupt onset, stepwise worsening with some partial remissions, and relatively prominent physical signs. The cognitive and other psychologic changes in multi-infarct dementia are so similar to those found in Alzheimer's disease that no easily administered, generally accepted neuropsychologic test can distinguish reliably between the two. Early in both conditions, the EEG is either normal or contains only some nonspecific slowing. Likewise, although the CT scan shows small areas of infarction in multi-infarct dementia, in both conditions the CT scan usually, but not necessarily, shows atrophy.

Cerebrovascular accidents of the cerebral hemisphere may cause psychomotor and other seizures because about 5 percent of cerebral infarctions become irritative scars. Therefore, in patients with cerebrovascular disease, brief mental aberrations may result from TIAs, transient global amnesia, cardiac arrhythmias, or partial complex seizures.

Another important and probably often overlooked psychologic manifestation of a CVA is depression. Above and beyond despair attributable to physical disabilities, many patients with CVAs have inordinate apathy, depressed mood, sleep disturbance, and appetite loss. In studies of these patients, the clinical diagnosis of depression has been confirmed by dexamethasone suppression test abnormalities. Thus, antidepressant therapy has been recommended for CVA patients who appear depressed.

On the other hand, some psychologic changes may be iatrogenic. Many antihypertension medications, such as Aldomet (methyldopa) and Inderal (propranolol), impair mental function by reducing cerebral blood flow, acting as false neurotransmitters, or otherwise creating neuronal aberrations. Likewise, diuretics can cause confusion and seizures if they deplete the serum sodium concentration below 120–125 mEq/mL. Also, when patients who are receiving these medications stand up, they suddenly receive less cerebral blood flow and therefore tend to feel lightheaded, vertiginous, and confused.

Locked-In Syndrome

In contrast to patients having predominantly psychologic impairment, patients with the *locked-in syndrome* are mute, quadriplegic, and apparently unable to respond; however, careful evaluation will reveal that not only are they alert and can move their eyes and eyelids, but their mental faculties are preserved. Their EEG may even be normal. This condition is the result of an infarction of the lower brainstem. Patients are mute because of bulbar palsy and quadriplegic because of bilateral corticospinal tract interruption. The cerebral cortex and upper brainstem remain intact. At least one patient with the syndrome responded to questions using eyelid blinks in Morse code. Patients with the locked-in syndrome can be confused with those in coma, in a vegetative state, or with profound dementia. If mute CVA victims can blink their eyes meaningfully, physicians should test their ability to see, hear, and then calculate. Further exploration may uncover a case in which an intact mind has been neglected.

Laboratory Tests in CVAs

In most cases the diagnosis of a CVA is made on the basis of the clinical evaluation and confirmed with CT (Chapter 20). Alternative diagnoses are brain tumor, abscess, subdural hematoma, and, rarely, systemic illness with neurologic complications, such as vasculitis (Chapter 19).

A CT scan will simultaneously indicate the existence and location of almost all CVAs, except those that are fresh and small. Subdural hematomas and the other structural lesions can also be excluded. Compared with CT, skull x-ray films are superfluous. An EEG is not helpful because it cannot reliably indicate the location or cause of most lesions.

Cerebral arteriography is done in selected cases after CT. It is mostly used for diagnosing carotid stenosis, cerebral aneurysms, and vascular malformations.

Examination of the CSF via a lumbar puncture is used to diagnose a subarachnoid hemorrhage when CT is unavailable or equivocal. It is also indicated when meningitis or encephalitis is suspected. However, it is not usually performed in CVAs and, except under special circumstances, it should not be performed if an intracranial mass lesion is present (see Transtentorial Herniation, Chapter 19).

Therapy of CVAs

During the initial phase of a CVA, careful attention must be paid to maintaining a patent airway and supporting vital bodily functions. Fluids should be given in liberal amounts and salts must be repleted in order to ensure adequate cerebral perfusion. There is no proven benefit to use of steroids, anticoagulants, oxygen, or vasoactive medicines. If the patient is not alert or the gag reflex is diminished, all nutrition should be provided intravenously, medications should be given parenterally, and nasopharyngeal secretions must be cleared by frequent suctioning.

Decubitus ulcers (bed sores) must be prevented because, in addition to being unsightly and malodorous, they lead to potentially fatal sepsis. The physician must order air mattresses, sweat-absorbent bed surfaces (e.g., artificial sheepskins), and foam rubber elbow and heel cushions. Nurses should reposition the patient every two hours. Since urinary incontinence adds to the likelihood of developing a bed sore, and also makes patients cold and wet and creates repugnant odors, indwelling or condom catheters should be used.

The patient's bed should be placed against the wall so that all visitors and staff must approach the patient from the side without perceptual impairment. For example, after suffering a left hemiparesis and a left homonymous hemianopsia, the patient should be placed with his or her left side against the wall so that people approach from the right, and important objects, e.g., call-buttons, television, clock, and pictures, can be seen and grasped.

The family should help by orienting the patient and bringing a luminous dial clock, a calendar, and a family picture. They should help reposition the patient and passively move paretic limbs to avoid contractures. The family might locate appropriate rehabilitation facilities.

The majority of physical and psychologic recoveries occurs spontaneously. Hemi-inattention and anosognosia resolve over a period of 1 to 3 weeks. Aphasias usually improve to almost their fullest extent in 3 to 6 weeks. Speech therapy will help with dysarthria and offer patients encouragement, but a scientific benefit or favorable cost-effectiveness ratio has not been established. "Cognitive and perceptual skill training" for impaired mentation, sensory impairment, and visual loss has not yet been fully evaluated.

Traditional physical therapy will maintain muscle tone, forestall bedsores, and prevent contractures. Therapy will usually help patients with simple hemiparesis to regain their ability to walk, circumvent some impediments, and avoid maladaptive but expeditious compensations.

Various psychologic aberrations may require medication. In particular, depression can be treated with antidepressants. Likewise, agitation, overwhelming anxiety, and hallucinations should be treated with neuroleptics. Control of these aberrations will orient the patient to the deficits, restraints, and therapies. When a patient's sleeping schedule is disrupted, mild hypnotics are necessary; however, phenobarbital and other barbiturates should be avoided because they tend to create agitation in brain injured patients, i.e., a paradoxical reaction.

SUMMARY

Signs of cerebrovascular disease can usually be attributed to TIAs or CVAs of either the carotid or vertebrobasilar (basilar) artery circulation. Carotid artery TIAs, which cause amaurosis fugax and cerebral dysfunction, often result from platelet emboli that originate at atherosclerotic plaques of the carotid artery bifurcation. Standard treatment, which depends upon the clinical situation, is either carotid endarterectomy or an antiplatelet agent, usually aspirin. Basilar TIAs, which usually cause vertigo, occasionally cause transient global amnesia. They are not amenable to surgery, but are also treated with aspirin.

Cerebrovascular accidents in the carotid circulation produce contralateral physical deficits, and depending upon which hemisphere is injured, specific psychologic disturbances. Such CVA patients have a tendency to have seizures and sometimes clinically significant depression.

Cerebrovascular accidents of the brainstem produce interesting combinations of cranial nerve palsies and motor dysfunction but usually not psychologic impairments. In particular, patients with the locked-in syndrome have devastating paresis but normal mental faculties.

On the other hand, multiple small cerebral infarctions lead to dementia. This multi-infarct dementia is similar to Alzheimer's dementia except that its onset is abrupt, its course intermittently progressive, and examination reveals more prominent motor and reflex abnormalities.

REFERENCES

Bresnihan G: CNS lupus. Clin Rheum Dis 8:183, 1982

Carter LT, Howard BE, O'Neil WA: Effectiveness of cognitive skill remediation in stroke patients. Am J Occup Ther 37:320, 1983

Finklestein S, Benowitz LI, Baldessarini RJ, et al: Mood, vegetative disturbance, and dexamethasone suppression test after stroke. Ann Neurol 12:463, 1982

Goodstein RK: Overview: Cerebrovascular accident and the hospitalized elderly—A multidimensional clinical problem. Am J Psychiatry 140:141, 1983

Hachinski V: Multi-infarct dementia. Neurol Clin 1:27, 1983

Hale G: The Source Book for the Disabled. Philadelphia, The Saunders Press, 1979

Keith L: A synthesis of studies on stroke rehabilitation. J Chron Dis 35:133, 1982

Perry J: Rehabilitation of the neurologically disabled patient: Principles, practice, and scientific basis. J Neurosurg 58:799, 1983

Robinson RG, Kubos KL, Starr LB, et al: Mood disorders in stroke patients. Brain 107:81, 1984

Ross ED, Rush AJ: Diagnosis and neuroanatomical correlates of depression in brain-damaged patients. Arch J Psychiatry 38:1344, 1981

QUESTIONS

1–10. Match the neurologic deficit with the most likely artery of infarction.

[Deficit]	[Artery]
1. Hemiparesis with relative sparing of leg	a. Right posterior cerebral
	b. Left posterior cerebral
2. Lower extremity monoparesis	c. Anterior cerebral
3. Monocular blindness from optic nerve ischemia	d. Middle cerebral
	e. Right middle cerebral
4. Left homonymous hemianopsia	f. Left middle cerebral
5. Left palate paresis, left limb ataxia	g. Ophthalmic
	h. Vertebral or posterior inferior cerebellar
6. Right third cranial nerve palsy with left hemiparesis	i. Perforating branch of basilar
7. Right hemiparesis with aphasia	j. Anterior spinal
8. Quadriplegia with intact position and vibration sensation	k. Basilar
9. Left sixth and seventh cranial nerve palsy with right hemiparesis	
10. Coma, quadriparesis	

11–20. Match the type of transient neurologic deficit with the artery involved (a, b, both, or neither).

[Deficit]	[Artery]
11. Transient global amnesia	a. Carotid
12. Amaurosis fugax	b. Basilar
13. Paresthesias of right arm and aphasia	
14. Vertigo, nausea, nystagmus, and ataxia	
15. Drop attacks	
16. Dizziness, malaise, headache	
17. Diplopia	
18. Dysarthria	
19. Transient hemiparesis	
20. Transient right hemiparesis without aphasia	

21–30. A 74-year-old man has had a left-sided headache for five days, a nonfluent aphasia, right hemiparesis with hyperreflexia, a Babinski sign, and right homonymous hemianopsia. Which of the following should be considered as likely possibilities?

21. Cerebral hemorrhage
22. Subarachnoid hemorrhage
23. Brain tumor
24. Subdural hematoma
25. Basilar artery occlusion

26. Carotid artery occlusion
27. Brain abscess
28. Conversion hysteria
29. Cerebral embolus
30. Multiple sclerosis

31–36. A 65-year-old man sustains a cerebrovascular accident, after which he is alert but mute and unable to move his arms or legs. He has paresis of the palate, bilateral hyperreflexia, and Babinski signs. He responds to verbal and written questions by blinking his eyelids.

31. Does this man have a fluent, nonfluent, or global aphasia?

32. In his vision impaired?

33. Is there evidence of cerebral damage?

34. How would the EEG appear?

35. If the EEG were normal, what would this syndrome be called?

36. Where is the lesion?

37–41. A 64-year-old man, who had sustained a right cerebral infarction the previous year, is admitted with the sudden, painless onset of right hemiparesis and mutism. After surviving the new insult, he has aphasia and bilateral paresis. While his eyes are frequently open, he fails to respond to either voice or gesture.

37. Where is the probable site of the recent injury?

38. What is the probable cause?

39. Would the EEG be normal?

40. If he were not paralyzed, would he be able to write?

41. Would he have bulbar or pseudobulbar palsy?

42–52. A 20-year-old woman awakens from sleep and finds that she has a mild left hemiparesis. Which are the possible causes of her deficit?

42. Cerebral thrombosis associated with oral contraceptives?

43. Cerebral vasculitis from lupus, drug abuse, etc.?

44. Cerebral embolus from mitral stenosis?

45. Cerebral embolus from drug abuse?

46. Rupture of a cerebral arteriovenous malformation?

47. Cerebral embolus from an atrial myxoma?

48. Compression of the right carotid artery during a stuporous sleep?

49. Infarction from sickle cell disease?

50. A prolonged postictal (Todd's) paresis?

51. A transient paresis of hemiplegic migraine?

52. Multiple sclerosis?

53–56. A 20-year-old woman is brought to the emergency room by her family because she is suddenly unable to speak or move her right side. She looks directly forward but does not follow commands. On inspection of her fundi, her eyes constantly evert. She seems to respond to visual images in all fields. The right arm and leg are flaccid and immobile, although her face is symmetrical. Deep tendon reflexes are symmetrical and no pathological reflexes are elicited. She does not react to noxious stimuli on the right side of her face or body.

53. Where is the apparent lesion?

54. (a) What pathologic features usually found with such a lesion are not present in the patient? (b) What nonpathologic features are present?

55. What is the most likely origin?

56. What readily available laboratory tests would lend great support to the diagnosis?

57–61. A 70-year-old man has the sudden onset of an occipital headache, nausea, vomiting, and an inability to walk. He has no paresis, but a downward drift of the right arm, and symmetrically active deep tendon reflexes with normal plantar response. He has dysmetria on right finger–nose and heel–shin movements and ataxia of gait.

57. Where is the lesion?

58. Which side?

59. What is its origin?

60. Why is there a "drift" of the right arm?

61. What is the consequence of increased size of the lesion?

62–65. A 75-year-old man has moderate, unremitting left-sided headaches and development of right-sided hemiparesis with hyperreflexia and a Babinski sign. On admission, he does not have either aphasia or visual field loss. During the initial three days in the hospital, however, he develops stupor with a dilated, unreactive left pupil and bilateral Babinski signs.

62. Where is the lesion?

63. What are the possible causes?

64. Which would be the most appropriate diagnostic test?

65. What is the origin of the pupillary abnormality?

66–67. Found wandering about in a confused manner, a 45-year-old woman is brought to the emergency room. She is lethargic, inattentive, and confused but not aphasic. Her pupils are equal and reactive, and her fundi are normal. Extraocular movements are full. All her extremities move well. She has hyperactive deep tendon reflexes and bilateral Babinski signs.

66. Where is the lesion?

67. What is the most likely cause?

68. Which of the following varieties of CVAs most often appears as patients awaken in the morning?

    a. Cerebral hemorrhage

    b. Cerebral thrombosis

    c. Cerebral embolus

    d. Subarachnoid hemorrhage

69. Which of the varieties of CVAs described in question 68 most often develop during sexual intercourse?

70. Which of the following CVA risk factors is the most important and correctable?

    a. Advanced age   d. Cigarette smoking

    b. High cholesterol diet   e. Hypertension

    c. Obesity   f. Lack of exercise

71. Which of the following is the standard therapy for vertebrobasilar artery TIAs?

    a. Endarterectomy

    b. Surgical anastomosis

    c. Coumadin

    d. Aspirin

72. Which of the following is thought to be the most important cause of multi-infarct dementia?

    a. Carotid bifurcation atherosclerosis

    b. Cerebral emboli

    c. Generalized atherosclerosis

    d. Hypertension

73. Which of the following is the greatest difference between Alzheimer's disease and multi-infarct dementia?

      a.   Quality of dementia
      b.   CT findings
      c.   EEG findings
      d.   Clinical course

ANSWERS

1. d	**11.** b (Posterior cerebral arteries)
2. c	**12.** a (Ophthalmic arteries)
3. g	**13.** a
4. a or e	**14.** b
5. h	**15.** b
6. i	**16.** Neither
7. f	**17.** b
8. j	**18.** a or b
9. i	**19.** a or b
10. k	**20.** b

21. No. Cerebral hemorrhages usually are suddenly occurring catastrophic processes.

22. No. The headaches would be sudden and incapacitating. Nuchal rigidity would be present.

23. Possibly, but the course is somewhat too rapid.

24. Unlikely. While the headache and hemiparesis are consistent, the aphasia and hemianopsia are rare with masses outside of the brain substance (i.e., extra-axial lesions).

25. No.

26. Good choice. This is a typical story of progressive carotid stenosis.

27. Possibly, but brain abscesses are rare.

28. No. There are objective neurologic findings: asymmetrical deep tendon reflexes and a Babinski sign.

29. No. These occur suddenly, but the deficit itself is compatible.

30. No. The headache and limited extent of the lesion are incompatible.

31. No. There is no evidence of aphasia. He can understand spoken language and respond appropriately.

32. No. He can read written questions.

33. No. The palatal and other motor pareses may be the result of brainstem damage. Cortical processes seem to be intact.

34. The EEG might appear normal since cortical functions are intact.

35. The locked-in syndrome.

36. The lesion is at the base of the lower brainstem.

37. The new lesion is in the left (dominant) hemisphere.

38. The sudden, painless onset suggests a thrombotic or embolic CVA.

39. The EEG will be abnormal because of extensive cerebral damage.

40. No. Aphasic patients generally have difficulty in all modes of communication.

41. He would probably have pseudobulbar palsy because of bilateral cerebral infarctions.

42–49. All yes. CVAs in young people are the result of diseases of the heart, blood, or blood vessels.

50–52. All yes. These other processes, not strictly cerebrovascular, may mimic strokes.

53. A patient who seems to have global aphasia and a right hemiparesis would usually have a left hemisphere lesion.

54. (a) She does not have the usual paresis of the lower (right) face, asymmetrical deep tendon reflexes, Babinski signs, or a right homonymous hemianopsia. (b) Eversion of the eyes during inspection is always a voluntary act. Inability to perceive noxious stimuli is rare in cerebral lesions and a sharply demarcated sensory loss (splitting the midline) is not neurologic.

55. Hysteria, malingering, or other psychogenic disturbance.

56. A normal EEG and CT scan.

57. The lesion is located in the cerebellum.

58. The abnormal findings are referable to the *ipsilateral* cerebellar hemisphere, in this case the right.

59. In view of the patient's age and the sudden onset, a CVA is most likely. Since it is painful, a cerebellar hemorrhage must be considered primarily.

60. The right arm drifts downward probably *not* on the basis of a mild paresis (because strength is normal and no corticospinal tract findings were elicited), but because damage to the cerebellar system disturbs coordination.

61. If the hemorrhage were to expand, the brainstem would become compressed. That would result in coma and death.

62. In view of the left-sided headaches and contralateral hemiparesis, the lesion would be on the "left side" of the CNS. Since there is no language or visual disturbance, the physician cannot initially be certain that the deficit is referable to the cerebral hemisphere rather than the brainstem. The development of transtentorial herniation makes it clear, however, that in retrospect the lesion was in the left supratentorial (cerebral) compartment.

63. The rapid demise with transtentorial herniation suggests that a mass lesion continued to expand. An occlusion of the internal carotid artery with subsequent cerebral swelling and herniation is possible, but a subdural hematoma is more likely. Tumors, arteriovenous malformations, and abscesses are less common causes (Chapter 19).

64. The most appropriate diagnostic test would be a CT scan. Presumably, routine history, physical examination, and initial hematologic and chemistry tests would have been done on admission. By the time he "herniates," however, emergency measures must be instituted and those preliminary studies postponed.

65. The dilation and unreactivity of the left pupil is caused by compression of the third cranial nerve as the subdural hematoma squeezes the temporal lobe through the tentorial notch.

66. The woman has delirium. Since she has no lateralizing signs or indications of increased intracranial pressure, one cannot say that she has a "lesion."

67. Causes of diffuse neurologic dysfunction are metabolic alterations (uremia, hypoglycemia), postictal confusion, infectious processes (encephalitis), and intoxications (alcohol, barbiturates).

68. b		**71.** d
69. d		**72.** d
70. e		**73.** d

12

Visual Disturbances

Because visual disturbances are so frequent, psychiatrists should be aware of the rudiments of ophthalmology, including those major ocular, neurologic, and systemic illnesses that may cause visual impairment.* This chapter will discuss several common clinical problems likely to occur in psychiatric patients, including decreased visual acuity, visual field loss, glaucoma, and certain psychologic aberrations affecting vision.

APPROACH TO THE PATIENT

The physician should use a history supplemented by inquiries referable to the visual system (Table 12-1) to establish the specific nature of any visual symptom. The initial examination (Table 12-2) includes inspecting the globe, or "eyeball" (Fig. 12-1); assessing visual acuity, visual fields, and optic fundi; and testing pupil reflexes and ocular movement. Examinations for special cases, such as psychogenic blindness and visual agnosia, are discussed later in the chapter.

DECREASE IN VISUAL ACUITY

Visual acuity is routinely determined by having the patient read from either a Snellen wall chart or a hand-held card (Fig. 12-2). A person with "normal" visual acuity is someone who can read 3/8-inch letters at a distance of 20 feet. This acuity, which is the reference point of the system, is designated 20/20. People who can see at 20 feet whatever a normal person can see as far as 40 feet are said to have 20/40 acuity, and so on.

---

*Patients with visual impairment may receive assistance from many organizations, including the America Foundation for the Blind, 15 West 16th Street, New York, New York 10011, (212) 620-2000.

Table 12-1
Salient Features of a Patient's History

Is the symptom in one or both eyes?

What is the primary symptom?
  Decreased visual acuity
  Visual field loss: one or both eyes
  Diplopia: direction(s)
  Visual distortions or hallucinations, including
    halos around lights

What associated symptoms are present?
  Ocular: pain, scintillations
  Neurologic: headache, paresis, ataxia, impotence
  Systemic: fever, malaise, nausea, excessive thirst

Is there a history of any of the following conditions?
  Diabetes, hypertension, syphilis
  Use of psychotropic, anticholinergic, antituberculous, or other medications
  Abuse of tobacco, alcohol, or methanol
  Exposure to hallucinogens or industrial toxins

Is there a family history of visual disturbances, especially glaucoma?

Table 12-2
Salient Features of a Patient's Examination

Gross evaluation of the globe (eyeball)
  Injection of conjunctival vessels*
  Clarity of cornea and lens
  Inspection for Kayser-Fleischer rings (Chapter 18)*
  Corneal reflex

Determination of visual acuity
  Naked eye
  Corrected with eyeglasses or lens

Determination of visual fields
  Confrontation (see Fig. 4-2)

Inspection of fundi
  Optic disk: color, clarity of margins
  Retina: color, hemorhages,* exudates,* pigment deposit*
  Vessels:arterial pulsations,* venous pulsations

Testing of pupils
  Size, shape, and equality
  Light reflex
  Accommodation

Measurement of extraocular movement
  Position at rest
  Position when looking horizontally or vertically (diplopia,* nystagmus*)
  Strength of orbicularis oculi (eyelids)
  Changes with fatigue

  *Abnormalities.

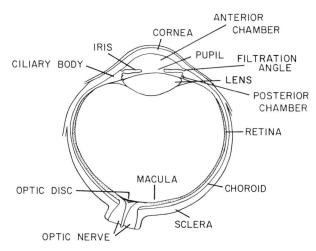

Fig. 12-1. The eye.

Optical Disturbances

In *myopia*, because of either too "thick" a lens or too "long" a globe, people have increasingly blurred vision at increasingly greater distances (Fig. 12-3). Myopia first becomes troublesome during adolescence when it causes difficulty with seeing blackboards, watching movies, and driving. Since reading and other close activities are unimpaired, people with myopia are said to be "nearsighted."

In its counterpart, *hyperopia* or hypermetropia (farsightedness), the lens is too "thin" or the globe too "short." People with hyperopia have increasing visual diffi-

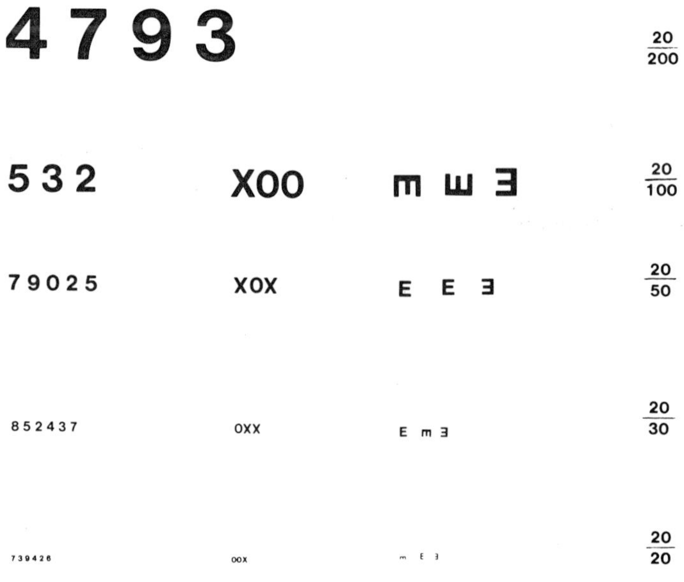

4 7 9 3			$\frac{20}{200}$
5 3 2	XOO	� origin origin	$\frac{20}{100}$
7 9 0 2 5	XOX	E E ⋺	$\frac{20}{50}$
8 5 2 4 3 7	oxx	E m ⋺	$\frac{20}{30}$
739426	oox	ᵐ ᵋ ᵌ	$\frac{20}{20}$

Fig. 12-2. This hand-held visual acuity chart should be held 14 inches from the patient. The acuity is that line which can be read without a mistake.

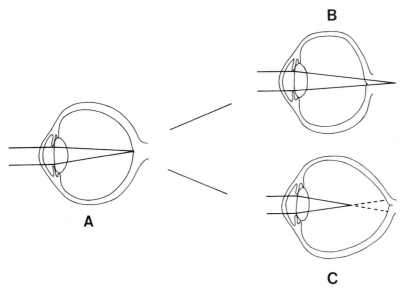

Fig. 12-3. Image focusing in myopic and hyperopic eyes. (A) In normal eyes, the lens focuses the image onto the retina. (B) In hyperopic eyes, the shorter globe or improperly focusing lens causes the image to fall behind the retina. (C) In myopic eyes, the longer globe or improperly focusing lens causes the image to fall in front of the retina.

culty at increasingly shorter distances. In *presbyopia,* a related optical condition, the lenses of elderly patients are not able to focus on closely held objects. Both patients with hyperopia and those with presbyopia have difficulty reading and sewing, and they tend to hold newspapers and needles away from themselves.

Besides these ocular conditions, use of certain medications can lead to important optical disturbances. The foremost is *drug-induced accommodation paresis* in which patients also have visual acuity impairment for closely held objects (Fig. 12-4). Normally, when a person looks at a closely held object, a parasympathetically mediated *accommodation reflex* contracts the ciliary body muscles, which thickens the lens to focus the image on the retina. However, medications with anticholinergic properties block this reflex and thus cause blurred vision. (They also occasionally precipitate glaucoma by causing pupillary dilation.) The tricyclic antidepressants and, to a lesser extent, the tetracyclic antidepressants have great enough anticholinergic strength to cause accommodation paresis without causing other side-effects. Even trazodone (Desyrel), which has a different chemical structure, causes blurred vision. In contrast, phenothiazines, butyrophenones, and the minor tranquilizers have little or no anticholinergic activity or associated blurred vision.

Abnormalities of the Lens, Retina, and Optic Nerve

Cataracts (loss of lens transparency) are found as complications of old age (senile cataract), trauma, diabetes, myotonic dystrophy (Chapter 6), and chlorpromazine (Thorazine). When this medication is given in large quantities, such as 300 mg daily for 2 years, it induces minute opacities in the sclera, cornea, and lens. Fortunately, they do not impair vision.

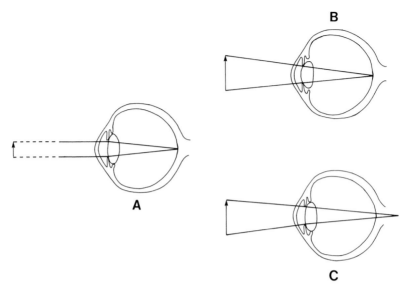

Fig. 12-4. Accommodation and accommodation paresis: (A) When looking at a distant object, parallel light rays are refracted little by a relatively flat lens onto the retina. (B) Accommodation: When looking at a closely held object, ciliary muscle contraction increases the curvature of the lens greatly refracting the light rays. (C) Accommodation paresis: If the ciliary muscles are paretic, the lens cannot form a rounded shape. Its weakened refractive power can only focus the light rays, from closely held objects, behind the retina; however, parallel light rays from distant objects are still focused on the retina. Therefore, with accommodation paralysis, closely held objects will be blurred, but distant ones will be distinct.

Changes in the retina that may interfere with vision can be manifestations of congenital injuries, degenerative diseases, or diabetes. Patients who have received thioridazine (Mellaril) in massive doses, such as 2,000 mg daily for 1 month, sometimes develop retinal pigment accumulations similar to those observed in retinitis pigmentosa (Fig. 12-5), but they too usually cause no visual loss.

In contrast, optic nerve injuries, some of which are liable to be encountered in a psychiatrist's practice, almost always produce marked visual loss. One example is olfactory groove or sphenoid wing meningiomas (Chapter 19), which compress the adjacent optic nerve and grow into the frontal or temporal lobe. Thus, these tumors may trigger partial complex seizures and also induce intellectual and personality changes. Another example is pituitary tumors, such as *adenomas* or *craniopharyngiomas,* which can grow upward to compress the optic chiasm or downward to damage the pituitary gland. Compression of the optic chiasm leads to optic atrophy and bitemporal hemianopsia, and pituitary compression to headache, decreased libido, loss of secondary sexual characteristics (i.e., eunuchism), and diabetes insipidus.

With the important inflammatory condition of the optic nerve, *optic* or *retrobulbar neuritis,* there is sudden, painful visual loss in one eye (Fig. 12-6). Since patients are usually otherwise in good health and the optic disk appears normal, they may be mistakenly diagnosed as suffering from a psychogenic disturbance (Chapter 3). In fact, about one third of optic neuritis patients ultimately develop multiple

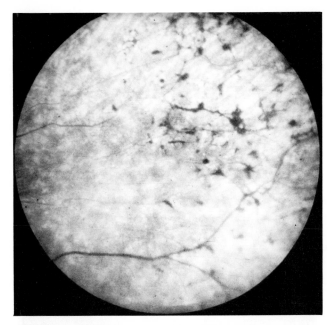

Fig. 12-5. Hyperpigmentation that appears like black bone spicules is seen in retinal changes induced by thioridazine (Mellaril).

sclerosis (Chapter 15). With recurrent optic neuritis attacks, whether or not part of multiple sclerosis, the optic nerve may become atrophic and the eye blind.

Another inflammatory condition of the optic nerve is *temporal*, or *giant cell*, *arteritis*. It affects old people and typically causes headaches, malaise, weight loss, and sometimes the appearance of depression. If temporal arteritis is not promptly treated with steroids, optic nerve and cerebral infarctions may ensue. Finally, methanol intoxication in alcoholics and chronic papilledema from untreatable brain tumors or improperly treated pseudotumor cerebri are associated with optic atrophy and blindness.

GLAUCOMA

Glaucoma is characterized by elevated intraocular pressure because of decreased outflow of aqueous humor through the *filtration angle* of the anterior chamber of the eye (Fig. 12-7). Two common varieties, based on the configuration of the angle, are recognized, and one of them occasionally results from psychotropic medications. If either variety is untreated, glaucoma will damage the optic nerve and cause irreparable visual loss.

Fig. 12-6. The long section of the optic nerve behind the eye, the retrobulbar portion, is subject to multiple sclerosis and other inflammatory conditions. Such abnormalities, *optic* or *retrobulbar neuritis*, cause loss of vision. However, in their early stages, they do not cause any observable change in the optic disk, which is the bulbar portion of the nerve.

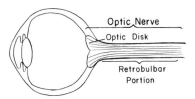

Optic Nerve

Optic Disk

Retrobulbar
Portion

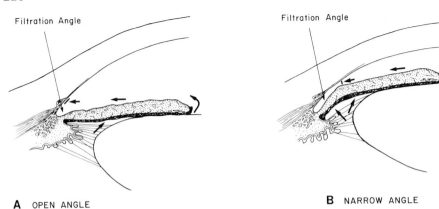

A OPEN ANGLE   **B** NARROW ANGLE

Fig. 12-7. (A) Open-angle glaucoma: the aqueous humor is not drained despite access to the absorptive surface of the angle. Impaired flow from the eye leads to increased intraocular pressure (glaucoma). (B) Narrow-angle glaucoma: When the iris is pushed forward, as may occur during pupil dilation, the angle is narrowed or even closed. Blockage of flow of aqueous humor leads to acute angle-closure glaucoma.

Open-angle or *wide-angle glaucoma* occurs far more frequently. It usually begins only after the age of 40 years. Initially, when symptoms are usually absent, it may be diagnosed only by detecting elevated intraocular pressure. Later, when some vision is lost, the optic cup is abnormally deep. Open-angle glaucoma is usually responsive to topical medications (eye drops), such as pilocarpine, that constrict the pupil and improve aqueous outflow from the filtration angle. Other suitable medications, such as timolol (Timoptic), reduce the production of aqueous humor. Marijuana reportedly lowers intraocular pressure, but standard topical medications are much more effective. Because of the effectiveness of medications, open-angle glaucoma seldom requires surgical treatment.

Psychotropic medications do not precipitate open-angle glaucoma, and people known to have it may be given heterocyclic antidepressants and other psychotropic medications as long as their glaucoma treatment is continued.

The other variety, *angle closure, closed-angle,* or *narrow-angle glaucoma,* is characterized by elevation of intraocular pressure caused when the iris blocks the outflow of aqueous humor at the angle. Patients with narrow-angle glaucoma usually are older than 40 years of age and have congenitally narrow angles. Only a few have had preceding symptoms, such as seeing halos around lights. In contrast to the relatively normal appearance of the eye in open-angle glaucoma, in acute angle-closure glaucoma, the vessels are engorged, the eye red, the pupil dilated, and the cornea hazy. Even more striking, the eye and forehead are painful and vision is markedly impaired.

Prompt treatment is mandatory. Topical and systemic medications open the angle (by constricting the pupil) and also reduce the production of aqueous humor. In addition, surgery or laser iridectomy is usually necessary to create a passage for the aqueous humor directly through the iris to the angle.

Besides developing spontaneously, angle-closure glaucoma is sometimes iatrogenic. For example, when the pupils are dilated for ocular examinations, the "bunched-up" iris can block the angle. Similarly, it may be precipitated by medications with anticholinergic properties, such as the heterocyclic antidepressants, because they also dilate the pupil. However, the incidence of glaucoma complicating antidepressant use is very low—far lower than the amount of discussion in the literature might lead one to expect.

Since measuring the intraocular pressure before medications are prescribed will not predict who will develop angle-closure glaucoma, few rules are practical. Clearly, everyone over the age of 40 years should have their intraocular pressure measured annually. Also, patients who are already treated for either form of glaucoma may continue to receive psychotropic medications as long as they remain under the observation of an ophthalmologist. Finally, patients with narrow angles should be given antidepressants cautiously.

Curiously, just as psychotropic medications can cause ocular problems, ophthalmologic medicines, when systemically absorbed, can cause psychiatric problems. In particular, medications that contain anticholinergic substances may induce frightening physical or psychologic symptoms, such as confusion or anxiety. Another example is the beta-blocker timolol (Timoptic), which can cause light-headedness, depression, or fatigue. Children are particularly susceptible. If they receive scopolamine and other atropine-like eye drops for ocular examination, they often develop agitation.

CORTICAL BLINDNESS AND ASSOCIATED PSYCHOLOGIC PHENOMENA

Patients with cortical blindness do not perceive visual stimulation because of bilateral occipital lobe (visual cortex) damage, usually from devastating cerebral injuries, such as bilateral occlusion of the posterior cerebral arteries, occipital head trauma, cerebral anoxia, multiple cerebral infarctions, or multiple sclerosis (Chapter 15). Notably, since the optic nerves and brainstem remain intact, the pupils of patients with cortical blindness are normal in size and reactivity to light.

In one frequently associated psychologic phenomenon, *Anton's syndrome,* patients with cortical blindness not only insist that their vision is intact, but with prompting they go on to "describe" their room, clothing, and various other objects. Its hallmarks are denial of blindness (similar to that in anosognosia) and the resultant confabulation. Anton's syndrome occurs most frequently in patients with preceding cognitive impairment, visual loss, and predominantly nondominant hemisphere damage.

Agnosia

Another associated phenomenon, *visual agnosia,* is a perceptual inability to identify an object by sight despite an intact visual system and absence of aphasia. For example, patients with visual agnosia are unable to write or say "key" when one is shown to them although they are able to make a drawing of it, describe its use, and say "key" if it is placed in their hand. Visual agnosia, which also results from cerebral cortical damage, differs from aphasia in that if vision is bypassed (when patients touch objects), language function is normal. Also, the site of the damage in visual agnosia is not as well established as in aphasia (see Fig. 8-1).

Visual agnosia is a major aspect of the infamous, experimentally produced

Klüver-Bucy syndrome (Chapter 16), which is produced by monkeys by resection of both temporal lobes. The loss of a good portion of their limbic system results in visual agnosia so severe that they not only touch all objects, they put any object they wish to identify into their mouth ("psychic blindness").

Color agnosia, a variety of agnosia that also results from unestablished damage to the cerebral cortex, is an inability to identify an object's color despite a normal ability to match colored cards, read Ishihara plates (pseudoisochromatic numbered cards), and say the colors of well-known objects, such as the sky. It differs from common color blindness, which is a sex-linked inherited retinal abnormality. In another variety, *prosopagnosia,* patients with bilateral occipito-temporal lesions cannot recognize familiar faces, although they can identify people by voice, dress, mannerisms, and other nonfacial characteristics (Chapter 8).

Psychogenic Blindness

A completely different situation is *psychogenic blindness*. Neurologists go to great lengths to diagnose this disorder even though it is usually self-limited, rare, and not indicative of major psychopathology. An uninhibited examiner simply might make childlike facial contortions or ask the patient to read some four-letter words. The patient's reaction to these provocations would reveal an ability to see. When only one eye is affected by psychogenic blindness, colored or polarized lenses will often confuse (or fatigue) a patient into revealing that vision is present. A vertically striped cylinder (drum) spun in front of any patient with a normal visual system will produce involuntary (*opticokinetic*) nystagmus. Likewise, looking at a large, moving mirror forces anyone with normal vision to follow visually the movement of their own image. Visual evoked response (VER) testing can show diagnostically helpful electrical potentials (Chapter 15). Alternatively, having patients wear lenses with negligible optical value may permit them to extract themselves from psychogenic blindness without embarrassment.

A special disturbance is *tubular or tunnel vision* (Fig. 12-8), a pattern inconsistent with the laws of optics, which dictate that the visual area expands with increasing distance. An important exception to this law, however, is classic migraines (Chapter 9), which can cause peripheral vision constriction and make it appear to patients that they are looking through tubes.

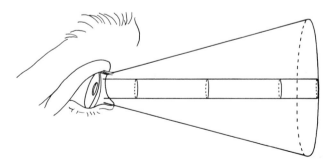

Fig. 12-8. The area seen by a person normally increases conically, proportionately to the distance from the object. In *tubular vision,* which defies the laws of optics, the visual area is constant despite increasing distance.

Nonpsychogenic Visual Hallucinations

Visual hallucinations may sometimes result from a seizure or other abnormal stimulation of the visual cortex. Alternatively, they may result from a lack of continuous stimulation of the visual cortex. Hallucinations from partial elementary seizures, which originate in the occipital lobe (Chapter 10), are "seen" in both eyes and usually consist of displays of brightly colored, slowly moving simple geometric forms lasting from a few seconds to several minutes. The displays may develop during sleep and appear within an area of hemianopsia.

On the other hand, complex partial seizures, which usually result from temporal lobe discharges, are apt to cause detailed visions in which objects appear distorted. In addition, these hallucinations are detailed, often accompanied by related sounds, thoughts, and emotions, and characteristically, impairment of consciousness.

Hallucinations, which can be associated with narcolepsy, are essentially dreams that have intruded into a patient's consciousness. They occur upon falling to sleep (hypnogogic) or awakening (hypnopompic) and are associated with the flaccid, areflexic paresis that is characteristic of dream-filled (REM) sleep (Chapter 17). The "hallucinations" are composed of varied sounds, thoughts, and emotions as well as visions. In comparison, although partial complex seizures may also occur during the twilight of sleep, they are stereotyped; more limited in sensory, cognitive, and affective composition; and associated with automatisms (Chapter 10).

Classic migraine headaches, in which the visual cortex may be irritated by ischemia, are usually preceded by crescentic scotomata with scintillating borders that enlarge and move slowly across the visual field (Chapter 9). In some cases, patients have tubular vision, homonymous hemianopsia, or other visual disturbances that are more often associated with nonmigrainous conditions. Most scotomata last from 1 to 20 minutes before yielding to the actual headache, but sometimes they are the sole manifestation of a migraine.

Many drugs, such as mescaline and lysergic acid diethylamide (LSD), and medicines such as scopolamine and L-dopa, cause visual hallucinations, presumably because they excite the cerebral cortical neurons. Likewise, DTs consist of visual hallucinations that are accompanied by agitated confusion (delirium), sweating, and tachycardia. Typically, in all these metabolic abnormalities, hallucinations are accompanied by psychologic and physical excitement.

Finally, visual hallucinations may be produced by any sudden visual loss. Those from cortical blindness, namely Anton's syndrome, are one example. Another is that of soldiers who, following eye wounds, have periods of "seeing" brightly colored forms and even entire scenes. Similarly, eye surgery in the elderly is occasionally followed by visual hallucinations, disorientation, and agitation. Some physicians suggest that this complication results from spontaneously discharging unstimulated cortical neurons, whereas others believe that it results from sensory deprivation superimposed on dementia. Whatever the reason, bilateral ophthalmologic surgical procedures in the elderly should be avoided.

VISUAL FIELD LOSS

Visual field loss patterns (Fig. 12-9) are a reliable guide to the location of a lesion. And the location, in turn, suggests the cause. In general, the following rules apply.

LEFT CENTRAL SCOTOMA   BITEMPORAL HEMIANOPSIA

BITEMPORAL SUPERIOR   LEFT HOMONYMOUS
QUADRANTANOPSIA   HEMIANOPSIA

Fig. 12-9. Uniocular *central scotomata* may be caused by migraine attacks, optic neuritis, or other ipsilateral optic nerve injuries. *Bitemporal superior quadrantanopsia* is usually caused by lesions of the optic chiasm such as pituitary adenomas. *Bitemporal hemianopsias* are caused by advanced compression of the optic chiasm. *Homonymous hemianopsias,* with or without macular sparing, are most often caused by contralateral cerebral lesions, such as infarctions.

Monocular quadrantanopsias, hemianopsias, scotomata, and blindness are usually the result of optic nerve injury.

Homonymous quadrantanopsias and hemianopsias are almost always the result of visual tract injuries between the optic chiasm and the occipital cortex (see Fig. 4-1). The most common situation is a middle cerebral artery infarction that results in a contralateral homonymous hemianopsia accompanied by hemiparesis and hemisensory loss. An homonymous superior quadrantanopsia (Fig. 12-10), while rare, is noteworthy because it may be the only physical manifestation of a contralateral temporal lobe lesion that produces partial complex seizures. Another loss that is noteworthy is an homonymous hemianopsia that excludes the center of vision (macular sparing) because it is said to be diagnostic of occipital lobe lesions. However, this rule has been challenged, and even if true, it is an impractical guide because such fine visual field determinations are beyond the ability of a nonspecialist.

Bitemporal quadrantanopsias and hemianopsias indicate a lesion at the optic chiasm. The vast majority are pituitary adenomas, which, as discussed previously, compress the optic chiasm, cause optic atrophy, and lead to hypopituitarism.

CONJUGATE OCULAR MOVEMENT

People's eyes move together in a paired, coordinated (*conjugate*) manner so that they can look laterally and can follow moving objects. Abnormalities in the conjugate ocular movement system are often prominent manifestations of neurologic injury. Also, subtle abnormalities have been associated with psychiatric illnesses.

Conjugate ocular movement originates in *cerebral conjugate gaze centers,* which

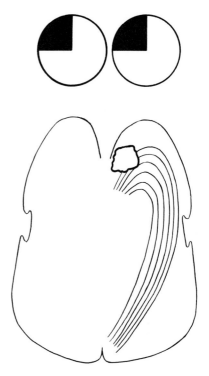

Fig. 12-10. Large anterior temporal lobe lesions may interfere with forward sweeping optic tract fibers. Thus, these lesions, which are rare, may cause a contralateral homonymous superior quadrantanopsia as well as partial complex seizures.

are located in the frontal lobes. When a person is at rest, each cerebral center continuously emits impulses that go through a complicated pathway to move the eyes contralaterally. Since the effect of each center is counterbalanced, the eyes remain midline (Fig. 12-11). When a person wants to look to one side, the contralateral cerebral gaze center becomes increasingly active. For example, if someone wants to look toward an object on the right, the impulses of the left cerebral gaze center are increased and, as if it pushes the eyes away, the eyes turn to the right. If this person also wanted to reach for the object, the left cerebral corticospinal center, which is adjacent to the gaze center, would mobilize the right arm.

The activity of the conjugate gaze center is increased during partial seizures. Not only do partial seizures cause the eyes to move contralaterally, but since they usually envelop the adjacent corticospinal tract, they may also deviate the head contralaterally and produce tonic-clonic activity of the contralateral limbs. By contrast, if patients have unilateral destructive cerebral injuries, such as cerebrovascular accidents (CVAs), the activity of the gaze center on that side is reduced, and the activity of the other center, being unopposed, pushes the eyes toward the injured side. For example, with a left cerebral infarction, the eyes deviate toward the left, and since the corticospinal tract is generally involved, the right side of the body is paralyzed. This example illustrates the sayings, "When the eyes look away from the paralysis, the stroke is cerebral" and "The eyes look toward the stroke."

Each cerebral gaze center actually works by stimulating a contralateral *pontine gaze center*. In contrast to the cerebral center, each pontine center pulls the eyes toward its own side (Fig. 12-12). Thus, a pontine infarction allows the eyes to be pulled toward the opposite side. For example, if the right pontine gaze center were damaged, the eyes would deviate to the left. In addition, because the right pontine

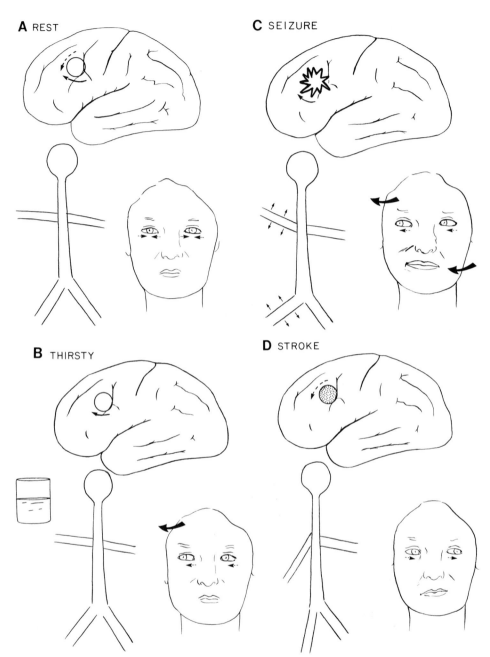

Fig. 12-11. (A) At rest, the eyes are midline because the impulses of each frontal lobe conjugate gaze center are balanced, each "pushing" the eyes contralaterally. (B) Voluntary increased activity of the left cerebral gaze center drives the eyes to the right (contralaterally). (C) Involuntary increased cerebral activity also drives the eyes contralaterally. With left cerebral seizure activity, the right arm and leg develop tonic-clonic activity. (D) A CVA destroys the left cerebral gaze center, permitting the right center to deviate the eyes toward the lesion. It also destroys the cerebral motor strip, causing contralateral paresis: The eyes are "looking" away from the hemiparesis.

232

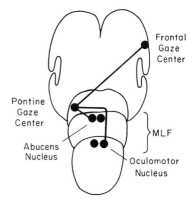

Fig. 12-12. When looking to the right, the left frontal conjugate gaze center stimulates the right (contralateral) pontine gaze center, which, in turn, stimulates the right (adjacent) abducens nerve nucleus and, through the left medial longitudinal fasciculus, the left (contralateral) oculomotor nerve nucleus.

corticospinal tract would be damaged, the left limbs would be paralyzed. With a pontine lesion, the eyes "look toward the paralysis."

Each pontine gaze center stimulates the adjacent abducens nucleus and, through the *medial longitudinal fasciculus* (*MLF*) (see Figs. 15-3 and 15-4), the contralateral oculomotor nucleus. Innervation of one abducens nucleus and the other oculomotor nucleus is necessary for conjugate lateral eye movement. If both abducens nuclei were simultaneously stimulated, both eyes would turn outward, and if both oculomotor nuclei were stimulated, both eyes would turn inward. When the MLF is injured, as often occurs in MS and brainstem CVAs, the *MLF syndrome* (*internuclear ophthalmoplegia*) develops. In this condition, the cranial nuclei and nerves are normal, but the eyes cannot move conjugately (Chapter 15).

Another important ocular movement abnormality is *nystagmus* (rhythmic eyeball oscillation). Although nystagmus is often caused by labyrinthitis, in many cases it is caused by various neurologic injuries, such as multiple sclerosis, brainstem infarction, Wernicke-Korsakoff syndrome, alcohol intoxication, and drug use. Therefore, the presence of nystagmus can suggest that patients are taking diazepam (Valium), barbiturates, or other hypnotic medications. Also, since nystagmus is routinely found in seizure patients who take therapeutic doses of phenytoin (Dilantin) or phenobarbital, its absence suggests noncompliance with an anticonvulsant regimen.

Ocular movement disturbances have also been described in patients with schizophrenia and, less frequently, affective psychosis. Such patients have been found to have abnormal conjugate ocular movements that effect their ability to follow moving targets visually in the normal way (*smooth pursuit*). The smooth pursuit abnormality, which does not appear to be caused by either inattention or medication, is postulated to originate in a disorder "above" the pontine gaze center.

Disordered ocular movements have also recently been reported in patients with Huntington's chorea (Chapter 18). In both this illness and oculogyric crises, ocular movement impairments can be linked to dopamine excess.

DIPLOPIA

Diplopia ("double vision") is rarely the result of ocular abnormalities, such as a dislocated lens. Instead, it is almost always caused by neurologic disorders, including oculomotor or abducens cranial nerve injury, brainstem infarction, or extraocular muscle disorders. Sometimes, however, it can be psychogenic.

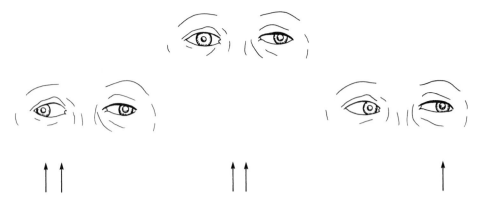

Fig. 12-13. Left oculomotor nerve palsy. in the center picture, a patient looks ahead. His left upper lid is lower, the pupil larger, and the eye deviated slightly laterally. Since the eyes are dysconjugate, the patient sees two arrows (diplopia) when looking ahead. In the picture on the left, the patient looks to the right. Since the paretic left eye fails to cross medially beyond the midline, the eyes are more dysconjugate and there is greater diplopia. In the picture on the right, the patient looks to the left. Here, the eyes are almost conjugate and there is little or no diplopia.

Oculomotor nerve injury results in ptosis, pupil dilation, lateral deviation of the eye, and diplopia that is greatest when the patient looks away from the resting position of the eyes (Fig. 12-13). Abducens nerve injury results in medial deviation of the eye and diplopia when looking laterally, but neither in ptosis nor pupil abnormality (Fig. 12-14).

While diplopia is frequently the result of cranial nerve injury, several conditions are important variations. When myopic adults read or drive while fatigued, they develop momentary diplopia because of ocular muscle fatigue. Also, myasthenia

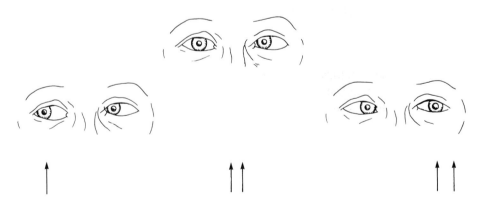

Fig. 12-14. A left abducens nerve palsy. In the center picture, a patient looks ahead. The patient's left eye is deviated medially. The eyes are dysconjugate and the patient sees two arrows when looking ahead. In the picture on the left, the patient looks to the right. The eyes are conjugate and the patient sees only a single arrow. In the picture on the right, the patient looks to the left. The paretic left eye fails to cross the midline. The exaggeration of the dysconjugate gaze increases the diplopia.

gravis causes diplopia, which is initially transient and never associated with pupil abnormalities (Chapter 6).

On the other hand, although congenital ocular muscle weakness, *strabismus*, causes dysconjugate gaze, children do not have diplopia because the brain is able to suppress the image from the weaker eye. However, with continuous suppression of the vision of that eye, the eye will become blind (*amblyopic*). Thus, babies and children with a "crossed" or "lazy eye" often have the "good" eye patched several hours each day to force them to use the visual and muscle systems of the weak eye.

Finally, patients may have psychogenic diplopia. Usually, it is "mild" and in all directions of gaze. There is, of course, no observable abnormality. Nonetheless, physicians must be careful not to overlook subtle neurologic conditions, especially myasthenia gravis and internuclear ophthalmoplegia. In another psychogenic disturbance, children or young adults, as if looking at the tip of their nose, fix their eyes in a downward and inward position. This ocular movement is a burlesque that can be overcome by inducing opticokinetic nystagmus.

HORNER'S SYNDROME AND ARGYLL-ROBERTSON PUPILS

Horner's syndrome, which consists of ptosis, miosis, and anhidrosis, should not be confused with an oculomotor nerve injury even though ptosis is the most prominent sign of both conditions (Fig. 12-15). In Horner's syndrome there is neither impairment of ocular motility nor diplopia, and the pupil of the affected eye is small. Moreover, the syndrome results from injury to the sympathetic tract anywhere along its roundabout course, which begins in the brainstem, descends in the cervical spinal cord, ascends through the chest, and, wrapped around the carotid artery, finally innervates the pupil, eyelid, and facial sweat glands. Thus, Horner's syndrome can be caused by lateral medullary infarctions (Wallenberg's syndrome); cervical spinal cord injury; apical lung (Pancoast's) tumors; and, because of a carotid artery abnormality, cluster headaches.

Argyll-Robertson pupils, which also must be differentiated from oculomotor nerve injury, are irregular, asymmetric, and small (1–2 mm). In addition, they are characteristically unreactive to light but do constrict normally when patients look at closely held objects, i.e., during accommodation. The impaired light reflex with intact accommodation has given rise to the saying, "Argyll-Robertson pupils are like prostitutes, they accommodate but do not react." While Argyll-Robertson pupils have historically been a manifestation of syphilis, in the vast majority of cases seen today they result from diabetic autonomic neuropathy.

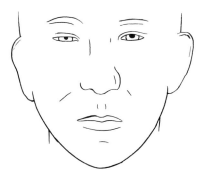

Fig. 12-15. Horner's syndrome, which may be found in brainstem, spinal cord, carotid artery, or thoracic lesions, consists of miosis (a small pupil), ptosis, and, with special testing, anhidrosis (loss of sweating).

REFERENCES

Abramowicz M (ed): Amoxapine (Ascendin). The Medical Letter 23:39, 1981
Abramowicz M (ed): Maprotiline (Ludiomil). The Medical Letter 23:58, 1981
Abramowicz M (ed): Trazodone (Desyrel). The Medical Letter 24:47, 1982
Damasio AR, Damasio H, Hoesen GWV: Prosopagnosia: Anatomic basis and behavioral
    mechanisms. Neurology 32:331, 1982
Keane JR: Neuro-ophthalmic signs and symptoms of hysteria. Neurology 32:757, 1982
Lipton RB, Levy DL, Holzman PS, et al: Eye movement dysfunctions in psychiatric patients:
    A review. *Schizophrenia Bulletin* 9:13, 1983
Reid WH, Rakes S: Intraocular pressure in patients receiving psychotropic medications. Psy-
    chosomatic 24:665, 1983
Rubens AB: Agnosia. In Heilman KM, Valenstein E (eds): Clinical Neuropsychology. New
    York, Oxford University Press, 1979

QUESTIONS

1. Which findings characterize Argyll-Robertson pupils?
    a. Miosis
    b. Ptosis
    c. Irregular shape
    d. Unreactivity to light
    e. Unresponsiveness to accommodation

2. Which medications are associated with transient visual impairment because of accommodation paresis?
    a. Butyrophenones
    b. Amitriptyline
    c. Imipramine
    d. Phenobarbital
    e. Phenytoin

3. Which of the following cause cataracts that interfere with vision?
    a. Myotonic dystrophy
    b. Diabetes mellitus
    c. Ocular trauma
    d. Chlorpromazine

4. A 20-year-old soldier develops loss of vision in the right eye. The eye is painful, especially when moved voluntarily. No ocular or neurologic abnormalities are found, except for a relative decrease in light reaction in the right eye. After 1 week, vision returns, except for a small central scotoma. What illness is he likely to have had?

5. What is the prognosis in the case presented in question 4?

6. Which laboratory procedure will identify dysfunction of the optic nerve in patients with clinical symptoms and signs indicative of multiple sclerosis and also help distinguish patients with visual impairments from those with psychogenic impairments?

7. What are the characteristics of open- or wide-angle glaucoma?
    a. Chronicity
    b. Acute onset
    c. Hereditary predisposition
    d. Onset after age 40
    e. Raised intraocular pressure
    f. Precipitated by tricyclic antidepressant medications
    g. Absolute contraindication to use of tricyclic antidepressant medications
    h. Usually responsive to ocular or systemic medical therapy or both

8. What are the characteristics of closed- or narrow-angle glaucoma?
- a. Chronicity
- b. Acute onset
- c. Hereditary predisposition
- d. Onset after age 40
- e. Painful eye
- f. "Steamy"cornea
- g. Headache
- h. Precipitated by antidepressant medications
- i. Surgical treatment

9. Should patients with closed- or narrow-angle glaucoma be given tricyclic antidepressant medications?

10–15. Match the usual field loss (10–15) with the underlying illness (a–f):

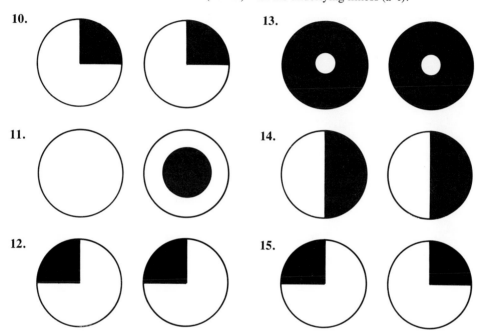

10.   13.

11.   14.

12.   15.

- a. 25-year old woman with paraparesis and ataxia
- b. 35-year-old woman with insidious onset of loss of peripheral daytime vision and all night vision. Her mother has a similar illness.
- c. 30-year-old man with episodes of seeing the American flag and hearing the first five bars of "America the Beautiful"
- d. 21-year-old man with loss of bodily hair, gynecomastia, and diabetes insipidus.
- e. 70-year-old man with global aphasia and right hemiplegia and hemisensory loss
- f. 75-year-old man with fluent (receptive, Wernicke's) aphasia

16–26. Match the characteristics of the visual hallucination with the source.

16. Associated musical hallucinations
17. Flashes of bright lights in the contralateral visual field
18. Associated olfactory hallucinations
19. Rotating blotches of color
20. Impairment of consciousness
21. Postictal aphasia
22. Throbbing unilateral headache
23. Nausea and vomiting
24. Simple blocks and stars of colors

- a. Seizures that originate in the occipital lobe
- b. Seizures that originate in the temporal lobe
- c. Classical migraine headaches

25. Twisting, complicated multicolored lights
26. Faces with distorted features or coloring

27-28. Match the symptom (27-28) with the possible origins (a-d).

27. Diplopia when looking to the right
28. Diplopia when looking to the left

a. Left third nerve palsy
b. Left sixth nerve palsy
c. Right third nerve palsy
d. Right sixth nerve palsy

29-30. Match the signs with the cause.

29. Third nerve palsy
30. Internuclear ophthalmoplegia

a. Ptosis
b. Miosis
c. Enlarged pupil
d. Nystagmus of abducting eye
e. Inability of affected eye to move
   medially, i.e., paresis of adduction

31. What are the common causes of ptosis?
   a. Third nerve palsy
   b. Sixth nerve palsy
   c. Pancoast's tumor
   d. Multiple sclerosis
   e. Myasthenia gravis
   f. Hysteria

32. What are the common causes of internuclear ophthalmoplegia?
   a. Multiple sclerosis
   b. Polio
   c. Muscular dystrophy
   d. Hysteria
   e. Heroin overdose
   f. Brainstem cerebrovascular
      infarctions

33. Which abnormality is reported to occur in patients with schizophrenia and, to a lesser extent, affective psychosis?
   a. Internuclear ophthalmoplegia
   b. Nystagmus
   c. Ptosis
   d. Conjugate gaze paresis
   e. Smooth pursuit abnormalities

34. A 70-year-old man awakens with a right hemiparesis, vertigo, and his eyes deviated to the right. Which of the following conditions will also be found?
   a. Aphasia
   b. Right homonymous hemianopsia
   c. Dementia
   d. Nystagmus

35. Which conditions indicate that the dopamine system is involved in conjugate eye movement?
   a. Internuclear ophthalmoplegia
   b. Nystagmus
   c. Pontine gaze center movement
   d. Oculogyric crisis

36. Which conditions have a predilection for people older than 65?
   a. Myopia
   b. Presbyopia
   c. Macular degeneration
   d. Classic migraines
   e. Temporal or giant cell arteritis
   f. Glaucoma
   g. Cataracts
   h. Optic neuritis

37. A 70-year-old man suffers a cerebral infarction. Afterwards, he has a right homonymous hemianopsia, right hemisensory loss, and a mild right hemiparesis. Although he can both say and write the names of objects that he feels, he has a peculiar inability to name objects that

he only sees, even when they are presented to his left visual field. What is the name of this condition and where is the lesion located? With which other conditions might this one reasonably be confused?

38. In which conditions are both pupils normally reactive to light?

a. Atropine poisoning
b. Psychogenic blindness
c. Cortical blindness
d. Optic neuritis
e. Acute angle-closure glaucoma
f. Argyll-Robinson pupils
g. Acute papilledema
h. Anxiety
i. Anton's syndrome
j. Classic migraine
k. Midbrain infarction
l. Transtentorial herniation
m. Pontine infarction
n. Internuclear ophthalmoplegia

39–46. Match the condition (39–46) with the neuropsychologic condition (a–j).

39. Cannot recognize familiar faces

40. Despite visual loss, (erroneously) describes hospital room and physician

41. Following cardiac arrest, blindness with with normal pupil light reflex. In addition, although alert, mental impairment is prominent

42. Cannot identify a red card, although able to match it to another red card and read a red-colored number on the Ishihara plates

43. Despite only a right homonymous hemianopsia, inability to read. Writing ability is normal.

44. Congenital inability to read Ishihara plates

45. Inability to name common objects under any circumstances

46. Cannot name objects when seen, but can name objects when described or felt

a. Cortical blindness
b. Visual agnosia
c. Color agnosia
d. Color blindness
e. Prosopagnosia
f. Anton's syndrome
g. Wernicke-Korsakoff syndrome
h. Alexia without agraphia
i. Congenital cerebral injury
j. Aphasia

ANSWERS

1. a, c, d

2. b, c

3. a, b, c

4. He probably had an episode of optic neuritis.

5. Most patients who have optic neuritis have no recurrences; however, about one third later develop multiple sclerosis. In other words, optic neuritis is usually not an early manifestation of multiple sclerosis.

6. Visual-evoked responses (VER), which are essentially analyses of the EEG when light is shown into the subject's eyes, will indicate the presence and location of impairment of the visual system. It is a sensitive procedure that permits detection of asymptomatic optic nerve lesions.

7. a, c, d, e, h

8. b, c, d, e, f, g, h, i

9. Patients with closed- or narrow-angle glaucoma may take tricyclic antidepressants once therapy for glaucoma has been instituted.

10. c. The patient may have partial complex (e.g., psychomotor) seizures and a right superior quadrantanopsia as the result of a left temporal lobe lesion. *or* f. The patient may have a left temporal lobe lesion giving him aphasia and a contralateral superior quadrantanopsia.

11.   a. The patient has spinal cord, cerebellar, and right optic nerve injury, probably as the result of multiple sclerosis.

12.   c. The patient may have psychomotor seizures and a left superior quadrantanopsia as the result of a right temporal lobe lesion.

13.   b. The patient has preservation only of the central vision during daytime, as did her mother. If examination of her fundi showed clumping of retinal pigment, the diagnosis of *retinitis pigmentosa* would be certain. Such a visual field examination also might be obtained with someone having tunnel vision.

14.   e. The patient probably has a dominant hemisphere cerebrovascular accident or tumor giving a right homonymous hemianopsia.

15.   d. The patient has a large pituitary tumor causing panhypopituitarism and bitemporal hemianopsia.

16. b	**22.** c	**28.** b, c
17. a, c	**23.** c	**29.** a, c, e
18. b	**24.** a, c	**30.** d, e
19. a	**25.** b, c	**31.** a, c, e
20. a, b	**26.** b, c	**32.** a, f
21. b	**27.** a, b	

33.   e. Such patients are reported to have smooth pursuit abnormalities, but since they are heavily medicated, they have oculogyric crises.

34.   d. This patient has an infarction in the left brainstem at the pontine level. Thus, he would not have signs of cerebral injury, such as aphasia, hemianopsia, or mental impairment. He would have nystagmus and also possibly injury to the left facial and abducens nerve nuclei which would result in left upper and lower facial paresis and medial deviation of the left eye.

35.   d. Oculogyric crises are precipitated by phenothiazines, including those used for nonpsychotic conditions, such as nausea and vomiting.

36.   b, c, e, f, g. These conditions, which are readily found in a large number of people, will become astronomical in numbers as the population ages. Combinations of these conditions may occur together in the same older person. Whatever the cause of visual impairment, it is a major threat to the mental well-being of the older person, especially to those with intellectual or emotional impairment.

37.   The patient has visual agnosia in which he cannot process visually acquired information. Aphasia would not account for his problem because the language function is normal as seen in his normal writing and speaking ability once vision is circumvented. In his case, the lesion is probably in the left parietal and occipital region. Additional testing might reveal Gerstmann's syndrome or alexia without agraphia (Chapter 7)—also found in posterior dominant hemisphere lesions.

38. b, c, g, h, i, j, m, n	**41.** a	**44.** d
39. e	**42.** c	**45.** j
40. f	**43.** h	**46.** b

13

Congenital Cerebral Injuries

Many common congenital neurologic disorders that cause lifelong physical and mental impairment can be readily diagnosed by routine clinical evaluation. Such disorders include varieties of cerebral palsy and various neurocutaneous disturbances. By contrast, the brain injuries said to cause hyperactivity and certain learning disabilities are often so difficult to detect that their existence has been questioned.

CEREBRAL PALSY

Cerebral palsy (CP)* is a nonscientific but generally accepted descriptive term for the permanent neurologic *motor system* impairments that result from cerebral injuries sustained in utero or during infancy. Characteristically, children and adults with CP suffer from spastic paresis of the limbs, a choreoathetotid movement disorder, or both. In addition, depending upon the variety of CP, they frequently, but not necessarily, have mental retardation, seizures, or other concomitants of cerebral injury. Whatever the particular handicap may be, it changes little as the child grows into adult life: after childhood, the CP deficits are static or nonprogressive. Although the cause of CP may be any condition that damages the brain from gestation through infancy, in most cases CP is associated with prematurity, low birth weight, anoxia during delivery, or neonatal hyperbilirubinemia (kernicterus). Recent medical developments that are effective in preventing or treating these conditions have been responsible for the fall in incidence toward 1 per 1,000 live births. Nevertheless, thousands of adults as well as children are handicapped by cerebral injuries that occurred perinatally.

In making a clinical evaluation, the physician might accept a history of perinatal cerebral injury followed by a permanent, relatively stable motor impairment as diagnostic of CP (Table 13-1). In such cases, it is not always necessary to perform CT,

---

*Patients with cerebral palsy and related disorders may receive assistance from the United Cerebral Palsy Foundation, 66 East 34th Street, New York, New York 10016, (212) 481-6300.

Table 13-1
Historical Features of Cerebral Palsy

Description of deficit
  Motor impairment
    Paresis: extent, degree
    Movement disorder: nature, age of onset
  Delayed acquisition of motor skills
  Associated conditions
    Mental retardation
    Seizures
Search for cause
  Maternal health
    Personal or familial neurologic illness
    Prenatal illness or abnormalities:
      Infections, medications, etc.
      Vaginal bleeding, paucity of fetal movements
  Delivery
    Prematurity
    Low weight for date
    Prolonged labor, fetal distress
    Obstetrical complications
  Neonatal period
    Low Apgar score
    Cyanosis, unresponsiveness
    Seizures
    Jaundice

EEG, and other tests. Rather, the physician should concentrate on the problem at hand and evaluate the patient's mental and physical abilities (Table 13-2). *Since many patients with CP have normal intelligence, despite major motor deficits, movement disorders, and hearing impairments, the physician should never conclude that a person has mental impairment or retardation without full, detailed, and specialized mental status evaluations.*

Varieties of CP

Of the many clinical varieties of CP, the two that occur most commonly and have the greatest descriptive value are *spastic* and *extrapyramidal* (choreoathetotic) CP. Each has a characteristic motor impairment and a predictable association with seizures and mental retardation.

Spastic CP, which accounts for approximately 70 percent of cases, is characterized by paralysis with marked muscular hypertonicity (spasticity). Since the paralysis results from cerebral damage, it is invariably accompanied by hyperactive DTRs, clonus, and Babinski signs. Characteristically, since cerebral damage has occurred before childhood growth, the affected extremities will be foreshortened, i.e., have *growth arrest*. Notably, spasticity and growth arrest create as much disability as the paresis alone.

Subcategories of spastic CP are based on the pattern of deficit—diplegic (paresis of both legs), hemiplegic (arm and leg), and quadriplegic (all limbs). Most important,

Table 13-2
Physical Findings of Cerebral Palsy (CP)

Motor deficits
  Signs of spastic CP
    Gross impairment: paresis/spasticity; growth arrest;
      pseudobulbar palsy
    Subtle impairment: unequal size of hands or feet; toe walking
      (from shortened heel cords); hand preference, e.g., right-
      handedness, before the age of 18 months.
  Signs of extrapyramidal CP
    Choreoathetosis
      Chorea: intermittent, rapid, jerky involuntary movements of
        the shoulders and hips
      Athetosis: continual, slow, writhing involuntary movements
        of the hands and feet
Associated conditions
  Intellectual impairment, i.e., mental retardation
  Seizures (generalized, focal motor or psychomotor)
  Impairment of special senses
    Visual: strabismus, myopia, blindness
    Auditory: deafness
    Vocal: dysarthria

with more extensive cerebral damage, there will be more extensive paresis, a greater incidence of seizures, and more severe mental retardation.

Diplegic CP is symmetric paresis, primarily of the legs (Fig. 13-1). Patients display toewalking and a scissors gait because the spasticity and short tendons keep the knees, ankles, and toes in a position in which they are straight, drawn together (adducted), and pointed downward (extended). Since cerebral damage is relatively

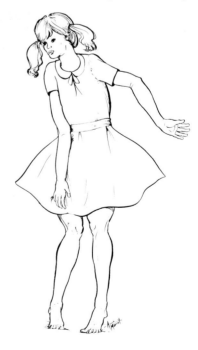

Fig. 13-1. Spastic diplegia. This 10-year-old girl with low-normal intelligence has straightening and inturning of the legs, a tip-toe stance, and scissors-like gait that could be alleviated somewhat by lengthening and transposing knee and heel tendons. She also has incoordinated, awkward movements of her arms (posturings).

mild and limited, seizures and mental retardation both occur in only about 25 percent of cases, which is much less frequent than in the other forms of spastic CP. The usual cause of spastic diplegia is prematurity and low birth weight, leading to periventricular injury that damages the corticospinal tract fibers of the legs (see Fig. 7-7). Recent developments in neonatal intensive care have greatly reduced the incidence of this form of CP.

Hemiplegic CP is usually spastic paresis of the face and the arm more than that of the leg (Fig. 13-2). Cerebral palsy patients resemble adults with middle cerebral artery occlusions but have growth arrest of the affected limbs. In particular, their thumb and great-toe nail beds will be smaller on the paretic side. Also, a contracted Achilles tendon forces them to walk on the toes of the affected short foot. Another feature of hemiplegic CP is abnormal early development of hand preference, e.g., right-handedness. Normally, this occurs only after two years of age: Exclusive use of one hand much before that time suggests palsy of the other.

More important, since the right hemisphere becomes dominant if the left is injured in infancy, people who have had congenital left hemisphere damage may become right hemisphere dominant and left-handed and have normal language development, even though they have right hemiparesis (Chapter 8). In contrast, adults who sustain left cerebral hemisphere injuries almost always have aphasia as well as right hemiparesis.

The cerebral damage in spastic hemiparesis is generally more severe and extensive than in spastic cerebral diplegia. Thus, seizures, including the psychomotor variety, or mental retardation develop in approximately 50 percent of cases.

Quadriplegic CP is paresis of all four limbs accompanied by pseudobulbar palsy. Since it results from severe, extensive cerebral damage, often caused by anoxia during delivery, 75 percent of cases suffer from seizures and mental retardation. In contrast,

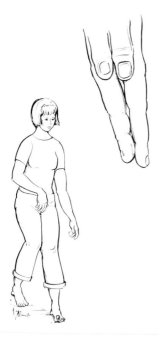

Fig. 13-2. Spastic hemiparesis. Since birth, this 28-year-old woman with normal intelligence has had weakness of her right arm and leg. She holds the arm, wrist, and fingers in a flexed posture. She has growth arrest. The right hand and fingers are foreshortened and the nail bed of the thumb is less broad. The right leg, especially the heel (Achilles) tendon is short, causing her to walk on her toes and circumduct her right leg. Her posture and gait are similar to those of adults who have suffered an infarction of the left middle cerebral artery (see Figs. 2-3 to 2-5).

there is a non-CP form of quadriplegia resulting from cervical spinal cord birth injury. In these cases, where there is no cerebral damage, there are no seizures, pseudobulbar palsy, or mental retardation.

Extrapyramidal CP, the other major category, accounts for 15 percent of cases. It is characterized by *choreoathetosis,* an involuntary writhing (athetosis) of the face, tongue, hands, and feet punctuated by jerking movements (chorea) of the trunk, arms, and legs (Fig. 13-3). Choreoathetosis is usually symmetric, but in some cases it is nearly unilateral. Like all involuntary movement disorders, it disappears during sleep and tends to be aggravated by anxiety (Chapter 18). Movements frequently prevent appropriate hand use and interfere with walking. They also affect the vocal mechanics of the larynx, pharynx, and diaphragm so that patients have marked dysarthria. In addition, deafness is a frequent complication.

Choreoathetosis is usually caused by either anoxia at birth or neonatal jaundice (hyperbilirubinemia) and resultant damage to the basal ganglia from kernicterus. Since the cerebral cortex may be relatively or entirely spared in kernicterus, this form of extrapyramidal CP is associated with the lowest incidence of cerebral cortical injury. Overall, only about 10 percent of patients have seizures and many have normal intelligence. Despite considerable impediments, many have completed college or other advanced education. These patients are liable to be underrated by a superficial social, academic, or medical evaluation.

Finally, *mixed forms* of CP—combinations of spastic paraparesis and choreoathetosis—account for about 15 percent of CP cases. The clinical patterns reflect the most

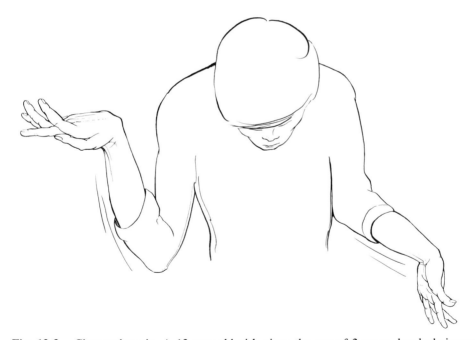

Fig. 13-3. Choreoathetosis. A 13-year-old girl, since the age of 3 years, has had sinuous movements of the wrist, hands and fingers. The movements force her hands into flexion at the wrist and her fingers into extension and overlapping positions. Quick, jerk-like movements are superimposed intermittently.

severe, extensive cerebral and basal ganglia damage, which is usually the result of a combination of jaundice, anoxia, and prematurity. As would be expected, this degree of damage is associated with the highest incidence of seizures or mental retardation— 95 percent.

In summary, seizures or mental retardation are found in increasingly greater incidence in choreoathetosis (10 percent), diplegia (25 percent), hemiplegia (50 percent), quadriplegia (75 percent), and mixed CP (95 percent).

Rehabilitation

Adequate assessment of the intellectual capabilities of patients is necessary, especially in the extrapyramidal forms of CP. Special schooling is required in many cases, but not all. Hearing aids will vastly improve the capabilities of some patients, and newly developed electronic typewriters permit some patients with severe dysarthria to communicate by (English or Spanish) print or voice output.

Attempts at physical rehabilitation must be made from many approaches. Braces and other mechanical devices may augment strength, and corrective surgery that transposes or lengthens tendons will ameliorate spasticity and contractures. Muscle relaxants, such as baclofen (Lioresal), may also reduce spasticity.

Although choreoathetosis is difficult to treat, neuroleptics and sedatives may suppress some movement. Experimental surgical procedures involving ablation of deep cerebral structures have been reported to reduce athetosis but with considerable risk and uncertain benefit.

Control of seizures is difficult. Often two or more anticonvulsants are required, causing patients to develop sedation, hyperactivity, or other side effects. Particularly when there is mental retardation, as is often the case, anticonvulsants may exacerbate behavioral disturbances.

Myelomeningocele, another congenital disorder, is a sac-like protrusion of the lower spinal cord, the cauda equina, and their meningeal coverings through a defect of the lumbar or sacral spine. Patients have areflexic paraparesis and incontinence. Moreover, myelomeningoceles are associated with comparable cranial abnormalities that cause hydrocephalus and mental retardation (Arnold-Chiari malformations). Unless defects are surgically corrected within several days after birth, fatal bacterial meningitis develops.

Myelomeningoceles result from neural tube closure defects that have been attributed to genetic abnormalities and exposure to toxins. After the birth of a child with myelomeningocele, there is a 10 percent chance the same abnormality will recur in future pregnancies. Affected fetuses can be detected by sampling amniotic fluid, testing maternal serum for alpha-fetoprotein, or with ultrasound examination. Cases have been the focus of debates about "fetal screening" and responsibility for mentally and physically impaired neonates who require extensive medical care.

NEUROCUTANEOUS DISORDERS

The neurocutaneous disorders are a group of illnesses, largely inherited in an autosomal dominant pattern, that cause a combination of neurologic and skin abnormalities. The brain and skin, sometimes together with the peripheral nerves, retina,

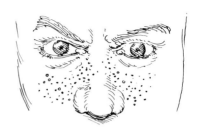

Fig. 13-4. Tuberous sclerosis. The cutaneous component, adenoma sebaceum, which is prominent on this patient's malar surface, are several millimeters in diameter, firm, and uniformly pale without surrounding inflammation.

and other organs, are affected together, presumably because they all derive from the ectodermal layer of the embryo.

The clinical manifestations of the neurocutaneous disorders are often not apparent until late childhood. Although these conditions are usually stable through adult life, in many cases the neurologic abnormality changes from a benign to a malignant condition. Of the many neurocutaneous disorders in the literature, only the three most clinically important ones—tuberous sclerosis, neuofibromatosis, and Sturge-Weber syndrome—are discussed below.

Tuberous Sclerosis

Tuberous sclerosis* is characterized by cutaneous *adenoma sebaceum* and, in most patients, the combination of epilepsy and progressive mental impairment. Lesions of adenoma sebaceum, which develops by puberty, are smooth, firm skin nodules over the chin, nose, and malar (cheek) region (Fig. 13-4). They resemble acne but can be distinguished by the fact that acne "pimples" have a liquid (pus) center, inflammation at the periphery, and are found on the chest and upper back as well as the face.

Dementia often begins in childhood and progresses slowly. It is associated with growth of cerebral *tubers,* which are brain nodules 1 to 3 cm in diameter that compress brain tissue, irritate the surrounding cortex to cause seizures, and occasionally undergo malignant transformation. In most cases, tubers cannot be removed because they are too numerous and too deep. The combination of progressive mental impairment, epilepsy, and poor prognosis forces many patients into institutions. However, about 30 percent of patients have a relatively benign form of the illness with few seizures and little or no mental retardation.

Neurofibromatosis

Neurofibromatosis† or Von Reckinghausen's disease, which seems to be inherited in only 50 percent of cases, is characterized especially by multiple *café au lait* spots and neurofibromas. Although as many as 40 percent of patients may have intellectual impairment, mental retardation may be present in only 2 to 5 percent.

---

*Patients with Tuberous sclerosis may receive assistance from the Tuberous Sclerosis Association of America, P.O. Box 44, Rockland, Massachusetts 02370, (617) 878-5528; or National Tuberous Sclerosis Association, P.O. Box 612, Winfield, Illinois 60190, (312) 668-0787.

†Patients with neurofibromatosis may receive assistance from The National Neurofibromatosis Foundation, 130 5th Avenue, New York, New York 10011 (212) 869-9034.

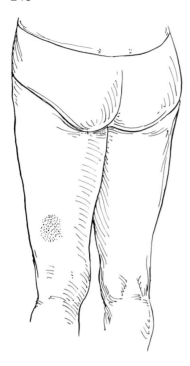

Fig. 13.-5. Café au lait spot. This flat, light brown skin lesion, when numbering six or more with each being greater than 1.5 cm, indicates neurofibromatosis.

Café au lait spots are flat and light brown (Fig. 13-5). They are found in at least 10 percent of normal people and indicate neurofibromatosis only if more than six are present and each is larger than 1.5 cm. Neurofibromas are subcutaneous, discrete or plexiform, papule-like growths measuring a few millimeters to several centimeters that generally emerge along peripheral nerves and are visible subcutaneously (Fig. 13-6). They can occur all over the body and reach grotesque proportions; David Merrick, the "Elephant Man," is an example.

Neurofibromas are usually begnign and create no functional impairment; however, occasionally they grow to compress the spinal cord, an important nerve root, or the cauda equina. Most important, they sometimes develop on the acoustic or optic cranial nerves, causing acoustic neuromas or optic gliomas.

Intracranial neurofibromas can be removed surgically, although sometimes the affected nerve must be sacrificed, but excision of peripheral neurofibromas is not feasible because virtually all peripheral nerves are involved. Café au lait spots can be blanched using lasers.

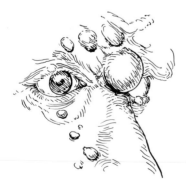

Fig. 13-6. Neurofibromas. While typically less than 0.5 cm, neurofibromas often grow to several centimeters on the face, trunk, and limbs.

Sturge-Weber Syndrome

Sturge-Weber syndrome, or *encephalo-trigeminal angiomatosis,* which is usually not hereditary, consists of vascular malformations of the face and ipsilateral cerebral hemisphere that cause a deep red facial discoloration (portwine stain) in one or more divisions of the trigeminal nerve distribution (Fig. 13-7). Since the first division is the one most often affected, the most common cutaneous abnormality involves the anterior scalp, forehead, and upper eyelid (see Fig. 4-11). By contrast, most people with small, patchy portwine stains and infants with small forehead or facial angiomas, such as strawberry nevi, do not have Sturge-Weber Syndrome.

The cerebral component of Sturge-Weber syndrome, which is both a vascular abnormality in the meninges and an underlying cerebral atrophy with calcification, is always a potent seizure focus. When cerebral damage is extensive, patients have homonymous hemianopsia, spastic hemiparesis, and sometimes mental retardation as well as epilepsy.

SUBTLE BRAIN INJURY

Attention Deficits and Hyperactivity

A refocused concept of minimal brain dysfunction (MBD), "attention deficit disorder (ADD) with or without hyperactivity," refers to a childhood condition characterized by inappropriate inattention and impulsivity. Despite the change in designation, however, many children with ADD, like those with MBD, are hyperactive. Moreover, as with MBD, their hyperactivity responds to stimulants such as amphetamine, which, however, do not improve either a shortened attention span or learning disabilities.

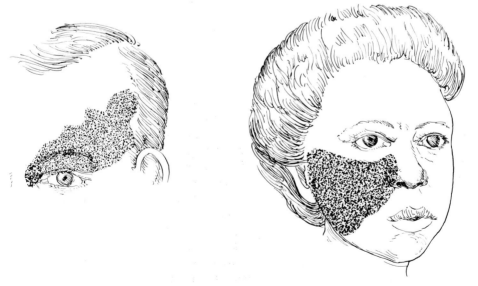

Fig. 13-7. The cutaneous deep red angiomatosis of Sturge-Weber Syndrome involves one or more divisions of the distribution of the trigeminal nerve (See Fig. 4-11).

Only 5 to 15 percent of ADD cases are associated with a diagnosable neurologic disease, which is almost always cerebral palsy or mental retardation. Most children with overt brain damage from cerebral anoxia or head trauma have reasonable attention spans and no hyperactivity. Also, any hyperactivity they do have does not appear to improve with stimulants.

Many ADD symptoms are undoubtedly manifestations of delayed cerebral maturation rather than brain injury. Slowed myelination of the frontal lobes and limbic system is said to retard age-appropriate fine and gross motor skills, intellectual ability, and socialization. Since maturation brings development of very important inhibitory influences, until the child with slow neurologic development is older, he or she may have uncontrollable diversions to newly presented stimulation, excessive motor and reflex activity ("disinhibition"), and unrestrained fears and fantasy.

Learning Disabilities

Learning disabilities are also often felt to be a manifestation of congenital brain injury and are often described in children with ADD or MBD. While they probably result from various social, emotional, or neurologic problems, several neurologic-based (neuropsychologic) learning disabilities have been described. Children with "developmental dyslexia" (reading impairment) frequently display right-sided hyperactive DTRs and other lateralized signs referable to dominant hemisphere congenital injury. In a disability that mimics Gerstmann's syndrome (dominant parietal lobe injury, Chapter 8), children have dyslexia with impairment of arithmetic skills (dyscalculia), impairment of left-right identification, and poor handwriting (dysgraphia). Overall, dyslexic children often have family members with a similar disorder and are disproportionately left-handed boys.

Neuropsychologic learning disabilities, which seem, in fact, to be childhood varieties of adult-onset syndromes, have also been associated with nondominant hemisphere injury. In particular, dyslexic older children and young adults have impaired spatial perception and a paucity of gesture and vocal emotion (prosody, Chapter 8) along with left-sided clumsiness, hyperactive DTRs, and other lateralized signs.

Physical Signs

Physical signs held by some to suggest subtle congenital brain injury—the "soft signs"—may, in fact, be merely manifestations of delayed cerebral maturation. Few soft signs have been statistically correlated with learning disabilities, and examiners' criteria for identifying these signs and determining their significance have been notably subjective and inconsistent. In addition, we are all aware from general observations (including observation of medical colleagues) that many people have excellent learning skills despite poor social graces, handwriting, and athletic abilities.

However, all this is still problematic. As noted previously, language impairments are found in boys much more often than girls, and left-handedness is disproportionately more frequent. Also, children with developmental dyslexia are reported to have slowed or irregular rapid alternating movements (dysdiadochokinesia, Chapter 2), incoordination, unsteadiness, and impaired fine motor movements, e.g., in buttoning clothing. In addition, children with delayed CNS maturation or actual injury often have "overflow" movements: excessive, unnecessary, or contralateral actions that usually occur when a skilled, repetitive task is attempted (Fig. 13-8). They also have persistent fidgety finger and body movements, called "adventitious" or "choreiform," that are similar to those seen in Sydenham's chorea, choreoathetotic CP, or mere restlessness. Curiously, frontal release signs (Chapter 7), which are often found in adults who sustain cerebral injuries, are not described in children with suspected brain injury.

Other commonly cited soft signs are unilateral "posturing" while walking on the sides of feet (Fig. 13-1), asymmetric DTRs, unsustained clonus, and inability to move the eyes without head motion. However, these movements may be manifestations of anxiety or disinhibition, rather than combinations of abnormalities of the basal ganglia and corticospinal tract.

Some childhood disturbances, which are occasionally considered soft signs, are in themselves especially important and in a different class from such problematic signs as left handedness. For example, speech difficulties (dysarthrias), whether or not they are associated with brain injury, possibly indicate a major pathologic condition and almost always interfere with school performance. Specific causes of dysarthria include pseudobulbar palsy, athetosis, cleft palate, and hearing impairment. Likewise, childhood gait impairments may be due to spastic diplegia (see above), Duchenne's muscular dystrophy (Chapter 6), and torsion dystonia (Chapter 18). Dysconjugate ocular gaze usually results from simple ocular muscle imbalance (strabis-

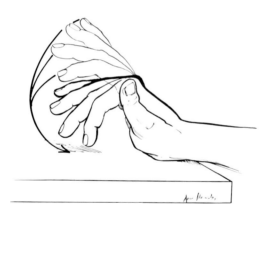

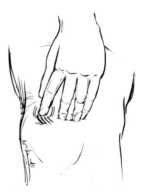

Fig. 13-8. Synkinetic overflow movements are revealed when all fingers move in unison after the child was asked to tap only his right index finger on the desk. In addition, "mirror" overflow movement is induced as his left fingers also begin to tap. Although mirror movements are normal before age 10 years, in children with hemiplegic CP they are first prominent in the "good" hand and eventually both hands.

mus); however, when it is found in combination with face, head, ear, and hand abnormalities, it is correlated with cerebral dysfunction. Moreover, persistent deviation of one eye will lead to loss of vision in that eye, i.e., *amblyopia*.

Laboratory Findings

Although some CT series report that dyslexic children have occipital lobe abnormalities or reversal of the usual planum temporale (language area) asymmetry, there are no specific CT abnormalities in ADD or MBD children. Routine EEG abnormalities, reportedly present in 25 to 75 percent of cases, include dominant frequency slowing, interhemispheric asymmetry, and sharp waves. However, these abnormalities, like soft signs, depend on the examiner, the patients studied, and the criteria applied. Also, the EEG changes are even more likely than the soft signs to be age-related, nonspecific, or even induced by movement, sleep, and medications.

Sophisticated studies, such as spectral analysis and evoked potentials, of children with learning disabilities have found only inconsistent, diffuse, or multifocal abnormalities that do not have a clear relation to cerebral language areas. In short, laboratory evaluation cannot provide confirmation of a diagnosis of either MBD or ADD.

Differential Diagnosis

Of the many possible causes of childhood neurologic impairments, the physician must give first consideration to congenital injuries: cerebral palsy, mental retardation, and visual or auditory impairments. In addition, several common conditions should also be considered, one being parent's giving various prescription or over-the-counter medications to children. For example, phenobarbital, cough medications, and antihistamines may cause hyperactivity. Migraines occasionally cause hyperactivity, as well as episodic behavioral disturbances that also mimic seizures, gastrointestinal difficulties, and mental alterations. Finally, both absence (petit mal) and partial complex seizures both may develop in childhood and cause inattentiveness and learning disabilities (Chapter 10).

MBD in Adults

Congenital mild brain injury is usually not a problem in adults. Childhood hyperactivity becomes controlled, if not by nervous system maturation, then by social constraints, and learning disabilities are avoided as appropriate occupations are chosen.

Nevertheless, some MBD children grow up to become MBD adults, in whom erratic behavior, poor organization, and inattentiveness may indicate subtle cerebral dysfunction. Many neurologists also feel that so-called rages, episodic dyscontrol, and idiosyncratic (pathologic) alcohol intoxication may partly result from congenital brain injury. Adults with MBD, like children with MBD, are clearly liable to have paradoxical reactions to barbiturates, other sedatives, and alcohol. Likewise, some have reportedly benefited from stimulants.

REFERENCES

Elliott FA: The episodic dyscontrol syndrome and aggression. In: Symposium on the Border-land Between Neurology and Psychiatry. Neurol Clin 2:113,1984

Golden GS: Neurobiological corelates of learning disabilities. Ann Neurol 12:409,1982

Haslam RHA, Dably JT, Johns RD, et al: Cerebral asymmetry in developmental dyslexia. Arch Neurol 38:679, 1981

Herskowitz J, Rosman PN: Pediatrics, Neurology, and Psychiatry—Common Ground. Behavioral, Cognitive, Affective, and Physical Disorders in Childhood and Adolescence. New York, Macmillan, 1982

Johnston RB, Stark RE, Mellits ED, et al: Neurological status of language-impaired and normal children. Ann Neurol 10:159, 1981

Nass R: Mirror movement asymmetries in congenital hemiparesis. Neurology 35:1059, 1985

Perkins WJ (ed): High Technology Aids for the Disabled. Boston, Butterworths, 1983

Riccardi VM: Von Recklinghausen neurofibromatosis. N Engl J Med 305:1617, 1981

Schwartz J, Kaplan E, Schwartz A: Childhood dyscalculia and Gerstmann syndrome: A clinical and statistical analysis. Neurology 31:81, 1981

Weintraub S, Mesulam MM: Developmental learning disabilities of the right hemisphere: Emotional, interpersonal, and cognitive components. Arch Neurol 40:463, 1983

Wender PH, Reimherr FW, Wood DR: Attention deficit disorder ("minimal brain dysfunction") in adults. Arch Gen Psychiatry 38:449, 1981

QUESTIONS

1–11. Match the neurocutaneous disorder with its manifestations:

1. Acoustic neuroma
2. Cutaneous lesions resembling rhinophyma
3. Progressive dementia
4. Neurofibromas
5. Adenoma sebaceum
6. Cauda equina syndrome
7. Intractable epilepsy
8. Café au lait spots
9. Facial angiomatosis
10. Optic glioma
11. Cutaneous lesions should not be mistaken for acne

a. Tuberous schlerosis
b. Von Recklinghausen's disease
c. Sturge-Weber Syndrome

12–17. Which of the following disorders causes episodic changes in mood or inattentiveness in children?

12. Migraines
13. Partial complex seizures
14. Antihistamines
15. Cerebral palsy
16. Sedative medications
17. Absences

18. In which of the following conditions will CT provide useful diagnostic information?
a. Attention deficit disorder   e. Sturge-Weber syndrome
b. Absences   f. Learning disabilities
c. Migraines   g. Tuberous sclerosis
d. Hydrocephalus   h. Tourette's syndrome

19. Which of the following procedures or developments has helped reduce the incidence of congenital brain injury or abnormality?
a. Prenatal chromosome analysis
b. Neonatal exchange transfusion
c. Fetal cardiac monitoring during labor
d. Amniocentesis
e. Ultrasound examinations
f. Prevention of RH incompatibility

20. Children who sustain brain injury of any sort until the age of 5 years are all eligible for assistance by most programs that serve CP children (True/False).

21. Which of the following is *not* usually found in children with mental retardation?
a. Dyslexia
b. Dysarthria
c. Hyperactivity

22. Which of the following is (are) *not* usually found in children with cerebral palsy?
a. Dyslexia
b. Dysarthria
c. Hyperactivity
d. Seizures

23. Adults with penetrating head injuries (e.g., gunshot wounds) frequently have:
a. Aphasia   d. Hyperactivity
b. Paresis   e. Seizures
c. Cerebral palsy   f. Mental retardation

24. A 1-year-old boy has a stroke because of sickle cell disease. This results in mild right hemiparesis. Which of the following will probably be additional consequences?
a. Chorea   d. Spastic cerebral palsy
b. Aphasia   e. Stunted growth of right arm
c. Seizures   f. Minimal brain dysfunction

25–30. Match the disorder with the cause.

25. Choreoathetosis   a. Cervical cord injury
26. Spastic quadriplegia   b. Kernicterus
27. Spastic hemiparesis   c. Cerebral anoxia
28. Deafness   d. Stroke in utero
29. Seizure disorder
30. Cortical blindness

31. List the following types of cerebral palsy in the order of increasing frequency of the likelihood of mental retardation.
a. Choreoathetosis
b. Spastic diplegia
c. Spastic quadriplegia
d. Spastic hemiplegia
e. Mixed spastic choreoathetosis

32. Which of the above types of CP has the lowest incidence of seizures?

33. Which of the above may not be apparent until as late as 2 years of age?

34. Which is the most commonly encountered form?

35. In which form are the legs affected more than the arms?

36. A 10-year-old boy is observed to have "fidgety" movements of the hands and feet and facial grimacing. Which of the following disorders may be present in childhood and may be manifested by such movement disorders?

    a. Cerebral palsy

    b. Minimal brain dysfunction

    c. Sydenham's chorea

    d. Wilson's disease

37–43. True or False

37. The predominent EEG frequencies are slower in young children than young adults.

38. Theta frequencies are slower than alpha frequencies.

39. Sleeping during EEG will alter the background activity.

40. Changes in attention will alter the EEG rhythms.

41. Changes in eye opening and closing will alter the EEG.

42. Some medications will alter the EEG.

43. Children will normally have scattered theta activity on an EEG.

ANSWERS

1. b	**16.** Yes	**30.** c
2. a	**17.** Yes	**31.** a, b, c, d, e
3. a	**18.** d, e, g	**32.** a
4. b	**19.** a, b, c, d, e, f	**33.** a
5. a	**20.** True	**34.** d
6. b	**21.** c	**35.** b
7. a	**22.** c	**36.** a, b, c, d
8. b	**23.** a, b, e	**37.** True
9. c	**24.** c, d, e	**38.** True
10. b	**25.** b	**39.** True
11. a	**26.** a or c	**40.** True
12. Yes	**27.** d	**41.** True
13. Yes	**28.** b	**42.** True
14. Yes	**29.** c or d	**43.** True
15. No.		

14

Neurologic Aspects of Pain

Newly discovered anatomic and biochemical information has led to considering pain as an entity as well as a symptom of different illnesses. Physicians can now offer more rational therapy for pain and its affective component, suffering. In particular, they can now more effectively treat patients who previously would have suffered intractable pain from stable bodily injuries, metastatic cancer, or chronic illnesses.

This chapter will first review the body's own *endogenous opiate* analgesic system. It then will trace anatomic "nociceptive pathways," which serve to convey pain (noxious stimulation) from injuries to the brain, and "antinociceptive pathways," which provide pain relief (analgesia). It will describe the ways in which analgesia is produced by the endogenous opiate pathway of the central nervous system, pain relieving medicines (analgesics), and certain surgical procedures.

ENDOGENOUS OPIATES

Endogenous opiates, often called *endorphins* (endogenous morphine-like substances), are mainly amino acid chains (polypeptides) synthesized in the central nervous system that bind onto and work through the same CNS receptor sites as the "exogenous" or "naturally occurring" opiates, such as morphine (Table 14-1). Experiments and several clinical trials in which endogenous opiates have been administered have shown that they produce the same effects as morphine, primarily analgesia, mood elevation (euphoria), sedation, and respiratory depression. Like morphine, repetitive administration leads to increasingly greater quantities being required to produce their effects (*tolerance*) and physical signs of withdrawal upon abstinence (*dependence*). In addition, naloxone (Narcan) reverses the effects of endogenous opiates just as it does the effects of morphine. Indeed, the narcotic antagonist effect of naloxone is so reliable that *naloxone-reversibility* is the criteria for determining whether the effect of an analgesic is mediated by the opiate pathways.

Many endogenous opiates and the adrenocorticotropin (ACTH) molecule appear

Table 14-1

Glossary

Beta endorphin: An endogenous opiate, concentrated in the pituitary gland, that consists of amino acid numbers 61–91 of beta lipotropin and gives rise to the enkephalins (Fig. 14-1).

Beta lipotropin: A 91-amino-acid polypeptide, which may be an ACTH fragment, that has no opiate activity itself but gives rise to beta endorphin.

Endogenous opiates: Polypeptides (amino acid chains) found within the CNS that create effects similar to those of morphine and other naturally occurring opiates. The effects of endogenous opiates and naturally occurring opiates are characteristically reversed by naloxone (Narcan).

Endorphins: Endogenous morphine-like substances that are a variety of endogenous opiates.

Enkephalins: Met-enkephalin, leu-enkephalin, and others, are 5-amino-acid polypeptides that are endogenous opiates found widely in the brain and dorsal horn of the spinal cord.

Naloxone (Narcan): A pure opiate antagonist that reverses all effects of endogenous and naturally occurring opiates.

Substance P: An 11-amino-acid polypeptide that is probably the primary pain neurotransmitter at the synapse of peripheral nerves with the lateral spinothalamic tract in the spinal cord.

---

to be derived from a large common precursor molecule (Fig. 14-1). The runners' "high," the painlessness of wounded soldiers, and effectiveness of placebos are all postulated to result from endogenous opiates secreted along with ACTH in such people who are under stress.

A large polypeptide fragment of the precursor molecule, *beta lipotropin,* which is concentrated in the pituitary gland, is not itself an endogenous opiate; however, *beta endorphin,* which constitutes amino acid sequence 61–91 of beta lipoprotein and is also concentrated in the pituitary, is an endogenous opiate. *Enkephalins* are short polypeptide endogenous opiates that include *met enkephalin,* which is a fragment of beta endorphin, and *leu enkephalin,* a fragment of a different precursor. Enkephalins, which may be even more potent than beta endorphin, are located in the amygdala, the brainstem, the spinal cord, and other areas of the CNS.

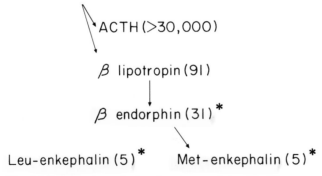

Fig. 14-1. The important endogenous opiates (*). The number of amino acid units in their polypeptide chain is noted within parentheses. A large precursor molecule (not pictured) gives rise to ACTH and beta lipotropin, which are often released together. Beta lipotropin gives rise to beta endorphin and met-enkephalin, but another precursor gives rise to leu-enkephalin.

PAIN AND ANALGESIA PATHWAYS

Peripheral Systems

Painful tissue inflammation liberates various chemicals, including prostaglandins and bradykinin, which stimulate certain peripheral nerve receptors (nociceptors). Pain may be alleviated at this very first step, while the process is still in the "periphery," with aspirin, acetaminophen (Tylenol), steroids, and nonsteroidal antiinflammatory agents, including ibuprofen (Motrin, Nuprin, Advil). These medicines are analgesic in part because they inhibit synthesis of prostaglandins or in other ways reduce tissue inflammation.

Pain, whether it originates from pressure, heat, or inflammation, is carried by two types of peripheral nerve fibers. *A delta* fibers, which are thinly myelinated fibers of small diameter, convey sharp or prickling sensations from the skin and mucous membranes. *C fibers,* unmyelinated but also small, convey nearly all painful sensations from the viscera and other tissues. Painful transmission along A delta and C fibers may be dampened by stimulation of large, heavily myelinated sensory fibers. This analgesic effect may be why people instinctually massage an injury at a proximal site. For example, a person spraining an ankle will rub the lower leg.

The famous "gate theory" of analgesia is based on this observation. It suggests that stimulation of large diameter, heavily myelinated fibers that carry vibration and position sensation, *A beta* fibers, inhibits pain transmission by the small fibers with little or no myelin. The gate theory has given rise to *transcutaneous electrical nerve stimulation (TENS),* in which electric current stimulation reduces pain.

Another way of reducing pain is to interrupt (block) the entire peripheral nerve by alcohol injection. *Nerve blocks* are useful in chest and abdominal pain because the thoracic and lumbar nerve roots can be injected with alcohol as they emerge from the vertebrae. However, this technique is usually not feasible for painful limbs because it will create paresis as well as analgesia. Nor is it practical with facial pain within the first division (V_1) of the trigeminal nerve, since analgesia involving the cornea leads to corneal ulcerations.

Sometimes sympathetic plexus or ganglia blockade is helpful. For example, in pancreatic carcinoma, the celiac plexus might be infiltrated with alcohol, and in the hand–shoulder syndrome, the cervical (stellate) ganglia can be infiltrated.

Central Systems

PAIN TRANSMISSION TO THE BRAIN

The peripheral nerve fibers enter the CNS at the dorsal horn of the spinal cord. They synapse either immediately or after ascending a few segments. At each synapse, the fibers release *substance P,* a small polypeptide, that is essentially the neurotransmitter for pain in the spinal cord (Fig. 14-2). After the synapse, a second neuron crosses to the other side of the spinal cord and ascends to the brain within the *lateral spinothalamic tract,* contralateral to the injury (see Figs. 2-6 and 2-14). There are also other, less well-defined tracts. Tracts carrying pain synapse primarily in the thalamus but also in the reticular activating system, other regions of the brainstem, and the limbic system.

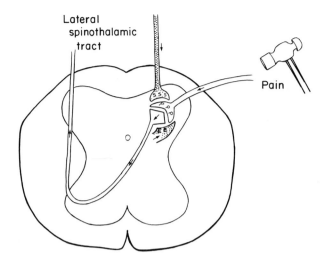

Fig. 14-2. Painful sensations are conveyed along the *A delta* and *C* fibers of the peripheral nerves to the dorsal horn of the spinal cord where, probably utilizing *substance P* (P), they synapse with the lateral spinothalamic tract, which ascends to the brain. Two (stippled) pain-dampening analgesic systems play upon the dorsal horn synapse: A tract that descends from the brain, which releases *serotonin* (S), and a spinal interneuron, which releases *enkephalins* (E).

To provide analgesia, usually in selected cases of malignant pain, the spinothalamic tract may be interrupted by severing the lateral portion of the spinal cord contralateral to the pain. This technique, called a *cordotomy,* is particularly useful when patients have intractable pain confined to a limb or one side of the trunk. However, it is not suitable for more generalized pain because bilateral spinal cord incisions can create respiratory drive difficulties (Ondiene's curse) and loss of bladder control.

In contrast to the analgesia produced by cordotomy, thalamic lesions usually do not create analgesia. In fact, both cerebrovascular accidents (CVAs) involving the thalamus and surgically created thalamic lesions often cause a distinctive burning sensation ("thalamic pain") that is felt on the contralateral side of the body. Also, while cerebral cortical injury from a CVA or a surgical procedure, such as a frontal lobotomy, reduces suffering, neither reduces the sensation of pain being present. As can commonly be observed, patients with CVAs still feel painful injuries in affected limbs but the affective component is blunted.

ANALGESIA PATHWAYS IN THE SPINAL CORD AND BRAIN

Not all peripheral nerves synapse in the dorsal horn and give rise to the lateral spinothalamic tract. Some synapse onto short neurons, *interneurons,* which play upon the lateral spinothalamic tract and block nociceptive transmission. These neurons release enkephalins, which provide analgesia that can be mimicked by intrathecal (intraspinal) injections of morphine and reversed by naloxone.

A descending spinal cord tract in the *dorsolateral funiculus* originates in the lower brainstem and relieves pain by playing on the lateral spinothalamic tract or other nociceptive pathways. Unlike other analgesic pathways, its neurons release *serotonin*. Some antidepressants, which have analgesic properties in addition to their mood-altering properties, presumably raise serotonin concentrations in this spinal cord pathway. Similarly, substances that deplete serotonin intensify pain.

Brainstem structures also give rise to short analgesic brainstem tracts. If these tracts are stimulated electrically, endogenous opiates are released, producing analgesia and euphoria.

THERAPIES

For patients with chronic, intractable pain due to undetermined or untreatable causes, a variety of medications and procedures can now be instituted alone or, preferably, in combination. While these treatments will not substitute for emotional support, they can be the physiologic basis for relief of the pain and suffering.

Mild Analgesics

Aspirin is one of the best analgesics. Two tablets (600 mg) have about the same potency as the standard dose of propoxyphene (Darvon), codeine, or oral meperidine (Demerol). Since aspirin and nonsteroidal anti-inflammatory agents are analgesic in large measure because they inhibit the synthesis of prostaglandins, they are more effective if taken before a painful injury. Also, since these analgesics act at the site of injury, i.e., *peripherally,* when they are given in combination with narcotics, which act on CNS opiate pathways *centrally,* they enhance narcotic analgesia. In short, taking two tablets of aspirin will increase the effectiveness of morphine.

Narcotics

Narcotics are the most potent analgesics. In addition, narcotics lessen suffering a great deal more than the peripherally acting analgesics. However, their use may be complicated by side effects and prescription difficulties. For example, patients routinely develop constipation, nausea, sedation, and those with lung disease, respiratory depression. Also, physicians, being fearful of the tendency of narcotics to produce tolerance and dependency, often prescribe them in too small or infrequent quantities and are subsequently reluctant to increase dosages appropriately during an illness.

If analgesics must be requested by the patient and given by nurses only after pain begins, the delay in treatment makes pain more difficult to alleviate. Moreover, the patient, worried about the recurrence of pain and about obtaining relief, becomes preoccupied and anxious. For practical purposes, narcotics should be given on a regular prophylactic basis, such as every two to three hours while the patient is awake, rather than at the onset of pain. They should be administered freely, frequently, and in large enough doses to preempt the pain.

As tolerance and dependency invariably develop, even more frequent and larger doses should be administered. Although the addition of psychotropic medicines might provide a synergistic effect, even moderate doses of narcotics can be given to patients in pain without causing respiratory depression or, unless desired, sedation. Moreover, not only is addiction an unrealistic consideration in seriously or terminally ill patients, it rarely occurs in patients with normal premorbid mental health who develop a brief, painful illness.

Constipation can be prevented with a combination of laxatives, such as Senokot, and stool softeners, such as Colace. Nausea, whether it is caused by the underlying illness, radiotherapy, chemotherapy, or the narcotics themselves, should be reduced with antiemetic suppositories, injections, or pills. (Since antiemetics are often composed of phenothiazines, doses that are too large can precipitate dystonic reactions [Chapter 18]).

Several narcotics are quite effective when given orally in a sufficiently large dose at frequent intervals. As initial medication and dosage, the following are suitable: morphine (30 mg q3h), hydromorphone (Dilaudid) (4 mg q3h), and levorphanol (Levo-Dromoran) (2 mg q4h). Methadone (Dolophine) is also satisfactory, especially since it is long-acting, but it is hard to obtain. For intramuscular use, morphine (10 mg q3h), hydromorphone (2 mg q3h), or levorphanol (2 mg q4h) are able to provide more substantial analgesia. These also can be given in an intravenous solution to provide continuous analgesia and decreased anxiety. However, since the effects of narcotics are dependent upon the route of administration, the same dose that is given orally may produce an overdose if given intramuscularly or intravenously. If the situation is reversed, undertreatment may precipitate narcotic withdrawal and recurrence of severe pain.

In special situations, narcotics may be administered either intrathecally or just outside the spinal cord covering (epidurally). These methods, which act directly on the spinal cord, may provide long-lasting relief of lower trunk, pelvic, and leg pain without producing mental changes. However, this method may be complicated by respiratory depression, which is naloxone-reversible, or by inflammation of the spinal cord covering (arachnoiditis).

Meperidine (Demerol), although probably the most frequently prescribed narcotic, is usually unsatisfactory. Since it is poorly absorbed when taken orally but well absorbed when given intramuscularly, changing routes of administration leads to complications. Moreover, when doses that are sufficient for analgesia are given for several days, especially in patients with renal insufficiency, accumulation of meperidine metabolites, e.g., normeperidine, can cause mental aberrations and then tremulousness, myoclonus (Chapter 18), seizures, and stupor.

Another overrated analgesic is heroin. Not only is the effectiveness of heroin in relieving pain and improving mood no greater than an appropriate dose of morphine, its potential for abuse is much greater. In "Brompton's cocktail" and its variations, heroin is combined with cocaine, chloroform water (for flavor), phenothiazines (for nausea), and gin or another alcoholic beverage. Unfortunately, these preparations, which have received popular support, are no more effective or better tolerated than adequate doses of morphine and antiemetics.

Finally, narcotics that possess narcotic antagonist properties, such as pentazocine (Talwin) and butorphanol (Stadol) have limited use. They were developed, quite rationally, to prevent addiction by incorporating narcotic antagonist properties into narcotic analgesics. Nevertheless, they are addictive and have psychomimetic effects that may produce hallucinations. Also, chronic injection of pentazocine leads to skin and muscle necrosis. Moreover, because of their antagonistic properties, a change from morphine (or a similar narcotic) to one of these mixed agonist-antagonist drugs will produce pain recurrence and withdrawal symptoms.

Psychotropic Medications

Adding tranquilizers or sedatives to analgesics is often beneficial because they reduce anxiety, restore sleep, and reduce painful muscle spasms. They also reduce requirements for narcotics and hypnotics.

Antidepressants are particularly beneficial. Sometimes they alone are sufficient for chronic pain from low back pain, degenerative arthritis, and tension headaches (Chapter 9). Not only do antidepressants treat the affective components of the illness, restore sleep patterns, and reduce anxiety, they may also produce analgesia by increasing serotonin concentrations in CNS analgesic pathways. This analgesia is not considered to be mediated through the endogenous opiate system because naloxone does not reverse it.

Acupuncture

Scientific data suggest that acupuncture is an effective form of analgesia in some people with mildly to moderately painful injuries. The "meridians," which are the traditional areas in which needles are placed, have been shown to be less important than dermatomes (see Figs. 2-15 and 16-2) for securing analgesia. Since acupuncture is associated with a rise in CSF endorphins and the analgesia is naloxone-reversible, acupuncture is presumed to work through the endogenous opiate system.

Placebos and Hypnosis

Placebos, which are commonly given by physicians either deliberately or when they prescribe ineffectual medications, will produce a definite but brief period of analgesia in about 30 percent of patients. They are most effective for acute, severe pain and least effective for continual minor pain. Also, they are particularly effective when patients have marked anxiety. Contrary to popular notion, a beneficial response to placebo does not mean that a patient's pain is psychogenic; however, people with anxiety do respond better. Since the analgesic effect of placebos is partially naloxone-reversible, placebos presumably stimulate the endogenous opiate system.

Hypnosis is occasionally useful in a wide variety of chronic painful conditions for a brief period. It is different than placebo therapy because patients' ability to be hypnotized does not correlate with their response to placebos, and hypnosis-induced analgesia is not naloxone-reversible, i.e., "hypnosis is not a placebo."

Stimulation-Induced Analgesia

Transcutaneous electrical nerve stimulation (TENS) has become an accepted, frequently effective treatment. It is especially useful for causalgia and posttraumatic neuralgia, or whenever there is pain in the lower back or limbs. In this technique, an electric stimulus is applied to the skin just proximal to the painful region. Presumably, stimulation of the underlying large nerve fibers, which causes "gating," produces

Table 14-2
Analgesics Mediated by the Endogenous
Opiate System*

Acupuncture
Narcotics
Placebo
Stimulation
TENS (transcutaneous electrical nerve stimulation)
Dorsal column stimulation
Periaqueductal gray matter and other deep brain stimulation

*Since these analgesics are partially or entirely reversed by naloxone
(Narcan), their effects are considered to be mediated by the endogenous
opiate system. In contrast, analgesia induced by tricyclic antidepressants
and hypnosis is not reversed by naloxone.

analgesia. Transcutaneous electric nerve stimulation probably works through the
endogenous opiate system because it is naloxone-reversible in most cases and less
effective in patients who have had prior narcotic treatment.

In a method that was theoretically similar to TENS, *dorsal column stimulation,*
electrodes were inserted directly onto the dorsal columns of the spinal cord. While
stimulation of the dorsal column itself should have produced analgesia, not only was it
ineffective in 50 percent of patients, but the procedure was complicated by infection,
spinal cord trauma, and pain at the electrode site. When dorsal column stimulation
was effective, it was, like TENS, naloxone-reversible.

Stimulation of the CNS has been taken a step further in recent experiments.
Neurosurgeons have implanted electrodes into the periaqueductal gray matter and
other brainstem regions that contain endogenous opiates. Stimulation of these sites
presumably releases stores of powerful endogenous opiates. It produces profound
analgesia that, like that of morphine, is naloxone-reversible, associated with euphoria, and attenuated by tolerance.

SUMMARY

Pain is transmitted from A delta to C peripheral nerve fibers upward through
contralateral lateral spinothalamic tracts to the thalamus, the reticular activating system, and other brainstem regions. The body's own analgesic systems include descending spinal cord tracts that release serotonin, spinal interneurons that release
enkephalins, and brainstem tracts that release endogenous opiates. Endogenous opiates, which include enkephalins, are mostly polypeptides. Like ACTH, they appear to
be derivatives of a large precursor molecule.

Aspirin and nonsteroidal anti-inflammatory agents provide analgesia largely by
inhibiting prostaglandin synthesis. Narcotics, by binding to CNS opiate receptors,
provide analgesia and also reduce suffering, but physicans should anticipate and allow
for tolerance, dependence, and side-effects. Analgesia can also be provided, although
less reliably, by stimulating the endogenous opiate system with acupuncture, placebos, or TENS (Table 14-2). Antidepressants may improve mood, restore sleep, and,
in particular, provide analgesia. Combining psychotropic medicines with analgesics
that act peripherally and ones that act centrally is often best when attempting to
ameliorate pain and reduce suffering.

REFERENCES

Abramowicz M (ed): Drug treatment of cancer pain. The Medical Letter 24:95, 1982

Atkinson JH, Kremer EF, Risch SC, et al: Neuroendocrine function and endogenous opioid peptide systems in chronic pain. Psychosomatics 24:899, 1983

Barber J, Gitelson J: Cancer pain: Psychological management using hypnosis. Ca 30:130, 1980

Fields HL: Pain II: New approaches to management. Ann Neurol 9:101, 1981

Foley KM: The treatment of cancer pain. N Engl J Med 313:84, 1985

Jessell TM: Neurotransmitters and CNS disease: Pain. Lancet 2:1084, 1982

Levine J: Pain and analgesia: The outlook for more rational treatment. Ann Intern Med 100:269, 1984

Reich J, Tupin JP, Abramowitz SI: Psychiatric diagnosis of chronic pain patients. Am J Psychiatry 140:1495, 1983

Spiegel K, Kalb R, Pasternak GW: Analgesic activity of tricyclic antidepressants. Ann Neurol 13:462, 1983

QUESTIONS

1–7. Match the substance with its effect on the pain pathways.

1. Morphine
2. Endogenous opiates
3. Serotonin
4. Substance P
5. Enkephalin
6. Beta endorphin
7. Nonsteroidal anti-inflammatory agents

a. Reduced tissue inflammation and reduced fever
b. Interfere with prostaglandin synthesis
c. Provide analgesia by acting on the CNS
d. Pain neurotransmitter in the spinal cord
e. Liberated in a spinal cord descending analgesic tract

8. Which properties of morphine are *not* shared with endogenous opiates?
    a. Tolerance
    b. Effectiveness in deep brainstem structures and spinal cord
    c. Causing mood changes as well as analgesia
    d. Reversibility with naloxone
    e. Commercial availability
    f. Causing respiratory depression

9–17. What is the composition of these substances?

9. Leu-enkephalin
10. ACTH
11. Morphine
12. Beta endorphin
13. Heroin
14. Beta lipotropin
15. Met-enkephalin
16. Serotonin
17. Substance P

a. 11-amino-acid polypeptide
b. 5-amino-acid polypeptide
c. Diacetyl morphine
d. Greater than 30,000 amino acid polypeptide
e. An indole
f. An alkaloid of opium
g. 91-amino-acid polypeptide
h. 31-amino-acid polypeptide

18. Which of these fibers do *not* carry pain sensation?
    a. A delta
    b. C
    c. A beta

19. In which spinal cord tract does almost all pain sensation ascend?
    a. Fasciculus gracilis
    b. Fasciculus cuneatus
    c. Lateral corticospinal tract
    d. Lateral spinothalamic tract

20. In which tract do pain-dampening fibers that utilize serotonin descend within the spinal cord?
    a. Lateral spinothalamic tract
    b. Dorsolateral funiculus
    c. Fasciculus gracilis
    d. Dentorubral tract

21. Which forms of analgesia are mostly naloxone- reversible?
    a. Acupuncture
    b. Narcotic administration
    c. TENS
    d. Aspirin
    e. Hypnosis
    f. Placebo
    g. Stimulation of periventricular gray matter

22. Why would the addition of aspirin or acetaminophen increase the effectiveness of narcotics?
    a. They are also narcotics
    b. They actually do not increase analgesia
    c. They stimulate endogenous opiate release
    d. They reduce painful inflammation at the site of injury
    e. They increase serotonin reuptake

23. Why are tricyclic and other antidepressants sometimes helpful in treatment of chronic pain?
    a. They treat depression
    b. They help restore restful sleep patterns
    c. They increase serotonin levels, which act to decrease pain
    d. They alter autonomic system activity
    e. They themselves are analgesics

24. What are the potential complications of mixed agonist-antagonist narcotics, such as pentazocine (Talwin)?
    a. Normeperidine accumulation
    b. Addiction
    c. Delirium
    d. Respiratory depression
    e. They can precipitate withdrawal in patients previously using meperidine (Demerol)

25. What are the potential complications of meperidine (Demerol) use?
    a. Marked undertreat when the same dose is given orally as intramuscularly.
    b. Normeperidine toxicity
    c. Overdose when the same dose is given parenterally as orally
    d. Stupor
    e. Seizures
    f. Tremulousness

ANSWERS

1.	c	10.	d	19.	d
2.	c	11.	f	20.	b
3.	e	12.	h	21.	a, b, c, f, g
4	d	13.	c, f	22.	d
5.	c	14.	g	23.	a, b, c, e
6.	c	15.	b	24.	b, c, d, e
7.	a, b	16.	e	25.	a, b, c, d, e, f
8.	e	17.	a		
9.	b	18.	c		

15

Multiple Sclerosis Episodes

Multiple sclerosis (MS),* called "disseminated sclerosis" in the United Kingdom, is important because it is the most common disabling neurologic illness of North American and European young adults. It is characterized by multiple episodes of multiple neurologic deficits. In its early stages only subtle, evanescent disturbances are present. Multiple sclerosis may then be confused with other neurologic conditions or psychologic aberrations. In its later stages, various mental disturbances, induced by combinations of neurologic and psychologic factors, complicate the illness. Overall, despite new tests, the diagnosis of MS and its complications rests on clinical grounds.

ETIOLOGY

A condition of unknown etiology, MS occurs when 1 mm to 3 cm patches of "white matter," the myelin sheaths of CNS axons, become inflamed, then sclerotic, and eventually stripped of myelin. Demyelinated patches, called *plaques*, are scattered (disseminated) throughout the optic nerves, brain, and spinal cord. Even though the body and axon of the nerves are relatively spared, demyelination impairs impulse transmission and causes neurologic deficits. These deficits seem to resolve as the inflammation subsides, but as plaques develop with repeated attacks, neurologic deficits accumulate.

Multiple sclerosis occurs 50 percent more frequently in women than in men and about ten times more frequently in close relatives of MS patients than in the general population. Spouses, however, are not especially vulnerable. The mean age of onset is 33 years, with virtually all cases developing between 15 and 50 years. Some patients suffer their first or subsequent attacks following pregnancy, delivery, infection, physical trauma, electrical injury, or psychologic stress, but there is no significant evidence that any of these factors cause MS.

---

*Patients with MS may receive assistance from the National Multiple Sclerosis Society, 205 East 42nd Street, New York, New York 10017, (212) 986-3240.

Immunologic abnormalities have been found. Patients with MS have increased frequency of particular HLA antigens and decreased suppressor T lymphocytes. Also, as in subacute sclerosing panencephalitis (SSPE) and several other debilitating neurologic illnesses, the CSF often has a high measles antibody titer. Moreover, there is a tendency for MS patients to have contracted measles at an older age than other persons.

Epidemiologic studies have suggested that an infectious agent is responsible. They have shown that the incidence of MS is greatest in patients who have lived, at least through age 15, in cooler northern latitudes (above the 37th parallel). In particular, the incidence of MS is higher in Boston than New Orleans; extremely low in Central Africa, Latin America, and, curiously, Japan; and higher in Europeans who emigrated as adults to Israel than in those who emigrated in childhood. Moreover, epidemiologic studies have suggested that an infectious agent may be transmitted by dogs. Although MS had practically never been diagnosed in the Faeroe islanders, who live off the coast of Scotland, these people suffered a virtual epidemic after British troops and their canine mascots occupied the islands during World War II. Also, many American MS patients had dogs and other small indoor pets while children, but a statistical significance is unproven.

CLINICAL MANIFESTATIONS

Initial manifestations may range from trivial impairment over several days to a group of debilitating disturbances that last for several weeks and do not fully recede. On the average, 2 to 3 years elapse before a recurrence (exacerbation) develops. Then the initial symptoms, accompanied by additional ones, generally recur. Most patients have a course characterized by exacerbations, then partial remissions, and finally accumulated impairments. However, from the outset, about 10 percent have steady deterioration. Many patients reach a state in which they are partially or fully blind, confined to a wheelchair, unable to speak distinctly, and overwhelmed by seemingly unwarranted bouts of emotion. On the other hand, about one third of patients have no functional disability 10 years after the diagnosis.

While many symptoms may occur during the illness, the initial and more frequent ones result from demyelination of the heavily myelinated CNS (white matter) tracts in the spinal cord, brainstem, and optic nerves. Only when the voluminous cerebral white matter has accumulated extensive demyelination, late in the course, does MS produce significant mental impairment. Since the unmyelinated cerebral cortical "gray matter" is relatively spared, MS patients do not develop signs of cerebral cortical dysfunction, such as seizures or aphasia. Likewise, since the basal ganglia are unmyelinated, involuntary movement disorders (Chapter 18) are virtually never manifestations of MS.

The most frequently encountered symptoms, alone or in combination, are paresis, sensory disturbances, ataxia, ocular impairments, bladder and sexual dysfunction, and mental disturbances (Fig. 15-1). Almost all MS patients develop paresis, if not at the onset of illness, then soon afterwards. They usually have paraparesis from spinal cord involvement (see Fig. 2-17), but sometimes hemiparesis from cerebral involvement. In both cases, since the CNS is damaged, patients have hyperactive DTRs and Babinski signs (Chapter 2). Spinal cord involvement is indicated by a characteristic

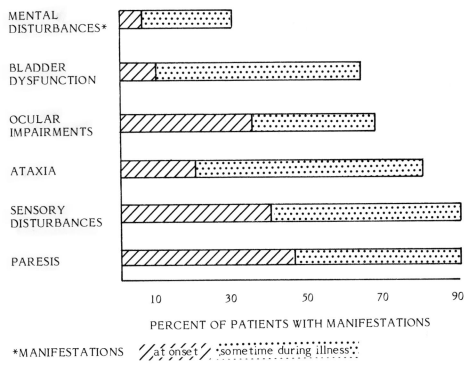

Fig. 15-1. Initial and cumulative manifestations of multiple sclerosis.

electrical sensation that extends from the neck down the spine when the neck is flexed (*Lhermitte's sign*). More important, spinal cord demyelination causes muscle spasticity that leads to gait impairment, painful leg spasms, and bladder and sexual disturbances.

Multiple sclerosis patients almost always also develop ataxia and other manifestations of cerebellar injury. Typically, they have gait ataxia (see Fig. 2-13) that causes them to spread their feet widely apart and lurch forward. When the ataxia is subtle, it can only be elicited by having the patient walk heel-to-toe (*tandem gait*). Other manifestations of cerebellar involvement are intention tremor (see Fig. 2-11), dysdiadochokinesia, and arrhythmic, disconcerting head rocking (*titubation*).

In addition, since their voice production is impaired by both ataxia and paresis, MS patients have dysarthria, typically manifested by irregular voice cadence and inability to separate adjacent sounds (*scanning speech*). For example, when asked to repeat a pair of short syllables, such as "ba . . . ga . . . ba . . . ga . . . ," the patient might place unequal emphasis on each syllable, blur them together, or fail to alternate them.

Sensory disturbances, which are a prominent feature of MS, result from cerebral or spinal cord plaques. Patients have hypalgesia or paresthesias in scattered limb or trunk areas, or below a particular spinal cord level. Since patients' descriptions of their sensory disturbances often overshadow objective findings and do not conform to commonplace neurologic patterns, those patients with only sensory disturbances are liable to be misdiagnosed as suffering from a psychogenic condition.

Ocular impairments, which are often early MS manifestations, include impaired visual acuity and disordered ocular motility. Visual acuity impairment results from attacks of *retrobulbar (optic) neuritis,* which is an inflammatory condition of the retrobulbar portion of the optic nerve (see Fig. 12-7). Optic neuritis causes both an irregular area of visual loss in one eye, a *scotoma* (Fig. 15-2), and pain when the eyes are moved. Since the optic disk is unaffected, ophthalmoscopic examination reveals no abnormality. This discrepancy between visual loss and normal ophthalmoscopy has given rise to the saying, "The patient sees nothing and the physician sees nothing." As an optic neuritis attack subsides, the pain leaves and most, if not all, vision returns. However, with repeated attacks, progressive visual loss ensues and the disk becomes atrophic.

About 25 percent of patients have had overt optic neuritis as their initial symptom, and the majority have had it at some time during their illness. New electrophysiologic studies have shown not only that the majority of MS patients have had optic neuritis attacks, but that almost all patients have had asymptomatic, if not symptomatic, optic neuritis. On the other hand, only 20 to 40 percent of young adults who develop optic neuritis as an isolated condition will later develop MS. Therefore, although optic neuritis is a common MS symptom, a single, simple attack of optic neuritis is not diagnostic of MS.

Multiple sclerosis also causes two ocular movement disturbances: *nystagmus* and the characteristic *internuclear ophthalmoplegia (INO),* which is also called the *medial longitudinal fasciculus (MLF) syndrome.* Nystagmus results from brainstem or cerebellar MS involvement. While MS-induced nystagmus is clinically indistinguishable from nystagmus caused by other conditions (Chapter 12), it frequently occurs in combination with tremor from ataxia and scanning speech (*Charcot's triad*).

Internuclear ophthalmoplegia, which causes diplopia on lateral gaze, results when demyelination or other MLF damage interrupts nerve impulse transmission to the oculomotor nuclei (Figs. 15-3 and 15-4). Although it may result from lupus in young adults and from basilar artery infarctions in elderly patients, INO is virtually pathognomonic of MS. Only botulism may create a confusingly similar picture of ocular motility.

Bladder dysfunction, which is usually a sign of spinal cord MS, in addition to impairing the functional capabilities of patients, causes psychologic repercussions and, even when mild, is associated with sexual impairment (Chapter 16). It results from a combination of spasticity and paresis of the external sphincter of the bladder (Fig. 15-5), paresis of the lower abdominal muscles, and bladder and sphincter incoordination (*dyssynergy*). Affected patients initially have frequent, small, and precipitous urinations, and also incontinence during sleep and sexual intercourse. Later in the illness, patients often develop urinary retention and more frequent incontinence. Many require intermittent or continuous catheterization, which burdens them with risk of infection, as well as esthetic problems.

Sexual impairment (Chapter 16), with or without bladder dysfunction, plagues

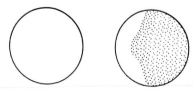

Fig. 15-2. Optic (retrobulbar) neuritis causes impaired vision in a large, irregular area (a *scotom*), which typically includes the center of vision, and pain on eye movement.

MEDIAL LONGITUDINAL
FASCICULUS (MLF)

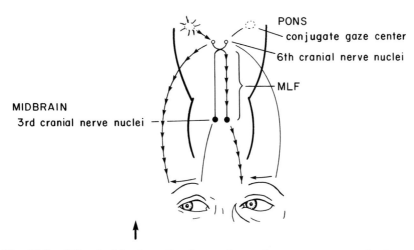

Fig. 15-3. When looking laterally, the pontine conjugate gaze center stimulates the adjacent abducens (sixth) nerve nucleus and, through the *medial longitudinal fasciculus (MLF)*, the contralateral oculomotor (third) nerve nucleus. Thus, when looking to the right, the right abducens and the left oculomotor nuclei are both stimulated (also see Fig. 12-12).

about 85 percent of MS patients. Men may have premature or retrograde ejaculation and impotence. They also have reduced fertility, partly because of sexual impairment and partly because spinal cord MS leads to lowered and abnormal sperm production. Women with MS tend to become unarousable and anorgasmic. Although they remain fertile, pregnancy is associated with exacerbations, and physical impairments make childbearing especially difficult.

MENTAL ABERRATIONS

Disturbances in emotional state and intellectual capacity, which arise from combinations of psychologic and neurologic factors, are frequent. As would be expected, depression in reaction to onset of illness is the most common disturbance; however, patients in remission may be troubled less by depression than by somatic complaints, social impairments, and anxiety.

In some respects, depression is not simply a psychologic response to the illness but a manifestation of cerebral involvement. Depression is found more frequently in MS patients than in those with other chronic neurologic and nonneurologic conditions that yield similar physical impairments. It is especially frequent during exacerbations, late in the course of the illness, or when intellectual function is compromised.

In view of the consequences of MS, the apparent elevation of mood in some patients, so-called "euphoria," has been a striking unexplained paradox. Certainly, some euphoric patients have been masking depression, and others simply have been feeling relief as an MS attack subsides. Besides these psychodynamic mechanisms,

INTERNUCLEAR OPHTHALMOPLEGIA

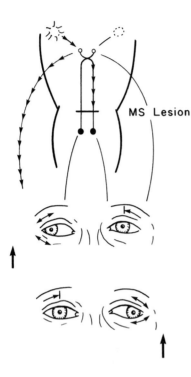

MS Lesion

Fig. 15-4. In *internuclear ophthalmoplegia (INO)*, interruption of the MLF prevents impulses from reaching the oculomotor nuclei. Since the oculomotor nuclei themselves are intact, the pupils and eyelids are normal in both eyes. When looking to the right, because the oculomotor nuclei are not stimulated, the left eye fails to adduct. The right eye abducts, but nystagmus develops. With bilateral INO, which is characteristic of MS, neither eye adducts and the abducting eye has nystagmus.

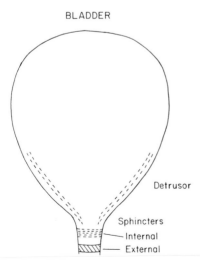

BLADDER

Detrusor

Sphincters
— Internal
— External

Fig. 15-5. Urinary bladder emptying (urination) occurs when the detrusor (wall) muscle contracts and *both* sphincter muscles relax. Voluntary urination requires parasympathetic stimulation (to contract the detrusor and relax the internal sphincter) and also voluntary action (to relax the external sphincter). Urinary retention occurs with either anticholinergic medications or excessive sympathetic activity. Both inhibit detrusor contraction and internal sphincter muscle relaxation. Retention occurs with spinal cord injury because the external sphincter is then spastic and paretic and also because, when the detrusor contracts, the sphincters fail to relax (dyssynergy).

euphoria may also be induced by high-dose ACTH, prednisone, or other steroid MS therapy. Also, laughing and other superficial aspects of euphoria may be manifestations of pseudobulbar palsy (Chapter 4). Since euphoria is associated with physical deterioration and subtle, if not overt, intellectual impairment, it probably results partly from extensive cerebral demyelination. Among the known effects of mood on MS are that emotional conflicts have been associated with exacerbations and that hospitalizations, which presumably remove patients from stress, are associated with remissions.

Intellectual impairments clearly result from extensive cerebral demyelination. Although the cerebral cortical gray matter is usually spared in MS, with long-established disease it may be extensively undercut, irritated by numerous plaques, or damaged in other ways. Thus, overt intellectual impairment does not appear until late in the course of the disease, when physical incapacity is pronounced. Until then, only subtle, nonspecific intellectual changes can be detected. Demonstrating them requires complex neuropsychologic tests, such as the Wechsler Adult Intelligence Scale (WAIS) and the Halstead Category Test.

By contrast, in Alzheimer's disease, which affects the gray matter virtually exclusively, intellectual impairment occurs first and becomes pronounced before any physical impairment develops. Another contrast is with CVAs, which typically damage both gray and white matter and thus cause combined intellectual and physical impairment, such as right hemiparesis and aphasia. Even with multi-infarct dementia, intellectual and physical deficits progress together (Chapter 11).

Sometimes the mental disturbances of MS mimic psychosis. However, the incidence of such pronounced disturbances is much less than that found in other neurologic illnesses, including Alzheimer's disease, head trauma, and partial complex epilepsy. In MS, psychotic disturbances probably originate from intellectual impairment and sensory deprivation. Other causes may be steroid therapy, which can lead to "steroid-induced psychosis," delirium from systemic infection, or other illness. In general, physicians should assume that psychotic behavior and even less pronounced mental aberrations are manifestations of cerebral demyelination or another physical condition.

LABORATORY TESTS

The diagnosis of MS, like such common illnesses as migraine headaches and herniated intervertebral disks, can be based on the patient's history and neurologic examination. Laboratory tests, although potentially useful in some respects, are often superfluous as well as expensive. They are indicated, however, when symptoms are vague, few objective signs are present, or, more important, when only a single overt attack has occurred or a single CNS area is involved. Some tests indicate exacerbations of MS, quiescent as well as active disease, or prior asymptomatic attacks. Unfortunately, no single test is diagnostic, and many false-negative and false-positive results occur.

The "hot-bath test," which still has historic interest, has fortunately fallen into disuse. In this test people who were suspected of having MS were immersed in a very warm bath for about 30 minutes. If the warmth precipitated neurologic deficits that resolved as the patient's temperature returned to normal, a diagnosis of MS was strongly supported. However, the test occasionally produced disabilities from which patients did not recover.

Routine CSF protein analysis during an MS attack will often reveal that while protein concentration is normal (40 mg/100 mL) or only slightly elevated, the gamma globulin portion will be elevated (17 percent or greater). In contrast, in other chronic inflammatory CNS illnesses, including fungal meningitis, neurosyphilis, and SSPE, the CSF is characterized by marked elevations in total protein concentration as well.

A more specific diagnostic indicator is the presence of CSF *oligoclonal bands*. The substance constituting these bands is actually a discrete IgG protein, similar to an antibody, that is found in more than 90 percent of MS patients with either quiescent or active disease. It may, however, also be found in chronic inflammatory CNS illnesses. Another diagnostically important CSF substance is *myelin basic protein*. It is not found either normally or in chronic MS, but presumably because of myelin breakdown, in MS exacerbations and several rare neurologic illnesses, such as leukodystrophies and central pontine myelinolysis. The cost (in 1985) of such CSF analyses, which require a lumbar puncture, is about $250.

Although routine EEGs are not diagnostically helpful, new electrophysiologic *evoked response tests* can reveal visual, auditory, or sensory pathway impairment. The tests are based on repetitive stimulation of these heavily myelinated pathways, which produces (evokes) a characteristic electrical response that may be detected with electrodes similar to those used for EEGs. With any injury, the delay (*latency*) between the stimulus and response is prolonged and often abnormal in form. Evoked response tests are particularly useful in demonstrating asymptomatic demyelinating lesions, the presence of which would indicate that a neurologic illness has affected multiple CNS areas. For example, if a patient has deficits referable only to the spinal cord, but evoked response tests reveal an optic nerve injury, the physician would know that at least two CNS areas were injured, and therefore MS would be a likely diagnosis. The cost of evoked response testing is about $300 to $800.

Visual evoked responses (VERs), which are the most important of these tests, reveal any optic nerve abnormality whether or not the patient or physician is aware of visual impairment. Visual evoked responses are performed by recording the latency as a patient looks at a rapidly flashing television test pattern. Prolonged and otherwise abnormal latencies are found in virtually all cases of MS with optic neuritis. Abnormal results are also found with other optic nerve lesions, such as optic gliomas (Chapter 19), congenital injury (Chapter 13), and optic neuritis when it occurs apart from MS. Visual evoked responses are also helpful in distinguishing ocular from cortical blindness and in identifying psychogenic visual loss (Chapter 12).

Brainstem auditory evoked responses (BAERs) measure responses to a series of clicks in each ear. They are helpful not only in indicating MS brainstem involvement, but in characterizing hearing impairments, diagnosing acoustic neuromas, and evaluating hearing in people unable to cooperate, such as infants and those with autism or psychogenic disturbances.

Somatosensory evoked responses involve application of various stimuli to a patient's arms or legs. Multiple sclerosis or other spinal cord injury will cause latencies to be prolonged or abnormal.

Computed tomography (CT) can demonstrate areas of demyelination that are indicative of MS plaques in either the cerebral or cerebellar white matter. In addition, since asymptomatic as well as symptomatic areas can be demonstrated, CT can show that a neurologic disease is disseminated. However, CT does not demonstrate abnormalities in the location or quantity that would be predicted by the clinical examination. In the near future, magnetic resonance imaging will be the best test to identify optic nerve, spinal cord, or brain demyelination.

Although MS patients have immunologic impairments, the appropriate tests are technically difficult and the results imprecise. For example, although CSF measles antibody titers can be measured, elevated levels are a nonspecific reaction that are found in SSPE and other neurologic conditions. Likewise, HLA antigens and suppressor T lymphocytes are not specific enough markets to be diagnostic.

THERAPY

Systemically administered high-dose ACTH, prednisone, or other steroids may foreshorten an MS attack or even reduce the final deficits. Although such steroid treatment may lead to euphoria or pronounced psychologic changes (steroid-induced "psychosis"), it is rarely complicated by opportunistic infections, such as TB or cryptococcal meningitis, as happens in lupus or renal transplantation treatment. Immunosuppressants besides steroids have been used, but their benefit is equivocal.

Physical therapy helps to preserve muscle tone, prevent decubitus ulcers, and provide maximum mobility. Depending upon the patient's bladder function, appropriate treatment might be medication, such as imipramine (Tofranil), catheterization, or external sphincter removal. Spasticity, another major problem, usually requires baclofen (Lioresal), diazepam (Valium), or other muscle relaxants.

Since depression is so common, physicians are justified in using antidepressant medications. In addition to their mood-elevating effects, these medications may improve sleep and reduce some of the pain associated with immobility and spasticity; however, since the heterocyclic antidepressants have anticholinergic effects, they may precipitate urinary retention and sexual impairment. Almost all patients with established MS can benefit from MS "clubs," clinics, or self-help groups that provide psychologic support and practical information.

CONDITIONS THAT MIMIC MS

Even with CSF analyses and electrophysiologic tests, MS may be difficult to diagnose. Several physically incapacitating conditions that frequently develop in young people may resemble it.

One such condition, the Guillain-Barré syndrome, is a demyelinating disorder of the peripheral nervous system (PNS) that generally strikes young and middle-aged adults (Chapter 5). Patients may have paraparesis or quadriparesis, mild sensory loss, and in severe cases respiratory insufficiency. Since Guillain-Barré syndrome affects PNS myelin, its paresis, unlike that of MS, is symmetric, accompanied by flaccidity and areflexia, and likely to disappear completely. In addition, since Guillain-Barré syndrome is a PNS illness, it does not cause optic neuritis, INO, or mental disturbances.

Brainstem gliomas, which occur in children as well as young adults, mimic MS because the corticospinal, cerebellar, and sensory tracts, and also the MLF, are injured. Cerebral astrocytomas, another neoplastic condition that occurs in young adults, cause cerebral hemisphere impairments, such as hemiparesis, and signs of increased intracranial pressure, such as headaches and papilledema. However, both illnesses produce steadily worsening symptoms and signs referable to a single CNS area, and each can be diagnosed with CT or other radiologic tests.

Although *acquired immune deficiency syndrome (AIDS)* usually begins with signs of systemic illness, such as fever, malaise, and lymphadenopathy, it often later produces combinations of seizures, hemiparesis, and dementia that are usually caused by multiple cerebral lymphomas or brain abscesses from toxoplasmosis or cryptococcosis (Chapter 7). AIDS-induced neurologic illness should not be confused with MS because it has a typically unremitting course and is associated with prominent signs of systemic illness. Also, almost all AIDS patients are found to have serum antibodies to human T-lymphotropic virus type III *(HTLV-III)*, and many of them with neurologic complications have CT, magnetic resonance imaging, and CSF abnormalities that indicate neoplasms or opportunistic infections of the CNS.

Neurologic complications of lupus and other vascular inflammatory diseases may also be confused with MS because they, too, produce multiple CNS abnormalities. Although lupus rarely appears as a neurologic illness, it eventually can cause the "three S's" of lupus: seizures, strokes, and psychosis.

In patients with paraparesis only, alternative diagnoses are spinal cord disorders that include combined system disease (B_{12} deficiency), cervical spine degeneration, and spinal meningiomas. Thus, spine x-rays, myelograms, and serum B_{12} level determinations are often used for differential diagnosis.

Probably the most common condition with which MS is confused is a psychogenic disorder (Chapter 3). Both people with MS and those with psychogenic disorders may have blurred vision, clumsiness, sexual impairments, and atypical sensory losses. If the neurologic examination fails to reveal definitive, abnormal neurologic signs, further investigation with VERs, CSF analysis, and other tests is indicated.

REFERENCES

Baretz RM, Stephenson GR: Emotional responses to multiple sclerosis. Psychosomatics 22:117, 1981

Baum HM, Rothschild BB: The incidence and prevalence of reported multiple sclerosis. Ann Neurol 10:420, 1981

Dalos NP, Rabins PV, Brooks BR, et al: Disease activity and emotional state in multiple sclerosis. Ann Neurol 13:573, 1983

Hallpike JF, Addams CWM, Tourtelloutte WW (eds): Multiple Sclerosis: Pathology, Diagnosis and Management. Baltimore, Williams & Wilkins, 1983

Korn-Lubetzki I, Kahana K, Cooper G, et al: Activity of multiple sclerosis during pregnancy and puerperium. Ann Neurol 16:229, 1984

Levy RM, Bredesen DE, Rosenblum ML: Neurologic manifestations of the acquired immunodeficiency syndrome (AIDS): Experience at UCSF and review of the literature. J Neurosurg 62:475, 1985

Marsh GG: Disability and intellectual function in multiple sclerosis patients. J Nerv Ment Dis 168:758, 1980

Peyser JM, Edwards KR, Poser CM, et al: Cognitive function in patients with multiple sclerosis. Arch Neurol 37:577, 1980

Poser CM: Exacerbations, activity, and progression in multiple sclerosis. Arch Neurol 37:471, 1980

Reisner T, Maida E: Computerized tomography in multiple sclerosis. Arch Neurol 37:475, 1980

Scheinberg LC (ed): Multiple Sclerosis: A Guide for Patients and Their Families. New York, Raven Press, 1983

Schiffer RB, Caine ED, Bamford KA, et al: Depressive episodes in patients with multiple sclerosis. Am J Psychiatry 140:1498, 1983

Snider WD, Simpson DM, Nielsen S, et al: Neurological complications of acquired immune deficiency syndrome: Analysis of 50 patients. Ann Neurol 14:403, 1983

Whitlock FA, Siskind MM: Depression as a major symptom of multiple sclerosis. J Neurol Neurosurg Psychiatry 43:861, 1980

QUESTIONS

1–5. A 25-year-old policeman develops paraparesis and markedly impaired visual acuity in his left eye over four days. Aside from a delayed light reaction in the left eye and lower extremity hyperactive deep tendon reflexes with Babinski signs accompanying the paraparesis, his neurologic examination is normal.

1. Which of the following disorders are possible causes of his disturbances?
   a. Spinal cord tumor
   b. Hysteria
   c. Multiple sclerosis
   d. Postvaccination encephalomyelitis
   e. Wilson's disease

2. Which areas of the nervous system are most likely to be involved?
   a. Right occipital lobe and thoracic spinal cord
   b. Thoracic spinal cord and left optic nerve
   c. Sacral spinal cord and left optic nerve

3. After 3 weeks, he becomes ambulatory and finds that his vision is almost normal. One year later, however, he develops dysarthria, ataxia, and tremor of the arms. Where is the new lesion?
   a. Cerebrum
   b. Cerebellum
   c. Brainstem
   d. Spinal cord

4. While a diagnosis cannot be made with complete assurance, this patient's illness is typical of a certain disorder. What is it?

5. A year after the episode of cerebellar dysfunction, he develops paraparesis, urinary and fecal incontinence, and complete loss of sensation below the umbilicus. What diagnostic procedure is indicated?
   a. Cranial computed tomography
   b. Visual evoked responses
   c. Myelography
   d. None of the above

6. Use of which of the following substances is associated with optic neuritis?
   a. Tobacco
   b. Oral contraceptives
   c. Ethyl alcohol
   d. Methyl alcohol
   e. Penicillin
   f. Heroin

7. With which of the following conditions is optic neuritis associated?
   a. Rubella   d. Combined system disease
   b. Gonorrhea   e. Sarcoidosis
   c. Multiple sclerosis   f. Vasculitis

8. Which of the following conditions may lead to internuclear ophthalmoplegia?
   a. Multiple sclerosis   d. Lupus erythematosus
   b. Subdural hematoma   e. Pontine gliomas
   c. Hysteria   f. Brainstem infarctions

9–12. A 60-year-old man has difficulty walking, lower back pains that radiate to the trunk and legs, loss of position sense (but intact pain and touch sense) in the feet, and pupils that are small and unreactive to light. Strength in the lower extremities is normal, but deep tendon reflexes are absent. He walks with a broad-based gait.

9. What is the origin of the gait disturbance?
   a. Cerebellar disturbance
   b. Spinal cord compression
   c. Multiple sclerosis
   d. Hysteria
   e. Dysfunction of tracts of the spinal cord

10. Although the pupils were small and unreactive to light, they were found to accommodate, i.e., become smaller when the patient looks at a closely held object. What is the pupillary disturbance called?

11. While the patient had dysfunction of two parts of the nervous system, he did not have multiple sclerosis. What disease is he most likely to have?

12. What laboratory test would be most helpful in confirming the clinical impression?

13–17. A 32-year-old man develops blindness and weakness and sensory loss of the right arm and leg. Deep tendon and plantar reflexes are normal. Pupils are equal and reactive to light. He recovers spontaneously after two days and is asymptomatic for one month, when he develops paraparesis. Although he cannot perceive pain below the umbilicus, he can distinguish warm from cold and perceive vibration and position sense. Deep tendon, plantar, anal and cremasteric reflexes are normal.

13. If the patient's right-sided weakness has been the result of cerebral multiple sclerosis or other lesions, with which of the following would his condition be associated?
   a. Weakness of the lower face on the right
   b. Weakness of the lower face on the left
   c. Alterations in the deep tendon reflexes on the right
   d. A flexor plantar response
   e. An extensor plantar response

14. In the second episode, the preservation of temperature sensation despite loss of pain sensation indicates that:
   a. The lateral spinothalamic tract is impaired
   b. The posterior columns are impaired
   c. There is a peripheral neuropathy
   d. None of the above

15. In multiple sclerosis, blindness is usually the result of retrobulbar or optic neuritis that often leads to optic atrophy. Under these circumstances, what are the pupillary reactions?
   a. The pupils are normally reactive to light
   b. The light reflex is impaired

16. With spinal cord injuries, how are the cremasteric and anal reflexes altered?

17. What is the origin of the patient's multiple symptoms that have occurred multiple times?

18–24. Match the ocular movement disorder with the cause(s).

18. Pupillary dilation, ptosis, and paresis of adduction

19. Bilateral ptosis

20. Bilateral horizontal nystagmus

21. Bilateral horizontal nystagmus, unilateral paresis of abduction, and areflexic DTRs

22. Nystagmus in abducting eye and paresis of adduction of other eye

23. Ptosis bilaterally, paresis of adduction of one eye, and normal pupils

24. Nystagmus in adducting eye and paresis of abduction of other eye

a. Wenicke's encephalopathy
b. Labyrinthitis
c. Psychogenic disorders
d. Myasthenia gravis
e. Multiple sclerosis
f. Midbrain infarction
g. None of above

25–28. With which conditions are the following laboratory results associated?

25. Anti-ACh receptor antibodies

26. CSF oligoclonal bands

27. CSF myelin basic protein

28. Antistriational antibodies

a. MS in its chronic phase
b. MS in its acute phase
c. Psychogenic disorders
d. Generalized myasthenia gravis
e. Fungal meningitis
f. Myasthenia with underlying thymoma

29. Of the natives of the following cities, who would have the highest and the lowest MS incidence?

    a. New Orleans
    b. Boston
    c. Tokyo

30. Which of the following people have the highest and lowest incidence of MS?

    a. Native Israelis (Sabras)
    b. All European immigrants to Israel
    c. Black Africans

31. In which situations do visual evoked responses (VERs) show prolonged or otherwise abnormal latencies?

    a. Asymptomatic optic neuritis
    b. Retrobulbar neuritis
    c. Almost all patients with longstanding MS
    d. Patients with psychogenic blindness
    e. Optic nerve gliomas

32. In MS patients, with which finding(s) is urinary incontinence associated?

    a. Leg spasticity
    b. Ataxia
    c. Spasticity of the external sphincter of the bladder
    d. Sexual impairment
    e. Internuclear ophthalmoplegia (MLF syndrome)

33. Which symptoms may develop only late, if at all, in the course of MS?

    a. Pseudobulbar palsy
    b. Internuclear ophthalmoplegia
    c. Optic neuritis
    d. Bladder dysfunction
    e. Neurologic-induced mental changes
    f. Depression
    g. Sexual dysfunction
    h. Dementia

34. Which of the following conditions often leads to multiple CNS lesions in young adults?

    a. Lupus

    b. Acquired immune deficiency syndrome (AIDS)

    c. Myasthenia gravis

    d. Bacterial endocarditis

    e. Postvaccination demyelination (encephalomyelitis)

35. Which of the following conditions may lead to "euphoria" in MS patients?

    a. Pseudobulbar palsy

    b. Medications

    c. Cerebral cortex demyelination

    d. Extensive cerebral demyelination

    e. Depression

    f. Remission of an acute attack

    g. Partial complex seizures

    h. Extensive periventricular demyelination

36. While the geographic studies suggest that an environmental factor causes MS, they may also reflect that certain genetic pools (races) are more susceptible to MS. Which of the following factors can suggest a genetic predilection?

    a. VER studies

    b. HLA studies

    c. Israeli immigrant studies

    d. Failure of spouses to contract MS

37. Which of the following conditions are said to precipitate MS exacerbations?

    a. Pregnancy

    b. Depression

    c. Hot baths

    d. Lack of exercise

    e. Hyperthyroidism

    f. Anxiety

    g. Cold weather

    h. Electric injury

38. In a patient who suddenly developed paraparesis, urinary incontinence, and a T_{10} sensory level, which test is the best in indicating that the illness affects a CNS area besides the spinal cord?

    a. CSF oligoclonal bands

    b. CSF myelin basic protein

    c. EEG

    d. CT of the head

    e. VERs

    f. Hot bath test

ANSWERS

1. a. No. Spinal cord tumors would create spastic paraparesis, but they would be unable to cause visual impairment.

    b. No. Hysteria might lead to visual and motor complaints; however, people with hysteria cannot mimic abnormal light, DTR, or plantar reflexes.

    c. Yes. The policeman might have multiple sclerosis affecting the optic nerve and spinal cord.

    d. Yes. Inflammatory reactions to vaccinations, especially for smallpox and rabies, leads to CNS demyelination syndromes that mimic multiple sclerosis.

    e. No. Wilson's disease produces movement disorders and changes in mental status.

2. b. The patient has retrobulbar neuritis and impairments of the thoracic spinal cord.

3. b

4. Multiple sclerosis

5. d. With another episode of neurologic deficit, the diagnosis of multiple sclerosis can be made with even greater assurance. Although the current event is also compatible with spinal cord compression by a tumor as well as another episode of multiple sclerosis, the possibility of such a young man developing a second neurologic illness is so remote that a myelogram is unjustified. The other diagnostic procedures are clinically irrelevant.

6. a. Yes; b. No; c. Yes; d. Yes; e. No; f. No

7. a. No; b. No; c. Yes; d. Yes; e. Yes; f. Yes

8. a. Yes; b. No; c. No; d. Yes; e. Yes; f. Yes

9. e. The gait disturbance is entirely explainable by loss of proprioception in the lower extremities. Loss of reflexes and pupillary abnormalities suggest that the disease is not psychogenic.

10. Argyll-Robertson pupils

11. Tabes dorsalis from syphilis

12. Positive serology, e.g., VDRL, on the spinal fluid

13. a, c, e

14. d. Pain and temperature sensation both travel in the spinothalamic tract. Their dissociation defies the usual laws of neurology.

15. b. With optic nerve injuries that cause blindness, the pupils are unreactive to direct light. Moreover, in acute optic neuritis, attacks are accompanied by pain.

16. Cremasteric and anal reflexes, both superficial reflexes, are suppressed by both central and peripheral nervous system injuries. Their presence is evidence that the nervous system is physiologically intact.

17. Few illnesses cause recurring symptoms and signs. This patient does not, however, suffer from multiple sclerosis since he has no objective evidence of neurologic dysfunction. On the contrary, he has evidence of a psychogenic disorder.

18. f	**22.** e	**26.** a, b, and e
19. d	**23.** d	**27.** b and e
20. a, b, e	**24.** g	**28.** f
21. a	**25.** d	

29. Highest—Boston; lowest—Tokyo

30. Highest—European immigrants; lowest—Black Africans

31. a, b, c, e	**34.** a, b, d, e	**37.** a, b, c, f, h
32. a, c, d	**35.** a, b, d, e, f, h	**38.** e
33. a, e, h	**36.** b, c, d	

16

Neurologic Aspects of Sexual Function

Sexual function requires a fully working neurologic system. Many patients with neurologic illness have sexual impairments despite relatively normal libido, whereas those with some neurologic illnesses, even incapacitating ones, may have no impairment whatsoever. In many cases, patients' sexual potential and limitations should be known by both the patients and their physicians.

NEUROLOGIC FUNCTION

Erection and clitoral engorgement (genital "arousal") may be initiated by either cerebral or genital stimulation. Two main neurologic pathways, one originating in the brain and the other in the genitals, convey such stimulation. Both involve the central nervous system (CNS), the peripheral nervous system (PNS), and the autonomic nervous system (ANS).

In one pathway, various cerebral stimuli, such as pictures, sleep-related events, and emotional responses, are converted to neurophysiologic excitatory impulses. Most of these impulses travel down the spinal cord (part of the CNS) and leave at its sacral region to form the *pudendal nerve* (part of the PNS). Branches of the pudendal nerve supply the genital muscles and skin. Among their many functions, they relay genital tactile (touch) sensations to the spinal cord, which conveys them upward to the brain (Fig. 16-1).

Some excitatory impulses, as if diverted to a subsidiary pathway, leave the spinal cord at the T-12–L-4 region to join ANS *sympathetic* ganglia and at the S-2–S-4 region to join ANS *parasympathetic* ganglia. The ANS innervates the genitals, reproductive organs, bladder, sweat glands, and artery wall muscles. Stimulation of the ANS induces vascular distention, which results in genital arousal, and then a complex series of ANS-mediated events produce orgasm. The sympathetic and parasympathetic components depend on different neurotransmitters: acetylcholine in the parasympathetic and monoamines in the sympathetic. They also have different actions in arousal, orgasm, and ejaculation. However, since their roles are complementary and

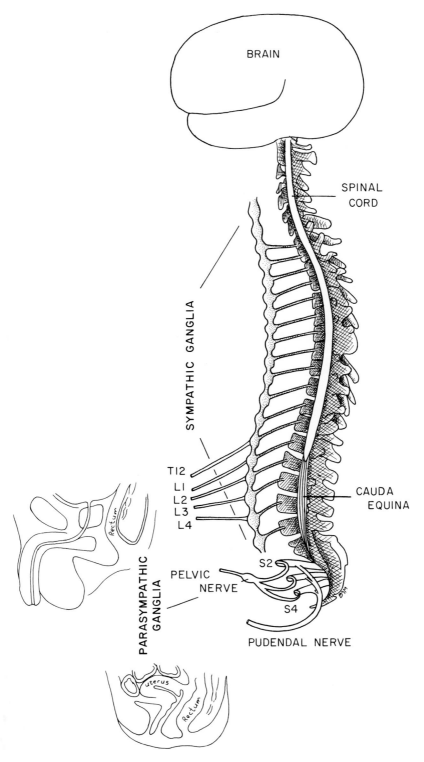

Fig. 16-1. The genitals are innervated by the sacral (S2–S4) spinal cord segments and also, in a virtually parallel and complementary manner, by the sympathetic and parasympathetic components of the autonomic nervous system.

vulnerable to the same injuries, medications, and psychologic inhibition, it seems impossible to make meaningful distinctions between them.

The other pathway, which is shorter and less complicated, is initiated by stimulation of the genitals and surrounding skin. Some sensory impulses pass upward through the pudendal nerve and spinal cord to the brain. Others, in the *genital-spinal cord reflex* synapse in the sacral region of the spinal cord and return, via the ANS, to the genitals. Stimulation of this pathway readily produces arousal and orgasm.

NEUROLOGIC IMPAIRMENT

The patient's history indicates a neurologic cause for sexual impairment when no arousal or orgasm occurs during any sexual activity, including masturbation and extramarital sex; men have no erections on awakening; or patients have certain neurologic illnesses (Table 16-1).

Physical signs of a neurologic cause should be sought not only on the routine neurologic examination (see Table 1-1), but also on examinations of sexually related (extrasexual) functions (Table 16-2). Since ANS function is crucial, signs of its impairment are important. Orthostatic hypotension, usually defined as a fall of 10 mm Hg in blood pressure on standing, is strong evidence of diabetic, medication-induced, or spontaneous ANS impairment. Anhidrosis, lack of sweating, in the groin and legs, which is usually accompanied by hairless and sallow skin, is another sign. It can be documented if necessary with the elaborate and messy "starch-iodine" test. Urinary incontinence is usually a manifestation of severe ANS impairment; however, more common causes, such as prostatism or stress incontinence, are often responsible. Finally, retrograde ejaculation, another sign, may be detected by examining a urine sample obtained after orgasm. Such urine will appear cloudy to the naked eye and, with a microscope, sperm will be seen.

With either spinal cord or PNS injury, weakness and a sensory loss below the waist or one confined to the genitals, anus, and buttocks, the "saddle area" (Fig. 16-2) may be present: Plantar and deep tendon reflex testing will indicate which system is responsible. With either CNS or PNS impairment, the scrotal, cremasteric, and anal ("superficial") reflexes (Fig. 16-3) will be absent.

The most important laboratory tests are *nocturnal penile tumescence (NPT) stud-*

Table 16-1
Indications of Neurologic Sexual Impairment

Continual Impotence
   Absence of morning erections
   No erection or orgasm during masturbation or sex with partners
Related Somatic Complaints
   Sensory loss in genitals, pelvis, or legs
   Urinary incontinence
Certain Neurologic Conditions
   Spinal cord injury
   Diabetic neuropathy
   Multiple sclerosis
   Herniated intervertebral disk
   Use of medications

Table 16-2
Signs of Neurologic Sexual Impairment

Signs of Spinal Cord Injury
    Paraparesis or quadriparesis
    Leg spasticity
    Sensory level
    Urinary incontinence
Signs of ANS* Injury
    Orthostatic hypotension or lightheadedness
    Anhidrosis in groin and legs
    Urinary incontinence
    Retrograde ejaculation
Signs of PNS† Injury
    Loss of sensation in the genitals, "saddle area," and legs
    Paresis and areflexia in legs
    Scrotal, cremasteric, and anal reflex loss‡

    *Autonomic nervous system.
    †Peripheral nervous system.
    ‡Also found with spinal cord injury.

ies, in which erections are monitored during one to three nights and correlated with rapid eye movement (REM) sleep.* Normal males, from infancy to old age, have erections and other manifestations of ANS activity, such as tachycardia, during more than 90 percent of REM sleep regardless of its overt dream content. Since NPT studies are a direct test of sexual function, they are probably more accurate than the traditional, indirect clinical evaluation. During NPT studies, impotent men, when

    *NPT studies are polysomnographic recordings performed in sleep disorder centers (Chapter 17) and cost about $1,000 in 1985.

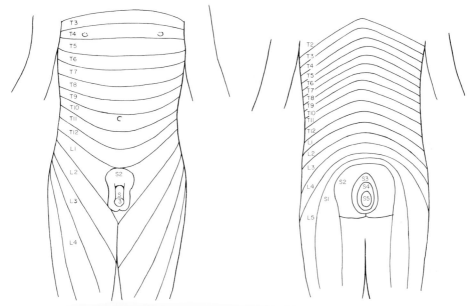

Fig. 16-2. The sacral dermatomes (S2–S5) innervate the skin overlying the genitals and anus, but lumbar dermatomes innervate the legs.

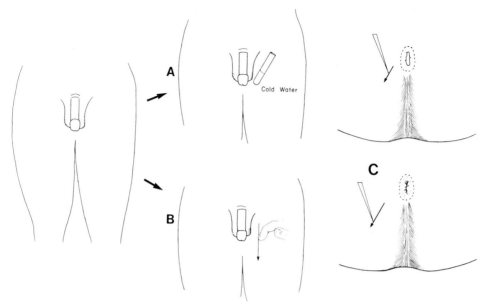

Fig. 16-3. (A) The *scrotal reflex:* When a cold surface is applied to the scrotum of a normal man, the testicles retract and the skin surface contracts. (B) The *cremasteric reflex:* When the inner thigh is stroked, the testicles of a normal man retract and the skin surface contracts. (C) The *anal reflex:* When the perianal skin is scratched, the anus tightens.

freed from social and psychologic influences, are sometimes shown to be capable of having erections. Contrary to traditional assertions, impotent men much more often are found to have neurologic or other physical abnormalities.

NEUROLOGIC ILLNESSES ASSOCIATED WITH SEXUAL IMPAIRMENT

Sexual function, being dependent on CNS, PNS, and ANS, is vulnerable to various neurologic illnesses. Some textbooks, while technically correct, list dozens, but only several are responsible for the vast majority of cases. As a general rule, if a neurologic illness associated with sexual impairment is present, the physician should initially assume that the sexual impairment has a neurologic rather than a psychologic basis. Equally important, many illnesses that are physically incapacitating do not cause sexual impairment.

Spinal Cord Injury

Unfortunately, thousands of people suffer spinal cord injuries. Such injuries usually result from automobile, horseback riding, diving, and trampoline accidents; penetrating knife or bullet wounds; or multiple sclerosis (MS) (Chapter 15).* Sexual impairment, as well as other manifestations of spinal cord injury—spastic paraparesis

---

*Patients with spinal cord injury may receive assistance from veterans associations, The National Multiple Sclerosis Society (see Chapter 15), or the March of Dimes, 1275 Mamaroneck Avenue, White Plains, New York 10605, (914) 428-7100.

or quadriparesis, urinary incontinence, and sensory loss (Chapter 2)—depends on the site of the injury and its completeness. The patient's libido should remain intact; however, sexual impairment often leads to diminished libido and other psychologic problems.

CERVICAL OR THORACIC (UPPER) SPINAL CORD INJURY

When the upper portion of the spinal cord is transected, ascending sensory and descending excitatory impulses are completely interrupted. Also, since such injuries are located above the level from which the ANS emerges, genital ANS innervation is lost. When the cervical spinal cord is injured, quadriparesis develops, and when the thoracic spinal cord is injured, paraparesis. In both cases, the injury prevents the patient from feeling genital tactile stimulation. With lower thoracic spinal cord injuries, however, breast stimulation may be appreciated.

Although both CNS and ANS innervation is lost, the genital-spinal cord reflex remains intact. Therefore, in response to genital stimulation, patients can occasionally have physical arousal and orgasm without being able to feel either. If erections develop, they are usually too weak for intercourse. If orgasms occur, they may be neither pleasurable nor exciting. Moreover, orgasms may even produce an excessive, almost violent response, *autonomic hyperreflexia,* in which patients have hypertension, bradycardia, nausea, and lightheadedness.

In addition to losing genital touch sensation, patients lose sensation for bladder fullness and generally require catheters. With upper spinal cord injuries caused by transection, men become infertile because of inadequate and abnormal sperm production, but women continue to ovulate, menstruate, and retain their capacity to conceive and bear children.

With incomplete spinal cord injuries, as in MS and many nonpenetrating injuries, sexual and extrasexual deficits are less pronounced and autonomic hyperreflexia is not a problem. However, inappropriate erections and premature ejaculation plague men, and varying degrees of anorgasmy affect both men and women.

Sexual therapy offers several options. The strength of erections can be increased by constricting the penis with a condom. Plastic or other penile prostheses can be implanted. Orgasms may be induced with mechanical vibrators in the partner and sometimes the patient.

LUMBAR OR SACRAL (LOWER) SPINAL CORD INJURY

When the lower spinal cord is transected, the critical genital-spinal cord reflex is interrupted and no form of stimulation can produce pleasurable sensation, arousal, or orgasm. Also, as in upper spinal cord transection, patients have paraparesis and urinary incontinence. Since the ANS continues to innervate the genitals, fertility in both men and women is preserved. Although lower spinal cord injuries are generally devastating, incomplete ones may permit some sexual function based on residual genital sensation and physical mobility.

Poliomyelitis and Other Exceptions

Before the Salk and Sabin vaccines were developed, many people suffered from poliomyelitis (polio), which is a motor neuron disease that causes only trunk and limb paresis. Characteristically, intellect, sensation, involuntary muscle strength, and ANS functions are spared (Chapter 5). Therefore, polio victims have full libido, genital sensation, bladder control, sexual function, and fertility. Another motor neuron disease that does not affect sexual or bladder function is amyotrophic lateral sclerosis (ALS). Extrapyramidal illnesses (Chapter 18), such as choreoathetosis, dystonia, Wilson's disease, Huntington's chorea, and parkinsonism, despite causing difficulties with mobility, also do not impair sexual desire, sexual function, or fertility.

Diabetes Mellitus

Sexual impairment, especially retrograde ejaculation and impotence, eventually affects almost 50 percent of diabetic men and is the first sign of diabetes in about 5 percent of patients. Diabetic sexual impairment results from ANS and PNS injury. Therefore, since the bladder and genitals have common ANS innervation, impotence and urinary incontinence coincide in diabetics. The bladders of affected patients are typically large, flaccid, and poorly controlled (Fig. 16-4). Patients also have anhidrosis and orthostatic hypotension, but curiously they do not necessarily have other complications of diabetes, such as retinopathy, nephropathy, or peripheral vascular disease. Although diabetic sexual impairment should not directly damage the libido, psychologic repercussions, as in spinal cord injury, can be debilitating. Some impotent diabetic men have low testosterone concentrations and some have hyperprolactinemia; however, testosterone therapy has only a placebo effect.

Descriptions of sexual impairment in diabetic women conflict. For example, Kolodny (see References) found that 35 percent of diabetic women had anorgasmy and that sexual impairment was related to neuropathy; however, Ellenberg found that diabetic women were no more prone than nondiabetic ones to sexual impairment, and that diabetic women, even with profound neuropathy, had full sexual function. All agree that vaginal infections are more common in diabetic women, and, while they remain fertile, pregnancies are more often complicated by miscarriages and fetal malformations.

Multiple Sclerosis

Intermittent or permanent sexual impairment in MS patients results from patches of spinal cord demyelination (Chapter 15). Sexual impairment can be the sole symptom, and when it is found with vague sensory disturbances, the patient may be misdiagnosed as hysteric. Worse, MS often eventually brings about devastating deficits, of which sexual impairment is only one aspect.

Multiple sclerosis causes premature ejaculation, impotence, unarousability, or anorgasmy. In its early stages, patients may have few extrasexual deficits, but if episodes develop repeatedly, the incidence of sexual impairment, urinary incontinence, and extrasexual deficits all rise dramatically. Although fertility is preserved in women, pregnancies are associated with exacerbations. The fertility of men is impaired because of decreased sperm production, impotence, and retrograde ejaculation.

Medication-Induced Impairment

While hundreds of medications are implicated, only a few categories consistently impair sexual function, and in most cases, in view of their pharmacology, this effect is

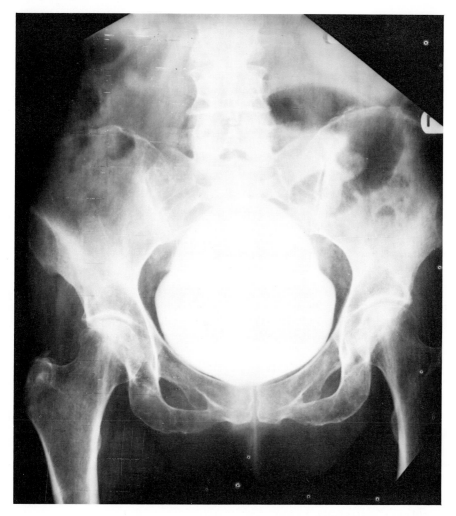

Fig. 16-4. This intravenous pyelogram (IVP) reveals a distended bladder, which is the large white circular area. The patient had diabetes mellitus that required insulin, complicated by urinary incontinence and impotence, which are typically associated with a large, flaccid bladder.

expectable. Antihypertensive medications cause erection, ejaculation, and orgasm problems because they interfere with sympathetic ANS function. While some exceptions are claimed, antihypertensive effects and sexual impairment side-effects usually coincide.

The tricyclic and, possibly to a lesser extent, almost all other antidepressants also create sexual impairment (Table 16-3). The anticholinergic action of heterocyclic antidepressants interferes with parasympathetic activity. Likewise, anticholinergic medications, which are often given to counteract the parkinsonian side-effects of phenothiazines, cause sexual impairment. All these medicines tend to cause dry mouth, orthostatic hypotension, accommodation paresis (see Fig. 12-4), and urinary hesitancy (see Fig. 15-5). Phenothiazines themselves and butyrophenones cause sexual impairment, also probably because of anticholinergic properties. That they increase prolactin levels also may be contributory.

Libido can be diminished by numerous medications, particularly those that are

Table 16-3
Psychiatric Medications
Associated with Impotence

Antidepressants
    Amitriptyline (Elavil†)
    Amoxapine (Asendin)
    Desipramine (Pertofrane†)
    Imipramine (Tofranil†)
    Isocarboxazid (Marplan)
    Lithium (Eskalith†)
    Nortriptyline (Aventyl†)
    Phenelzine (Nardil)
Antipsychotics
    Haloperidol (Haldol)
    Phenothiazines (Thorazine†)

According to Abramowicz M (ed):
Drugs that cause sexual dysfunction.
The Medical Letter 25:73–76, 1983.
†And other brands.

narcotic, hypnotic, or tranquilizing. Again, antihypertensive medications, which affect the CNS as well as the ANS, are apt to impair libido. In this group, reserpine, propranolol (Inderal), and methyldopa (Aldomet) are the most commonly cited medications, but package inserts or the *Medical Letter* (see References) should be consulted.

Miscellaneous

Sexual impairment can be caused by atherosclerosis of the arteries that supply the genitals. Similarly, if surgery of aortic aneurysms or the coronary arteries damages either the lower portion of the aorta or the dorsal artery of the penis, sexual impairment can result. To detect such vascular disease, men can have penile blood pressures measured. If these indicate penile vascular disease, various arterial reconstructive procedures, including grafting, can be attempted. However, in cases where vascular disease or surgery has caused spinal cord infarction, the prognosis is poor and surgery would not be helpful.

Another problem is sexual impairment after prostate surgery. In the past, such surgery led to impotence because it damaged the pudendal nerves, which are adjacent to the prostate; however, with the current procedures, transurethral prostatectomy (TURP) and suprapubic prostatectomy, these nerves are undamaged. Only radical prostate surgery, usually done for prastatic carcinoma, might be injurious enough to cause impotence.

Finally, herniated lumbar intervertebral disks occasionally compress the sexually important sacral nerve roots (S-2–S-4) within the spinal canal (Chapter 5). When this occurs, patients develop highly distressful, radiating low back pain. Examination will usually reveal signs of extensive nerve root compression that include ankle paresis, urinary retention, and Lasègue's sign (see Fig. 5-7). Thus, when sexual impairment results from a herniated disk, it is an obvious but minor part of the patient's problem.

Patients are difficult to evaluate when they have sexual impairment that they attribute to chronic but mild low back pain. Their pain must be considered carefully, but physicians should be reluctant to accept it as a cause of sexual impairment. On the other hand, patients who have undergone myelography, laminectomy, spinal fusion, and related operations of the lower spine may have developed nerve root injury from surgical trauma or postoperative *arachnoiditis* (inflammation of the covering of the nerve roots). These patients will often have unarousability and anorgasmy, aching chronic low back pain, and signs of nerve root compression.

LIBIDO

The limbic system and hypothalamic hormone secretions probably instill the basic, inherent sexual drive. These structures interact with the cerebral cortex through neuronal feedback loops and endocrine changes. Isolated limbic system injury, however, is rarely encountered because congenital, traumatic, vascular, and other common injuries damage the overlying temporal or frontal cerebral cortex as well as the limbic system.

The closest example is the experimentally produced *Klüver-Bucy syndrome,* in which increased heterosexual, homosexual, or autosexual activity and other behavioral changes are produced in rhesus monkeys after bilateral anterior temporal lobectomies that remove both amygdalae. The increased sexuality is accompanied by placidity (loss of fear, anger, and similar strong emotions), continual tactile activity, and "psychic blindness" (oral rather than visual exploration, similar to visual agnosia, Chapter 12). A modified form of this syndrome has been observed in humans with posttraumatic bilateral temporal lobe injury, Herpes simplex encephalitis, and rare cases of Alzheimer's and Pick's diseases. These patients, like the experimental monkeys, become placid and have a tendency to eat excessively and place inedible objects in their mouths (oral exploration). Heterosexual and masturbatory activity, in contrast, are increased in only about one half of the patients, and many only make suggestive gestures. Overall, they are more impaired by aphasia, memory impairment, dementia, and other manifestations of cerebral cortex injury than by sexual changes.

Although pituitary, hypothalamic, and diencephalic lesions have been associated with hypersexuality, most cases are characterized by hyposexuality and appetite changes. Curiously, Wernicke-Korsakoff syndrome and transient global amnesia, conditions in which portions of the limbic system are injured, are characterized by temporary memory impairment but no libido changes.

Possibly because the amygdala, hypocampus, and other limbic system structures are contained within the temporal lobe, partial complex (e.g., psychomotor) epilepsy, which often originates in temporal lobe dysfunction, is associated with changes in sexuality. During such seizures, patients may initiate rudimentary masturbatory activity or even partially undress, but they will not engage in heterosexual or planned violent activity.* During interictal periods patients are prone to hyposexuality and other personality aberrations (Chapter 10).

Increased libido may result from cerebral excitatory substances, including Sinemet, hallucinogens, and amyl nitrate. Similarly, several neurologic illnesses, in which cerebral "inhibitory centers" are damaged, are associated with an unrestrained libido. For example, people with mild mental retardation, Alzheimer's disease, parkinsonism, CVAs, cerebral palsy, or merely old age all may have a normal but uninhib-

---

*"Limbic seizures" have not been accepted by neurologists.

ited sexual drive. Sometimes parkinsonism patients who begin medical treatment suddenly develop an unexpected burst of sexual activity because the medications provide physical mobility and cerebral stimulation (Chapter 18). On the other hand, sexual and other desires may be impaired by conditions that cause extensive cerebral injury, such as multiple CVAs, Alzheimer's disease, and multiple sclerosis. The libido is also vulnerable to neurologic sexual impairments since lack of sexual satisfaction, as though through a "negative feedback loop," leads to decreased demand. For example, men with MS or diabetic impotence often lose their libido. Thus, the classic question posed to people with sexual dysfunction, "Is the problem decreased libido or impotence?" is sometimes like asking them about the chicken and the egg.

The patient in chronic pain who has decreased libido may, of course, be suffering from depression and may also be consuming potent analgesics; however, pain does affect spinal cord and brain opiate receptors and possibly interferes with pleasure from any source. Although libido persists despite a variety of other discomforts, including mild fatigue, hunger, and fear, the dampening effect of pain is popularly acknowledged as the classic refusal "Not tonight, honey, I have a headache."

REFERENCES

Abramowicz M (ed): Drugs that cause sexual dysfunction. The Medical Letter 25:73, 1983

Boller F, Frank E: Sexual Dysfunction in Neurologic Disorders: Diagnosis, Management, and Rehabilitation. New York, Raven Press, 1982

Bradley WE: Etiology of impotence in diabetes mellitus. Neurology 33:101, 1983

Comfort A (ed): Sexual Consequences of Disability. Philadelphia, George F. Strickley Co, 1978

DeLeo D, Magni G: Sexual side effects of antidepressant drugs. Psychosomatics 12:1076, 1983

Ellenberg M: Diabetic neuropathy. In Ellenberg M, Rifkin H. Diabetes Mellitus: Theory and Practice, 3rd ed. New York, Medical Examination Publishing Co, 1983

Hale G (ed): Sex Instruction for the Physically Handicapped. Philadelphia, Saunders Press, 1979

Karacan I: Nocturnal penile tumescence as a biologic marker in assessing erectile dysfunction. Psychosomatics 23:349, 1982

Kolodny RC, Masters WH, Johnson VE: Textbook of Sexual Medicine. Boston, Little, Brown, 1979

Lilly R, Cummings JL, Benson DF, et al: The human Klüver-Bucy. Neurology 33:1141, 1983

Monat RK: Sexuality and the Mentally Retarded: A Clinical and Therapeutic Guidebook. San Diego, College-Hill Press, 1982

Mooney TO, Cole TM, Chilgren RA: Sexual Options for Paraplegics and Quadriplegics. Boston, Little, Brown, 1975

Spark RF: Neuroendocrinology and impotence. Ann Intern Med 98:103, 1983

QUESTIONS

1. A 40-year-old man complains of longstanding intermittent impotence. He has severe low back pain, mild hypertension, and borderline diabetes. Which conditions should be considered as possible causes of his sexual dysfunction?

    a. Herniated lumbar intervertebral disk
    b. Antihypertensive medications
    c. Diabetic neuropathy
    d. Psychogenic factors
    e. All of above

2. A 24-year-old man, who complains of premature ejaculation, had episodes of unsteady gait, diplopia, and paraparesis. Neurologic examination may reveal which of the following?
    a. Internuclear ophthalmoplegia
    b. Absent abdominal reflexes
    c. Ataxia of gait
    d. Babinski signs
    e. Hyperactive deep tendon reflexes

3. Retrograde ejaculation may result from which of the following conditions?
    a. Ovarian dysfunction
    b. Diabetic autonomic neuropathy
    c. Psychogenic influence
    d. Use of guanethidine (Ismelin)
    e. Sexual inexperience

4. The physician might assume that patients with neurologic illness will have sexual dysfunction. With which illnesses is the assumption valid?
    a. Dominant hemisphere infarctions
    b. Nondominant hemisphere infarctions
    c. Parkinsonism
    d. Poliomyelitis
    e. ALS

5. Medications as well as particular illnesses cause impotence and other forms of sexual dysfunctions. In which illness is iatrogenic sexual dysfunction likely to be encountered?
    a. Psychosis
    b. Migraine headache
    c. Hypertension
    d. Low back pain
    e. Duodenal ulcer

6. During sleep, when do erections and emissions occur?

7. With which situations is fertility lost?
    a. Women with cervical spinal cord transection
    b. Men with cervical spinal cord transection
    c. Men with diabetes mellitus and neuropathy
    d. Women with diabetes mellitus and neuropathy

8. With which conditions are erections still possible?
    a. Severe diabetic autonomic neuropathy
    b. Use of Ismelin (guanethidine)
    c. Sacral spinal cord transection
    d. Cervical spinal cord transection
    e. Upper thoracic spinal cord transection
    f. MS

9. With which conditions are cremasteric reflexes lost?
    a. Severe diabetic autonomic neuropathy
    b. Psychogenic difficulties
    c. Sacral spinal cord injury
    d. Frontal meningiomas

10. A 35-year-old man suffers low back pain after falling down a flight of stairs at work. Among his complaints a month later is impotence. Examination reveals loss of pinprick sensation from the waist down to the toes but intact position, vibratory, and warm–cold sensation. Deep tendon and cremasteric reflexes are intact and plantar reflexes are flexion. To what could the impotence be attributed?

    a. Spinal cord injury
    b. Autonomic nervous system dysfunction
    c. Peripheral neuropathy
    d. Multiple sclerosis
    e. None of the above

11. In monkeys, with which of the following is the Klüver-Bucy syndrome associated?

    a. Psychic blindness
    b. Apathy
    c. Frontal lobectomy
    d. Loss of amygdalae
    e. Increased homosexual, heterosexual, and autosexual activity

12. In humans who have had bilateral temporal lobe damage, which of the following conditions are almost always found?

    a. Memory impairment, aphasia, or both
    b. Placing food and inedible objects into their mouths
    c. Hypersexuality
    d. Rage attacks

13. Which of the following conditions is likely to lead to transient or permanent temporal lobe or limbic system damage?

    a. Herpes simplex encephalitis
    b. Alcoholism
    c. TIAs of the posterior cerebral arteries
    d. Herpes zoster

14. With which of the following are pituitary tumors associated?

    a. Headaches
    a. Hyperprolactinemia
    c. Optic atrophy
    d. Homonymous superior quadrantanopsia

15. In normal males, with which alterations are REM-induced erections associated?

    a. Dreams with no overt sexual content
    b. Most dreams with even frightful or anxiety-producing content
    c. Increased pulse and blood pressure
    d. Increased cerebral blood flow
    e. An EEG that appears, aside from eye movement artifact, as though the patient were awake

ANSWERS

1. e. This man might have sexual impairment because of the various medical or psychogenic disorders.

2. a, b, c, d, e. The patient is likely to have MS with cerebellar, brainstem, and spinal cord involvement. Between episodes, when the patient is likely to have residual neurologic signs (a–e), he may also have sexual dysfunction. Premature ejaculation and impotence are often a manifestation of quiescent MS that has affected the spinal cord.

3. b, d. In retrograde ejaculation, semen is propelled by involuntary mechanisms into the bladder instead of the urethra. It is always the result of neurologic or local muscular dysfunction.

4. None of these answers is correct. Each condition may cause bodily weakness; however, sexual drive, genital sensation, and orgasmic reactions are all preserved.

5. a, c, e. Medications that cause impotence and similar sexual difficulties are usually those with anticholinergic properties, such as antipsychotic and ulcer therapy medications, or those with antihypertensive properties.

6. During REM-stage sleep, when dreams usually occur, erections and orgasm take place. Erections are also characteristically present on awakening.

7. b. Men with upper spinal cord injury have low sperm counts and produce abnormal sperm. Women are able to conceive and bear children despite spinal cord injury. Both men and women with diabetes retain fertility.

8. b, d, e, f. Erections are possible as long as the lumbosacral spinal cord and the sacral autonomic nervous system are intact. Thus, the men with severe diabetic autonomic neuropathy (a) and sacral spinal cord damage (c) will not be able to have erections. If the spinal cord damage is incomplete, as in patients with MS (f), or located in the upper region, as in patients with transection of the upper cord (d,e), potency may be preserved. Impotence with use of medications is inconstant and often incomplete. Most men who use Ismelin (b) should still be able to have erections.

9. a, c. Cremasteric reflexes require that the pudendal nerves, autonomic nervous system, and lower spinal cord be intact. When impotence and anorgasmy are accompanied by a loss of these reflexes, neurologic impairment must be considered.

10. e. Since the patient has no objective neurologic deficit, none of the neurologic illnesses are indicated. In fact, the dissociation of pinprick and warm–cold sensation is not possible anatomically, since both sensations travel in the same nerve pathways.

11. a, b, d, e. The monkeys, which undergo temporal lobectomy with removal of the amygdalae, have oral exploratory behavior and, although their vision is intact, they cannot identify objects by their appearance, i.e., they have *visual agnosia*. The monkeys characteristically lose fear and extreme emotion, sometimes appearing fearless although they are actually apathetic. Most striking, they have increased, indiscriminate sexual activity.

12. a, b. The human variety of the Klüver-Bucy syndrome is characterized by impaired language function and memory, the tendency to eat excessively, and, like monkeys, placing inedible objects in their mouths. Possibly contrary to expectations, they have little increased sexual appetite or violent outbursts.

13. a, b, c. Herpes simplex has a predilection for the frontal and temporal lobes and thus this variety of encephalitis often leads to memory impairment and the psychomotor variety of partial complex seizures. Herpes zoster usually does not involve the CNS, although, when it does, its effects are inconsistent. Instead, it usually causes painful postherpetic neuralgia. Posterior cerebral TIAs cause ischemia of the temporal lobes and are associated with confusion and memory impairment, the so-called syndrome of "transient global amnesia." Alcoholism leads to the Wernicke-Korsakoff syndrome, which is associated with hemorrhage into the mammary bodies and other parts of the limbic system.

14. a, b, c, d

15. a, b, c, d, e

17

Sleep Disorders

The incidence of sleep disorders is so high that they should qualify as a public health problem. For example, about 10 percent of Americans are unhappy about the quality or quantity of their sleep, and 3 to 10 percent use sleeping pills (sedatives or hypnotics). Moreover, surveys have revealed that when people habitually have too little sleep (less than four hours) or too much (greater than ten hours), they have increased morbidity and mortality.

In the last two decades, the study of sleep and its disorders has given rise to an entirely new branch of medical practice.* Using the *polysomnogram* (*PSG*), which is a recording of the electroencephalogram (EEG), electromyogram (EMG), ocular movements, and vital signs of sleeping people, investigators have studied normal patterns, variations, and disorders of sleep. In addition, they have examined biologic correlates of dreaming, nighttime behavior, and psychologic status. This chapter will review their findings and emphasize those conditions that cause sleep disruptions, too little sleep (insomnia), and too much sleep (excessive daytime sleepiness).

NORMAL SLEEP

Two phases of sleep vary and recur throughout a normal night. Their most salient difference is that dreaming and rapid, conjugate, horizontal movement of the eyes take place together in one phase, called *rapid eye movement* (*REM*) *sleep*. The other phase, *non–rapid eye movement* (*NREM*) *sleep*, which is longer, has other distinctive qualities (Table 17-1). A possible explanation for the pattern is that the locus ceruleus and the median raphe, two deep brainstem structures, have reciprocal functions and their cyclic activity alternately triggers REM and NREM sleep.

---

*Patients with sleep disorders may receive assistance from the Association of Sleep Disorders Centers, TD-114, Stanford University School of Medicine, Stanford, California 94305.

Table 17-1
Stages of Normal Sleep

| Stage | Gradation | Movement | | EMG | EEG |
		Somatic	Ocular		
NREM					
1	Light sleep	Persistent facial tone and repositioning movements of body every 15–20 minutes	Slow, rolling eye movements	Continual activity	Loss of alpha activity
2	Intermediate sleep	Same	Absent	Slight reduction	Sleep spindles and K complexes
3	Deep sleep	Same	Absent	Further reduction	Increased proportion of slow-wave (1–3 Hz) activity
4	Deepest sleep	Same	Absent	Further reduction	Greatest proportion of 1–3 Hz activity
REM	Activated or paradoxical sleep	Absence of all muscular movement and tone, except for brief episodes of facial and limb movement	Rapid, conjugate, eye movements	Silent	Low-voltage activity, ocular movement artifacts

REM Sleep

Since most people who are awakened during a REM period report that they were having a dream, REM sleep has become synonymous with dreaming. The dreams that occur during REM sleep are intellectually complex, on a superficial level at least, and rich in visual imagery. The vigorous eye movements are attributed to people watching or feeling themselves participating in a dream.

Aside from the eye movements and uninterrupted breathing, there is virtual absence of muscle movement and tone in the head, trunk, and limbs. The muscles are paretic and flaccid, and their deep tendon reflexes (DTRs) are areflexic. An EMG shows absent electric activity in the chin and limb muscles (Fig. 17-1).

Despite the sleeping person's motionlessness, so much autonomic nervous system activity takes place in REM sleep that it has been called "activated" or "paradoxical" sleep. For example, there is an increase in pulse, blood pressure, intracranial pressure, cerebral blood flow, and muscle metabolism. Also, regardless of the content of dreams, penile erections occur (Chapter 16).

The EEG, which is also relatively active, is composed of eye-movement artifact superimposed on asynchronous, low-voltage, high-frequency activity. Aside from the artifact, it is similar to EEGs in wakefulness. Overall, in REM sleep, the bodily activities and EEG, but not the EMG, are more similar to those in wakefulness than to those in NREM sleep.

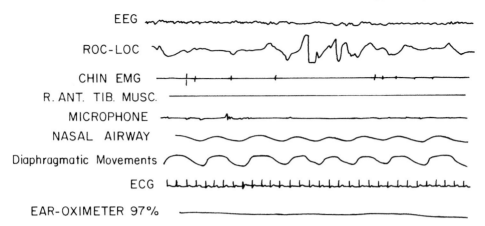

Fig. 17-1. Polysomnography (PSG) of REM sleep characteristically shows that the EEG channel has low-voltage, fast activity and the channel referable to ocular movement (ROC-LOC) indicates rapid eye movement (REM) by the large-scale, quick movements. Electromyography (EMG) of the chin and right anterior tibialis muscles shows virtually no activity, which indicates absence of muscle movement and tone. The microphone channel indicates a little noise, which may be a snore. The airway and diaphragm channels indicate normal breathing and air movement.

NREM Sleep

NREM sleep is divided into four stages that are distinguished by progressively greater depths of unconsciousness and slower and higher voltage EEG patterns. In all stages of NREM sleep, the eyes have slow, rolling motions, and people form only brief, rudimentary thoughts. Also in contrast to REM sleep, muscle tone is present, DTRs can be elicited, and EMG activity is present in the chin and limb muscles (Fig. 17-2).

While there is a generalized decrease in autonomic nervous system function, important hypothalamic-pituitary (neuroendocrine) activity occurs. For example, growth hormone is secreted almost entirely about 30 to 60 minutes after sleep begins, and cortisol is secreted in five to seven discrete late nighttime episodes, which accu-

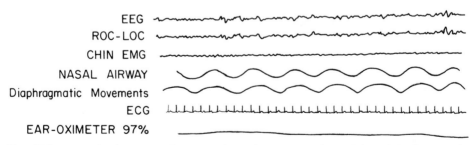

Fig. 17-2. A PSG of stage 1 of NREM sleep shows some slow EEG activity but not the higher-voltage, very slow EEG activity of deep or slow-wave NREM sleep. The PSG also shows, in the ROC-LOC channel, no substantial ocular movement, i.e., no REM activity. The chin muscles have tone as indicated by continual, low-voltage EMG activity. Breathing and cardiac activity are normal.

mulate to yield the day's highest cortisol concentration at about 8 AM. In addition, the third and fourth stages of NREM sleep, which are called *slow-wave* or *deep NREM sleep*, provide most of the physical recuperation derived from a night's sleep. As if the immediate role of sleep were to revitalize the body, these stages occur predominantly in the early night.

Patterns

People usually fall asleep five to ten minutes after retiring; however, this interval, *sleep latency*, is highly variable because it is influenced by a multitude of psychologic and physical factors. Once asleep, people enter NREM sleep and pass in succession through its four stages. After about 70 to 110 minutes of NREM sleep, they enter the initial REM period, which lasts for about ten minutes. The interval from falling asleep to the first REM period, *REM latency*, which normally averages 90 minutes, is critical in affective and sleep disorders.

The NREM–REM cycle repeats itself throughout the night with a periodicity of about 90 minutes. REM periods, which occur four or five times nightly, are progressively longer and more frequent (Fig. 17-3). In later sleep, body temperature falls to the day's lowest point (the nadir). The final REM period merges with awakening. Thus, people's final dream may be influenced by surrounding morning household activities, and when men awake they usually have erections.

Variations

EFFECTS OF AGE

As people grow older, they spend less time sleeping and dreaming. Neonates sleep 16 to 20 hours a day, with about 50 percent of that time in REM sleep. Young

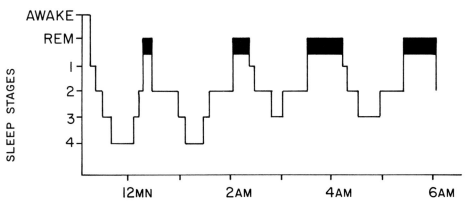

Fig. 17-3. In the conventional representation of a normal night's sleep pattern, REM periods start about 90 minutes after sleep begins, i.e., the REM latency is 90 minutes. REM periods then recur somewhat more frequently and in longer duration throughout the night. NREM sleep progresses through regular although less deep stages.

children spend 10 to 12 hours sleeping at night and during afternoon naps, with about 30 percent in REM sleep.

Adults average is six to eight hours, with 20 to 28 percent in REM. However, when adults are accustomed to relatively little sleep, the proportion of deep NREM sleep greatly increases, while that of REM remains constant. Therefore, in these cases, the *quantity* of deep NREM sleep tends to be preserved at the expense of REM sleep.

The elderly, who sleep somewhat less than young adults, have sleep that is fragmented, especially in its later half, by multiple brief awakenings. These people obtain part of their sleep in daytime naps that occur not only after meals and in the late afternoon, which are times of normal sleepiness, but irresistibly at any time, including during social activities. Their REM periods, instead of being longer and more frequent in the later night, change neither in duration nor frequency. Sleep onset and awakening times are usually earlier, (i.e., are *phase advanced,*) so that elderly people typically both go to sleep and awaken early. In the elderly, unlike other adults, reductions in sleep are taken at the expense of stage 4 NREM sleep. In addition to these variations, the elderly have an increased incidence of inadequate sleep because of medication-induced insomnia, various sleep disorders, and medical illnesses.

SLEEP SCHEDULES

For most adults, social and occupational demands determine a morning awakening time and, indirectly, an evening bedtime. These external considerations usually override emotional makeup, early conditioning, physical activities, and possibly an intrinsic sleep mechanism.

However, some people, "night owls" or "owls," prefer to remain awake late into the night and sleep until early afternoon. They gravitate to entertainment industries and other nighttime work, and form friendships with other "owls." These people, who are well-adjusted, must be distinguished from those who, handicapped by their daytime sleep schedule, are said to have "delayed sleep phase syndrome" (see below). In contrast, "larks" arise early in the morning. Their work, which is more conventional, is decidedly more productive in the morning than in the afternoon.

SLEEP DEPRIVATION

Important changes occur during the night following sleep deprivation, as might be caused by an adult working all night or children skipping their customary afternoon nap. In such conditions, both sleep latency and REM latency are shorter, and sleep time lengthened. Also, there is *REM rebound*, in which the first REM period occurs earlier or even immediately (*sleep onset REM*), and subsequent REM periods, compared with normal ones, are generally longer and thus occupy a greater proportion of sleep time. In short, as is commonly known, after missing sleep, the normal person will immediately fall deeply asleep, dream a great deal, and sleep late the next morning.

REM rebound also occurs following withdrawal from sedatives, hypnotics, and alcohol—substances that selectively suppress REM sleep. Sleep onset REM, which is often associated with REM rebound, is also found in a variety of disorders (see below).

DYSFUNCTIONS ASSOCIATED WITH SLEEP

Night Terrors, Sleepwalking, and Bedwetting

Parasomnias are behavioral aberrations that disrupt sleep. The most common ones are *night terrors, sleepwalking,* and *bedwetting,* which all occur during deep NREM sleep and thus tend to occur during the first few hours of sleep when deep NREM sleep predominates. They are believed to be the result of a partial arousal rather than manifestations of dreams. Parasomnias usually begin in early childhood and cease before puberty. In children, they are not associated with psychiatric disturbances. However, when parasomnias persist or develop in adult life, they are associated with characterologic disorders and even psychosis.

Children are liable to have more than one variety of parasomnia. In these cases, parasomnias might be confused with partial complex seizures (Chapter 10); however, the seizures tend to be stereotyped, undergo secondary generalization, and be followed by (postictal) confusion. A PSG during attacks of either a parasomnia or seizure will be diagnostic.

Night terrors (pavor nocturnus) are a type of parasomnia in which children suddenly awake and behave as though they were in great physical danger. Children experiencing a night terror stare, moan, and sometimes speak a few words with their eyes fully open and their pupils dilated. They sweat, have tachycardia, and hyperventilate. Also, they thrash about and fight attempts to be held, often leaving their parents' arms to walk aimlessly. Parents are neither able to awaken them nor provide comfort. The episode lasts for several minutes and ends abruptly. The children, who are apparently terrified, suddenly return to a deep sleep. Despite the apparently vivid and awesome features of the episode, children surprisingly have no recollection of it in the morning.

Night terrors may occur as often as several nights a week but usually take place only a few times a month. They are apt to follow the excessive, deep NREM sleep resulting from sleep deprivation. They may be precipitated by noises or other disruptions that partially rouse children, but they are not related to frightening events of the day, and during the episode there is no REM activity.

Night terrors may be prevented in some children by enforcing an afternoon nap and avoiding sleep disruptions, such as loud noises, and not permitting a child too much to drink before sleeping, which would result in a need to urinate. Treatment of an individual episode is not feasible because of its brevity. When children suffer from night terrors several times a week, prophylactic medical therapy with diazepam (Valium) or imipramine (Tofranil) may be considered. The impact may be reduced by reassuring the parents that night terrors will cease by themselves and are not a result of pain, parental abuse, or emotional disturbance.

In contrast, *nightmares* are essentially dreams that have a frightening content, i.e., "bad dreams." They contain complex imagery that a child is able to recall if awakened during the nightmare or on arising in the morning. Nightmares are unaccompanied by bodily changes or vocalizations other than crying. Often a nightmare ends itself by awakening the child, but if not, parents may interrupt it by awakening the child.

Nightmares can occur throughout the night during any REM period. They often develop when REM activity is increased, as during REM rebound from sleep deprivation, and following frightening experiences. Therefore, treatment of frequent nightmares would include exploring the circumstances and content of the dreams and occasionally the use of medications. In adults, nightmares are not only a manifestation of psychologic processes, they are also notoriously precipitated by REM rebound associated with withdrawal from alcohol, barbiturates, or other drugs.

Sleepwalking (somnambulism) usually consists just of sitting or standing during deep NREM sleep. When people walk, they do so slowly with their eyes open, and they travel familiar pathways. Although they seem to be awake, if questioned, they are confused and inappropriate. Diazepam may be helpful in preventing sleepwalking.

Bedwetting (enuresis) is considered a parasomnia when it is present in children older than five years and in all adults. In children, bedwetting can be treated with imipramine (Tofranil) or with behavior modification therapy devices that complete a low-voltage electric circuit, which "alerts" a child who wets the bed. However, in adults, bedwetting can result not only from a sleep disorder or psychologic disturbance but from a variety of neurologic illnesses. For example, it can result from degenerative cerebral disease and thus be associated with dementia. In addition, it can result from seizures and be the only evidence of a nighttime seizure. Also, spinal cord damage, as with multiple sclerosis, or cauda equina injuries can lead to nighttime incontinence. Therefore, when bedwetting develops in older children or adults, a neurologic examination should be included in the evaluation.

Other Parasomnias

Another nighttime dysfunction, *periodic movements*, is characterized by regular, episodic leg and bodily movement. This condition may awaken the patient and his or her bed partner and lead to insomnia. Unlike the previously described parasomnias, periodic movements are not confined to a particular sleep phase.

Periodic leg movements are stereotyped, brief (1 to 3 second), bilateral dorsiflexion movements of the foot and toes. They take place at 20- to 40-second intervals, for periods of ten minutes to several hours, primarily but not exclusively during NREM sleep (Fig. 17-4). They can occur alone or be associated with other sleep disorders, use of antidepressants, or withdrawal from various medications.

Restless leg syndrome is a related condition in which people have an uncontrollable urge to move their legs. Even after they fall asleep, their legs continue to move in the same periodic fashion.

All these disorders are different from the generalized bodily jerk preceded by a sensation of falling that affects virtually all people at some time as they "fall" asleep. These movements, called *sleep starts, hypnic jerks,* or *somnolescent starts,* occur in the twilight of sleep and are not associated with parasomnias, periodic movements, or any illness.

More limited, nonperiodic movements can develop. *Bruxism,* grinding of the teeth, mainly occurs in the transition from wakefulness to sleep. It can lead to headaches, temporomandibular joint pain, and dental injury. Although daytime bruxism is felt to be psychogenic, the etiology of nocturnal bruxism is unknown. *Head banging,* usually found only in children younger than five years, is a rocking head

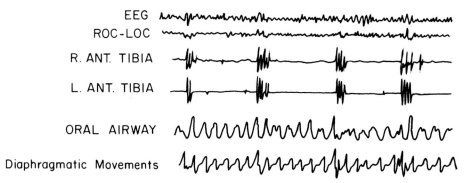

EEG
ROC-LOC
R. ANT. TIBIA
L. ANT. TIBIA
ORAL AIRWAY
Diaphragmatic Movements

Fig. 17-4. Periodic leg movements occurring during NREM sleep, which is typical, are revealed in this PSG. At about 30-second intervals, both anterior tibialis muscles contract synchronously—dorsiflexing the patient's ankles. Despite the movements, this patient remains asleep.

motion unconnected with any particular phase of sleep. In adults, it is associated with psychologic problems.

Neurologic and Medical Conditions Precipitated by Sleep

Some seizures seem to be precipitated by sleep (Chapter 10). For example, about 45 percent of patients with primary generalized epilepsy have seizures predominantly during sleep, and sleep deprivation precipitates seizures in epilepsy patients. Seizures tend to develop in deep NREM sleep, and therefore usually occur mostly toward the end of the night. However, those following sleep deprivation occur early in the night. The tendency for seizures to develop after sleep deprivation has led to the practice of obtaining an EEG after enforced sleep deprivation. This technique, which is quite harmless while being valuable, elicits sharp waves and a variety of spike-and-sharp wave activity in more than one third of epileptic patients who have no such abnormalities on routine EEGs.

In contrast to seizures that develop during sleep, classic involuntary movement disorders, such as Parkinson's disease and chorea (Chapter 18), are characteristically absent during sleep. Curiously, tics and palatal myoclonus persist during sleep.

Several cardiovascular disorders may occur during sleep. Angina pectoris and myocardial infarctions take place much more often during REM than NREM phases; asthma, congestive heart failure, and gastroesophageal reflux occur with equal frequency in either phase; and thrombotic cerebrovascular infarctions are more frequent during NREM sleep, when pulse and blood pressure are relatively low.

Another disorder clearly associated with sleep is vascular headaches (Chapter 9). Migraines and, even more so, cluster headaches are not only associated with sleep, they seem to be precipitated by REM phases. In rare persons, these headaches may occur only during REM periods, but in most people, they begin during early morning intense REM sleep and continue after awakening. Thus, excessive sleep or other conditions that increase REM sleep are associated with headaches. Also, in many cases, medications that suppress REM sleep reduce headaches.

INSOMNIA

Insomnia, the inability to fall or remain asleep, is characterized by shorter sleep time, lighter sleep, or frequent arousals. People may have insomnia because their sleep is interrupted by parasomnias or other disorders, such as nightmares, or because their sleep is prevented by psychologic or medical illness. Rather than suffering from excessive daytime sleepiness (see below), most patients with insomnia seem continuously wakeful. They do not complain of fatigue and do not nap during the day.

Drug and Alcohol Related Insomnia

Many people have insomnia because they take medicines, such as aminophylline or pseudoephedrine (Actifed), which have stimulant effects. Some may consume excessive caffeine, the most common stimulant, in coffee (which has 60 to 140 mg of caffeine per cup), cola drinks (25 to 55 mg per cup), and many headache medicines (e.g., 130 mg in two Excedrin tablets). Americans can easily and inadvertently ingest so much caffeine (250 to 500 mg per day) that it causes insomnia and other manifestations of caffeinism: agitation, tremulousness, palpitations, gastric distress, diuresis, and "caffeine-withdrawal headaches" (Chapter 9).

More troublesome than excessive coffee intake, of course, is abuse of sedatives, hypnotics, or alcohol. When used chronically, these substances disrupt sleep cycle periodicity. They also increase REM latency and shorten REM periods. Interference with REM sleep may be so great that it is completely suppressed. Deep NREM sleep is also reduced. Nevertheless, medication-induced sleep is, at least for limited periods, able to provide sleep and recuperation.

The elderly inadvisedly take inordinate quantities of both prescription and over-the-counter sleeping pills and are often psychologically dependent on them. Not only are hypnotics rarely effective if taken for more than one month, they can aggravate insomnia (*medication-induced insomnia*). Also, when people who have Alzheimer's disease or other brain damage take hypnotics, instead of being sedated they may, in a "paradoxical reaction," develop agitation, psychologic aberrations, and hallucinations.

People who suddenly abstain from chronic use of alcohol, sedatives, neuroleptics, or hypnotics, especially short-acting barbiturates, may develop *drug withdrawal insomnia*. In this condition, people have excessive daytime sleepiness that is often accompanied by physical and psychologic agitation. When they are able to fall asleep, they have REM rebound, as though their previously suppressed REM sleep were suddenly unleashed. Withdrawal from alcohol or barbiturates may also lead to seizures, usually of the generalized tonic-clonic variety.

Delayed Sleep Phase Syndrome

A particularly interesting, newly described variety of insomnia is the *delayed sleep phase syndrome*. Unlike most other forms of insomnia, this one often begins in adolescence. Patients cannot fall asleep until the early morning, but once asleep, they have normal sleep phases and, if not awakened, normal sleep length. They would be happy "owls," but their schedule prevents them from sleeping as long as necessary and they feel fatigued.

The unique aspect of the delayed sleep phase syndrome is that although medications are unsuccessful in making the patients fall asleep earlier, patients can *delay* their sleeptime without medication by 30 to 60 minutes successively each night. Thus, using "chronotherapy" to postpone their sleep onset through almost an entire day, eventually they fall asleep at 11 PM and, with effort, maintain that time.

Insomnia in Major Psychiatric Illness

In patients with endogenous depression, especially the elderly, PSGs show a short REM latency. Not only does the first REM period occur before 60 minutes, it is abnormally long and intense. Although the total amount of REM sleep is about the same in normal and depressed people, in those who are depressed, REM periods occur in relatively quick succession in the early night, leaving the later night almost devoid of REM. This preponderance of REM sleep in the depressed person's early night is similar to that in the normal person's later night.

Depressed people, as well as many others, also have increased sleep latency and then intermittent awakenings throughout the night. They tend to arise early in the morning, i.e., "early terminal awakening," which foreshortens their sleep. Unlike most normal people, when depressed people have a reduction in total sleep, deep NREM sleep is reduced.

Although the short REM latency is characteristic of depression, it is not diagnostic and about 15 percent of patients with depression have normal or even prolonged REM latency. Some patients with nonaffective psychiatric disorders have shortened REM latency, and, more important, it is also found in people with sleep deprivation; those who withdraw from alcohol, neuroleptics, and other medicines; those with narcolepsy (see below); and those with medical illness. In mania and acute agitation, REM sleep may be abolished and total sleep may be markedly reduced; however, in mania, when sleep does occur, REM latency is shortened.

Depressed people, in addition to abnormal sleep patterns, have related neuroendocrine abnormalities. Their body temperature nadir occurs several hours earlier than normal. Likewise, they have earlier excretion of cortisol and the norepinephrine metabolite MHPG. Overall, the earlier onset of first REM, the bulk of REM sleep, temperature nadir, and nocturnal hormone excretion are all a forward movement of the circadian rhythm of normal people, or a *phase shift advance*. It is as though when depressed people fall asleep, they leap ahead into the middle of the sleep and neuroendocrine cycles of normal people.

Schizophrenic patients vary in their sleep patterns according to the activity of the disorder. In acute schizophrenia, the total sleep time is decreased and sleep occurs in small segments throughout the day. Patients with chronic schizophrenia, in contrast, have essentially normal sleep patterns, and, interestingly, can distinguish their dreams from hallucinations.

A frequently occurring but underrecognized disorder is *pseudoinsomnia*. In this condition, people complain of not sleeping long or deeply enough, but PSGs show a normal pattern and duration of sleep. This discrepancy, along with other complaints, suggest that the symptoms originate from psychologic disturbances.

EXCESSIVE DAYTIME SLEEPINESS

Excessive daytime sleepiness is a feeling of fatigue and a tendency to nap one or more times throughout the day. Some cases are attributed to insomnia; however, aside from patients with psychologic or medical illness, the majority have *narcolepsy* or *sleep apnea*.

Narcolepsy

Narcolepsy is a condition in which multiple, brief, irresistible episodes (attacks) of sleep intrude into the waking hours of patients so that their days are dominated by sleepiness. Narcolepsy is the keystone of three other associated disorders, each of which are aspects of REM sleep: *cataplexy, sleep paralysis,* and *sleep hallucinations.* Together they form the *narcoleptic tetrad,* or *narcolepsy–cataplexy syndrome.*

Although some studies indicate that narcolepsy has a genetic basis, its cause is not yet established. It affects men and women equally, usually starting during adolescence, when the first symptom is excessive daytime sleepiness. Subsequently, narcolepsy is complicated by cataplexy and the other disorders.

Most narcolepsy attacks are preceded by a feeling of overwhelming fatigue, and they usually occur when the patient is comfortable and safe. Unlike boredom-induced naps, narcolepsy attacks sometimes occur when patients are standing or even engaged in activities that require constant attention, such as driving. Moreover, they typically occur about 12 times weekly at the onset of narcolepsy and 24 times weekly later in the illness. Each attack usually lasts 10 to 15 minutes, but it can be interrupted by noise or movement.

Attacks characteristically, but not invariably, begin with a REM period, a so-called "sleep-onset REM," rather than the normal preliminary NREM phases (Fig. 17-5). In other words, REM latency in narcolepsy is so short that it is virtually absent. Likewise, nighttime sleep, which is restless, has a sleep-onset REM and also multiple, brief, spontaneous awakenings.

Cataplexy, which usually begins about four years after the onset of narcolepsy, consists of episodes of sudden weakness that can be precipitated by heightened emotional states, most often laughter but also anger, surprise, or fright. These episodes last less than 30 seconds, and they occur about nine times weekly initially and 28 times weekly later. In cataplexy's most dramatic but rare form, the entire body musculature becomes limp and patients slump to the floor; however, unless there is a simultaneous sleep attack, they remain alert. Most often, patients have weakness limited to certain muscles. For example, the knees may buckle, the jaw drop open, or the head fall forward. Affected muscles also lose their tone and DTRs.

The flaccid, areflexic paresis of cataplexy with normal ocular movement, breathing, and other vital functions recreates the muscular state characteristic of REM sleep. Moreover, a PSG obtained during cataplexy demonstrates REM activity with absent EMG activity.

The other disturbances accompanying narcolepsy, sleep paralysis and sleep hallucinations, affect only about 10 percent of patients. They may be present on awakening (hypnopompic) or falling asleep (hypnogogic). Each has physical, psychologic, and PSG manifestations of REM sleep that have intruded into people's alert state. Like

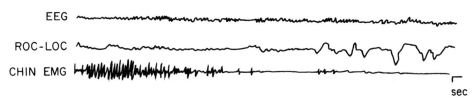

Fig. 17-5. A PSG during the start of a narcoleptic attack shows the characteristic, relatively immediate onset of rapid eye movements accompanied by loss of (chin) muscle activity.

cataplexy, they begin several years after the onset of narcolepsy, but they each occur only about six times weekly.

Patients with sleep paralysis are unable to move for several seconds on awakening or when falling asleep. As in cataplexy and normal REM sleep, they are able to breathe and move their eyes but otherwise they are virtually paralyzed. Similarly, patients with sleep hallucinations have vivid, dreamlike sensations on awakening or falling asleep. During both of these phenomena, PSGs reveal REM activity.

Medical treatment for narcolepsy and its associated disturbances relies on the use of stimulants in combination with medications that suppress REM sleep. Medicines suggested for daytime sleep attacks are pemoline (Cylert), methylphenidate (Ritalin), or amphetamines; for cataplexy, chlorimipramine, imipramine, or protriptyline (Vivactil); for nighttime sleep disturbances, imipramine or triazolam (Halcion).

Sleep Apnea Syndrome

The other major cause of excessive daytime sleepiness is the sleep apnea syndrome. This disorder results from multiple 10-second to 2-minute interruptions in breathing (apnea) that partially awaken the patient from nighttime sleep. In the *obstructive variety*, apnea is caused by blockages within the oropharyngeal portion of the respiratory pathway. The most common airway obstacles are congenital deformities, hypertrophied tonsils or adenoids, trauma, and other structural lesions (Fig. 17-6). The *nonobstructive*, or *central*, *variety* of apnea results from cessation of diaphragmatic movements because of inconsistent CNS respiratory effort.

Whatever the mechanism, apnea causes awakenings that are too brief and incomplete to be recognized by the patient or the patient's bed partner. However, they result in excessive daytime sleepiness that forces patients to succumb to multiple daytime naps. The naps associated with sleep apnea often occur under a variety of inappropriate conditions, such as when driving a car, and almost always follow fatigue, but individually they are similar to normal naps.

The apnea also leads to intermittent hypoxia (with oxygen saturation typically falling to 40 percent), cardiac arrhythmias, and pulmonary and systemic hypertension. Directly or indirectly, the apneic episodes also lead to morning headaches and, reportedly in many patients, intellectual and emotional impairment.

During sleep, a patient's breathing intermittently seems to cease. Then periods of loud, irregular snoring start as breathing resumes. The snoring is so characteristic that in the presence of daytime sleepiness, it is virtually diagnostic of sleep apnea.

Patients characteristically tend to be middle-aged, hypertensive, and overweight men. Children who have enlarged tonsils have also been reported to have the sleep

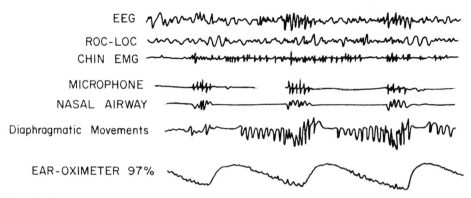

Fig. 17-6. A PSG during sleep complicated by sleep apnea shows that, during a period of NREM sleep, there is no diaphragmatic movement and the oxygen saturation falls. As diaphragmatic movements restart and reach a crescendo, loud snoring begins. After strenuous diaphragm movements, air moves through the nasal airway and oxygen saturation improves. During the obstructive phase, the EEG becomes faster and has higher voltage, which indicates a partial arousal.

apnea syndrome. The diagnosis of sleep apnea is indicated by a history of excessively loud, irregular snoring in a person who has sleepiness and an irresistible tendency to nap throughout the day. It can be confirmed by a PSG that shows periods of apnea, hypoxia, arousals, and respiratory abnormalities (Fig. 17-6). Because of REM sleep deprivation, REM latency is short. During the night, the episodes of sleep apnea occur in either phase of sleep, but they are more pronounced in REM sleep.

The initial treatment for this condition, in almost all cases, is to lose weight, stop smoking, and stop using sedatives, hypnotics, and alcohol. In the past, tracheostomies were performed to bypass the pharynx, but now simpler procedures, such as uvulopalatopharyngoplasty, are performed. When there is an element of central sleep apnea, a variety of medications, including protriptyline or medroxyprogesterone, have been reported to be useful. With effective treatment, patients have a dramatic reversal of their daytime sleepiness and cardiovascular abnormalities.

Other Disorders

The Kleine-Levin syndrome, *periodic hypersomnia,* is a rare sleep disorder. Patients are predominantly adolescent males. They have lengthy sleeps for periods of several days to two weeks, three or four times yearly. When the patients awaken between these episodes, they eat great quantities of food and display unusual behavior, including sexual disinhibition. At the same time they are slow, withdrawn, and apathetic. Some authors suggest that the disorder is akin to a burst of depression or the mirror image of anorexia nervosa. Others suggest that it is the result of encephalitis or a form of thalamic or hypothalamic damage. However, no consistent laboratory abnormality has been found that would determine that the disorder is clearly "organic," much less establish the site of abnormality.

In contrast, clear-cut cases of encephalitis, brain tumors, and hypothalamic injuries are often cited as causes of daytime sleepiness. Although these disorders might cause the appearance of sleep, in most cases patients are actually stuporous and have other signs of CNS dysfunction, such as intellectual impairment, hemiparesis, and abnormal reflexes. In addition, patients with hypothalamic injuries have endocrinologic disturbances. In virtually all of these cases, EEGs would reveal disorganized cerebral electrical activity rather than the usual pattern of REM or NREM sleep.

SUMMARY

Sleep may be interrupted by parasomnias, seizures, cardiovascular disturbances, and migraine and cluster headaches. Several disorders may be detected by considering features of the patient's history (Table 17-2), but in many cases a PSG is required. This technique will reveal that various disorders may be closely associated with either REM or NREM sleep.

Insomnia, besides being a problem itself, also rarely leads to excessive daytime sleepiness. It is often induced by stimulants, medications, drugs, and excessive alcohol. It is also a manifestation of the delayed sleep phase syndrome, in which patients fall asleep only in the early morning, but which can be corrected using chronotherapy, e.g., by further delaying their sleep until a conventional bedtime is reached. The

---

Table 17-2

Salient Historical Features of Patients with Insomnia or Excessive
Daytime Sleepiness*

A. Nighttime sleep
    1. What is the usual bedtime and time of falling asleep and awakening?
    2. What is the time spent sleeping compared with that spent in bed?
    3. What activities precede bedtime? (e.g., sex, food, medications, exercise)
    4. When asleep, is the patient apt to have any of the following interruptions?
        Nightmares or night terrors, sleepwalking, bedwetting
        Restless legs or generalized myoclonus
        Excessive snoring
        Headaches, chest pain, or other medical symptoms
B. Daytime sleep
    1. Are there afternoon or evening naps?
        Are they restful?
        Are they irresistible or not preceded by a feeling of fatigue
        Do they occur at inappropriate times?
    2. Are there episodes of loss of bodily tone?
        Does the patient slump suddenly and unexpectedly, especially following laughter or
          excitement?
        Does the patient have loss of tone in a single muscle group, such as those in the jaw
          or knees?
C. If left to his or her own schedule, would the patient be more alert and productive in the
    morning or night? And would such a self-determined schedule provide six to eight hours
    of continual, restful sleep?
D. General health
    1. Does the patient suffer from medical illness?
    2. Does the patient take any medication with a stimulating or sedating effect?
    3. Does the patient use alcohol habitually?
    4. Does the patient use coffee or other caffeine-containing beverage or food regularly or
       in the evening?

---

  *Proper history may only be obtained from a bed partner.

insomnia of depression is characterized by a short REM latency and an earlier onset, or phase advance, of body temperature nadir and neuroendocrine cycles. However, shortened REM latency is not an invariable manifestation of depression. It is also found in drug and alcohol withdrawal, narcolepsy, and nonaffective psychiatric illnesses.

Excessive daytime sleepiness, while often caused by insomnia, may be the result of narcolepsy or the sleep apnea syndrome. In the narcoleptic tetrad, narcolepsy is associated with cataplexy, sleep paralysis, and sleep hallucinations. All four are a manifestation of REM sleep. Sleep apnea syndrome is caused by airway obstruction or failure of respiratory drive. It characteristically results in snoring as patients attempt to overcome hypoxia and multiple partial arousals. Sleep apnea leads to hypertension, cardiac arrhythmias, and other disturbances that can be reversed with medical or surgical treatment.

REFERENCES

Akiskal HS, Lemmi H: Clinical, neuroendocrine, and sleep EEG diagnosis of "unusual" affective presentations: A practical review. Psychiatr Clin North Am 6:69, 1983

Carpenter S, Yassa R, Ochs R: A pathologic basis for Kleine-Levin syndrome. Arch Neurol 39:25, 1982

Ferriss G: Sleep disorders, Neurol Clin 6:51, 1984

Guilleminault C, Dement WC: Two hundred thirty-four cases of excessive daytime sleepiness: Diagnosis and tentative classification. J Chron Dis 29:733, 1976

Guilleminault C, Faull KF, Miles L, et al: Posttraumatic excessive daytime sleepiness: A review of 20 patients. Neurology 33:1584, 1983

Kales A, Cadieux RJ, Soldatos CR, et al: Narcolepsy-Cataplexy: I. Clinical and electrophysiologic characteristics; II. Psychosocial consequences and associated psychopathology. Arch Neurol 39:164, 1982

Kupfer DJ, Thase ME: The use of the sleep laboratory in the diagnosis of affective disorders. Psychiatr Clin North Am, 6:3, 1983

Moore-Ede MC, Czeisler CA, Richardson GS: Circadian time keeping in health and disease. N Engl J Med 309:469, 530, 1983

Orlosky MJ: The Kleine-Levin syndrome: A review. J Psychosomat 23:609, 1983

Wehr TA, Gillin JC, Goodwin FK: Sleep and circadian rhythms in depression. In Chase MH, Weitzman ED (eds): Sleep Disorders: Basic and Clinical Research. New York, SP Medical & Scientific Books, 1983, pp 195–225

Weitzman ED: Sleep and aging. In Katzman R, Terry R (eds): The Neurology of Aging. Philadelphia, F.A. Davis, 1983, pp 167–188

Weitzman ED, Czeisler CA, Coleman RM: Delayed sleep phase syndrome. Arch Gen Psychiatry 38:737, 1981

Zarcone VP: Sleep and alcoholism. In Chase MH, Weitzman ED (eds): Sleep Disorders: Basic and Clinical Research. New York, SP Medical & Scientific Books, 1983, pp 319–325

QUESTIONS

1–15. Is the statement true or false?

1. Normal sleep begins in the first stage of NREM sleep and progresses through the four NREM stages before the first period of REM sleep occurs.

2.   REM sleep usually begins about 90 minutes after the onset of sleep.

3.   The bulk of REM sleep occurs in the early evening, whereas the bulk of NREM sleep occurs in the early morning.

4.   The normal sequence of NREM–REM sleep recurs with a periodicity of 90 minutes.

5.   REM sleep is a period of decreased physical and mental activity.

6.   The third and fourth stages of NREM sleep can be considered deep sleep, during which there is great restfulness.

7.   Sleep always begins with the first stage of NREM sleep.

8.   Aside from the artifact caused by eye movement, the EEG obtained in REM sleep is similar to the one found in wakefulness.

9.   The EEG during NREM sleep is characterized by synchronous, slow activity.

10.   In general, the proportion of REM sleep remains constant from birth to old age.

11.   People's sleep–wake schedules are determined mostly by social and occupational factors rather than internal, physiologic mechanisms.

12.   Pseudoinsomniacs sleep four to five hours a night.

13.   Some productive, vigorous, and well-rested people sleep as little as five hours nightly.

14.   Fear of having a nightmare may cause insomnia.

15.   Infant boys have penile erections during REM sleep.

16.   In the night after sleep deprivation, which of the following can be expected to occur?
    a.   Sleep may begin with a period of REM activity
    b.   Epileptiform discharges may emanate from the temporal lobe of patients with partial complex (psychomotor) seizures
    c.   Total sleep time will increase
    d.   There will be an increase in time spent in REM sleep.
    e.   There will be a greater increase in the third and fourth stages of NREM sleep

17–24.   Which of the following characteristics are associated with night terrors (a), nightmares (b), both (c), or neither (d)?

17.   Onset during the first and second stage of NREM sleep

18.   Onset during the third and fourth stage of NREM sleep

19.   Onset during REM sleep

20.   Are a variety of common dreams

21.   Recall for content usual

22.   May be precipitated by loud noises during first NREM period

23.   Patients seem frightened

24.   Are associated with somnambulism

25–42.   Which of the following phenomena typically occur during REM sleep (a), NREM sleep (b), either phase (c), or neither phase (d)?

25.   Sleepwalking (somnambulism)

26.   Asthma

27.   Angina

28.   Bedwetting (enuresis)

29.   Night terrors

30.   Cluster headache

31.   Erections

32.   Migraine headache

33.   Nightmares

34.   Dreams

35.   Seizures

36.   Parkinson tremor

37.   Muscular contraction (tension) headaches

38. Hemiballismus

39. Complex motor activity

40. Tics

41. Complex intellectual activity

42. Head banging

43–47. Is the statement true or false?

43. Recent studies of the physiology of sleep have confirmed the clinical observation that neurotic or reactive depression is almost always associated with impaired ability to fall asleep, and endogenous depression is almost always associated with early morning awakenings.

44. Sleep apnea is a disorder only of adults.

45. Sleep apnea is sometimes associated with narcolepsy.

46. Sleep apnea leads to cardiovascular disturbances as well as excessive daytime sleepiness.

47. Hypnopompic refers to phenomena that occur on awakening and hypnogogic refers to phenomena that occur on falling asleep.

48. With which of the following is narcolepsy associated?
   a. Cataplexy
   b. Hallucinations
   c. Sleep paralysis
   d. Sleep-onset REM

49. A 27-year-old woman had the recent onset of lethargy, fever, temporal lobe seizures, and lymphocytic pleocytosis of the CSF. Which of the following illnesses is most likely?
   a. Hypothyroidism
   b. Schizophrenia
   c. Herpes simplex encephalitis
   d. Metastatic carcinoma

50. Which of the following can be causes of shortened REM latency?
   a. Narcolepsy
   b. Barbiturate withdrawal
   c. Depression
   d. Mania
   e. Sleep deprivation
   f. Neuroleptic withdrawal
   g. Sleep apnea
   h. Hypnotic use

51. Which characteristic(s) is (are) common to the sleep patterns seen in depression and following sleep deprivation?
   a. Lengthened sleep latency
   b. Shortened REM latency
   c. Early terminal awakening
   d. Interruptions in sleep

52. Which of the following are found in the night after sleep deprivation?
   a. Increase in total sleep
   b. Short sleep latency
   c. Increase in stage I and II NREM sleep
   d. In children, increased susceptibility for night terrors
   e. Normal REM distribution
   f. Shortened REM latency
   g. Increased deep NREM sleep

53. What is the relationship of seizures to sleep?
   a. Many patients have seizures prominently or exclusively during nighttime sleep
   b. Seizures occur only in deep NREM sleep
   c. EEGs obtained after sleep deprivation may reveal evidence without clinical signs of seizures
   d. Sleep deprivation can precipitate a seizure in a previously seizure-free individual

54. With which physiologic change is REM sleep associated?
   a. Absent respirations
   b. Lower pulse and blood pressure
   c. Increased intracranial pressure
   d. High voltage, slow EEG activity
   e. Absent limb and chin EMG activity
   f. Penile erections

55. In depressed patients, which of the following are typical?
   a. Delay in the nighttime body temperature nadir
   b. Advance of REM activity
   c. Advance of cortisol excretions
   d. Delay in MHPG excretion

56. What are the consequences of alcohol withdrawal?
   a. Hallucinations during the day
   b. Excessive dreaming
   c. Increased REM sleep
   d. Tendency to have seizures
   e. Decreased NREM sleep
   f. Agitation
   g. Insomnia

57. Which of the following conditions usually begin before 21 years of age?
   a. Delayed sleep phase syndrome   d. Sleep apnea syndrome
   b. Head banging   e. Narcolepsy
   c. Kleine-Levin syndrome   f. Cataplexy

58. Which of the following are effective treatments for the delayed sleep phase syndrome?
   a. Continually advancing the bedtime
   b. Continually delaying the bedtime
   c. Hypnotics
   d. Stimulants

59. Which of the following are accurate statements regarding the sleep of elderly people?
   a. Their sleep cycle is advanced
   b. They have a shortened REM latency
   c. REM periods are of equal length and distribution throughout the night
   d. Their sleep occurs partly during daytime as irresistible naps
   e. They sleep more than young adults

60. Which factor is (are) the major determinants of most people's sleep schedule?
   a. Early learning
   b. Social and occupational demands
   c. Neuroendocrinic excretion
   d. Personality type
   e. Physiologic "clocks"

61. What are the possible effects of withdrawal from medications that have hypnotic effects?
   a. Insomnia
   b. Excessive daytime sleepiness
   c. REM rebound
   d. Heightened awareness
   e. Vivid dreams
   f. Seizures

ANSWERS

1. True	22. a	42. c
2. True	23. c	43. False
3. False	24. a	44. False
4. True	25. b	45. True
5. False	26. c	46. True
6. True	27. a	47. True
7. False	28. b	48. a, b, c, d
8. True	29. b	49. c
9. True	30. a	50. a, b, c, d, e, f, g
10. False	31. a	51. b
11. True	32. a	52. a, b, d, e, f, g
12. False	33. a	53. a, c, d
13. True	34. a	54. c, e, f
14. True	35. b	55. b, c
15. True	36. c	56. a, b, c, d, f, g
16. a, b, c, d, e	37. d	57. a, b, c, e, f
17. d	38. d	58. b
18. a	39. d	59. a, c, d
19. b	40. c	60. b
20. b	41. a	61. a, b, c, e, f
21. b		

18

Involuntary Movement Disorders

The involuntary movement disorders* are a group of different symptoms or conditions, rather than illnesses, that are believed to result from abnormalities of the basal ganglia. Several of these disorders appear with or are complicated by mental abnormalities, such as dementia, depression, or psychotic behavior. Since, with few exceptions, diagnostic laboratory tests have not been developed, the diagnosis usually rests on the patient's history, the appearance of the movement, and the presence of mental abnormalities.

This chapter will briefly review the anatomy, physiology, and neurotransmitters of the basal ganglia. It will then describe classic disorders that are common and known to result from basal ganglia abnormalities: parkinsonism, athetosis, chorea, hemiballismus, Wilson's disease, and dystonia. Next, it will describe disorders that do not conform to classic patterns and where their origin is largely unknown: tremors, tics, Tourette's syndrome, and myoclonus. Finally, it will review tardive dyskinesia, other medication-induced conditions, and similarly appearing disorders.

THE BASAL GANGLIA

Anatomy and Physiology

Although some texts include additional structures, the basal ganglia are essentially composed of three elements:

---

*Patients with movement disorders may receive assistance from the following organizations: Benign Essential Blepharospasm Research Foundation, 755 Howell Street, Beaumont, Texas 77706, (409) 892-1339; Dystonia Medical Research Foundation, 2675 Henry Hudson Parkway, Bronx, New York 10463, (212) 549-7365; National Huntington's Disease Association, Suite 402, 1182 Broadway, New York, New York 10001, (212) 684-2781; Parkinson's Disease Foundation, 650 West 168th Street, New York, New York 10032, (212) 923-4700; Tourette Syndrome Association, 4102 Bell Boulevard, Bayside, New York 11361, (718) 224-2999; United Cerebral Palsy Foundation, 66 East 64th Street, New York, New York 10016, (212) 481-6300.

- The *corpus striatum* (*striatum*), which includes the *caudate nuclei*, the *putamen*, and the *globus pallidus*
- The *subthalamic nucleus* (*corpus of Luysii*)
- The *substantia nigra* (Fig. 18-1)

Extensive and intricate tracts link the basal ganglia to each other. The major one is the *nigrostriatal tract,* which projects from the substantia nigra to the striatum. Others link the basal ganglia to the cerebral cortex, the thalamus, and other areas of the brain and spinal cord.

The basal ganglia are the origin of the *extrapyramidal tract,* which is complementary to the *pyramidal* or corticospinal *tract* (Chapter 2). The pyramidal tract transmits commands for voluntary movements, and the extrapyramidal tract modulates the movements and maintains appropriate muscle tone. The extrapyramidal system functions through delicately balanced excitatory and inhibitory neurons, each of which utilize different neurotransmitters. It does not descend within the spinal cord, but plays predominantly upon the contralateral corticospinal tract through intracerebral pathways. Thus, unilateral injuries to the basal ganglia induce clinical abnormalities in the contralateral limbs.

Neurotransmitters

Although peptide neurotransmitters such as substance P and the enkephalins may have an important role, it is well known that the basal ganglia utilize three classic neurotransmitters:

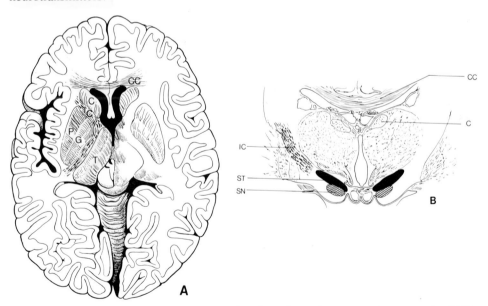

Fig. 18-1. (A) In this axial view, which is the plane shown in computed tomography (CT), the basal ganglia can be seen in relation to the brain. The head of the *caudate nuclei* (C) indent the anterior horns of the lateral ventricles. The *globus pallidus* (G) and *putamen* (P), which together are called the *corpus striatum* or *striatum,* are separated from the thalamus (T) by the (IC) posterior limb of the internal capsule. (B) In this coronal view, the *substantia nigra* (SN) and the *subthalamic nuclei* (ST) are in the midbrain, below the thalamus. Normally, the substantia nigra is black and large enough to be readily identified.

- *dopamine*
- *acetylcholine (ACh)*
- *gamma-aminobutyric acid (GABA)*.

DOPAMINE

Although dopamine is the neurotransmitter in many neurologic systems, about 80 percent of brain dopamine is concentrated in the striatum and the nigrostriatal tract. Dopamine in the nigrostriatal tract normally inhibits caudate activity. When dopamine depletion occurs, it leads to *akinesia* or *bradykinesia* (absent or slow movement). Dopamine excess, whether from illness or medicines, leads to *dyskinesias* (excessive, abnormal movements) and mental aberrations.

Dopamine is formed in sites outside of the brain, such as the adrenal gland, as well as in nigrostriatal neurons by decarboxylation of dihydroxyphenylalanine (dopa):

$$\text{dopa} \xrightarrow{\text{decarboxylase}} \text{dopamine}.$$

The concentration of dopamine can be artificially increased, as in the treatment of Parkinson's disease, by administering a precursor, L-dopa (Fig. 18-2). In this case, as long as some nigrostriatal (presynapic) neurons remain, enough L-dopa is metabolized to dopamine to reverse most symptoms of Parkinson's disease. Administering a dopa decarboxylase inhibitor, such as carbidopa, permits the brain dopamine concentration to rise without subjecting patients to systemic side-effects of L-dopa.*

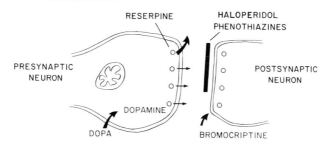

Fig. 18-2. In the presynaptic neuron, either naturally occurring dihydroxyphenylalanine (dopa) or medicines containing L-dopa, which are both dopamine *precursors,* are metabolized to the neurotransmitter dopamine. Amantadine (Symmetrel) and amphetamines can enhance dopamine activity by provoking its release from its storage sites or by blocking its reuptake into storage sites. In contrast, alpha-methyl-paratyrosine inhibits dopamine synthesis, and reserpine depletes dopamine storage sites. The postsynaptic neuron dopamine receptors can be triggered by dopamine *agonists,* such as bromocriptine (Parlodel), pergolide, and lergotrile. However, dopamine *antagonists,* such as phenothiazines, haloperidol, and other neuroleptics, which block the postsynaptic neuron dopamine receptors, reduce dopamine activity.

---

*Carbidopa is given along with L-dopa in Sinemet, a widely used antiparkinson medication. Since carbidopa does not enter the brain, it retards the conversion of dopa to dopamine only in sites outside the brain. Thus, the increased L-dopa-induced dopamine synthesis of the brain is protected.

Dopamine activity can be enhanced further by facilitating its release from presynaptic neuron storage sites by administering amantadine (Symmetrel) or blocking its storage by administering amphetamines–two other medicines useful in the treatment of Parkinson's disease.

Similar effects can be induced by giving dopamine *agonists,* which are chemically different than dopamine but act directly on the same postsynaptic receptors. For example, bromocriptine (Parlodel), an ergot alkaloid with powerful serotinin effects, is a dopamine agonist that also relieves symptoms of Parkinson's disease. It is effective even when the presynapic neurons have degenerated so much that they are incapable of metabolizing dopa to dopamine. Likewise, excessive dopamine agonist treatment also leads to dyskinesias and mental aberrations.

In contrast, many medicines reduce dopamine activity. Reserpine depletes dopamine concentration in the presynaptic terminals. Neurolepics, such as phenothiazines and haloperidol, which are dopamine *antagonists,* block the postsynaptic receptors. With the possible exception of reserpine, all these medicines induce signs of Parkinson's disease.

ACETYLCHOLINE

Acetylcholine (ACh), which is an excitatory neurotransmitter, increases caudate activity and thus opposes dopamine activity (Fig. 18-3). It is formed by the combination of acetyl Coenzyme A and choline utilizing the enzyme choline acetyltransferase (CAT):

$$\text{Acetyl CoA} + \text{choline} \xrightarrow{\text{CAT}} \text{ACh}$$

Attempts have been made to increase CAT and ACh concentrations because they are markedly reduced in some areas of the brain in Alzheimer's disease (Chapter 7), and also because of a postulated ACh deficiency in tardive dyskinesia. Increasing ACh activity has been attempted by providing ACh precursors, such as choline and

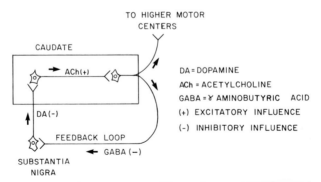

Fig. 18-3. The interaction of neurotransmitters can be viewed in terms of a feedback loop in which dopamine and gamma-aminobutyric acid (GABA) are inhibitory and acetylcholine (ACh) is excitatory. The physiologic terms "inhibitory" and "excitatory," however, are the opposite of the clinical situation. For example, too much dopamine is associated with chorea and too little with akinesia.

lecithin (phosphatidylcholine). Another strategy has been to administer physostigmine, which is an anticholinesterase (or a cholinesterase inhibitor) that retards CAT metabolism (see Fig. 7-5). By preserving the available CAT, physostigmine promotes ACh synthesis. Precursor and physostigmine treatments, which are complementary, often are given simultaneously. Although these maneuvers have increased concentrations, they have not produced the desired effects.

When decreased ACh activity is desirable, as in the treatment of Parkinson's disease, the well-known anticholinergic medicines are given (Table 18-1). In excessive doses, they too can cause mental aberrations.

GAMMA-AMINOBUTYRIC ACID

Gamma-aminobutyric acid (GABA) is essentially an inhibitory neurotransmitter that plays upon the nigrostriatal system. It is formed from glutamate by the enzyme glutamate decarboxylase (GAD):

$$\text{Glutamate} \xrightarrow{\text{GAD}} \text{GABA}$$

In Huntington's chorea, GAD and GABA concentrations in certain parts of the brain and in the cerebrospinal fluid (CSF) are reduced below normal levels. The GABA concentration is increased by the anticonvulsant, valproate.

GENERAL CHARACTERISTICS

The involuntary movement disorders have several common clinical features. The movements are increased by anxiety, exertion, fatigue, and stimulants, including coffee. They can be momentarily suppressed by intense concentration. Also, they are decreased by relaxation and, in some cases, by biofeedback. With the exception of palatal myoclonus and tics, they are absent during sleep.

When only extrapyramidal damage has occurred, patients have no signs of pyramidal (corticospinal) tract damage, such as paresis, spasticity, hyperactive reflexes, or Babinski signs (Chapter 2). Likewise, in this situation, they have no signs of cerebral cortical injury, the most important ones being dementia and seizures. These patients might be debilitated by uncontrollable movements and inarticulate speech, but they can be fully alert, intelligent, and, by using unconventional methods, able to communicate thoughtfully.

Another important consideration is that at the onset of illness, patients are liable to be misdiagnosed as having an "hysteric" or psychogenic disorder (Chapter 3). The error is usually made because the movements may seem bizarre, be apparent only

Table 18-1
Anticholinergic Medications

Brand Name	Generic Name	Usual Dosage
Akineton	Biperiden	1–2 mg tid
Artane	Trihexyphenidyl	2–4 mg tid
Cogentin	Benztropine	1–3 mg tid
Kemadrin	Procyclidine	2–5 mg tid

during anxiety, be willfully suppressed, and absent during sleep. Most important, when dementia is a component of the illness, it may appear to be a psychiatric disturbance and reinforce the misdiagnosis.

PARKINSON'S DISEASE

Clinical Features

Although the most prominent feature of this illness is a tremor, the most debilitating one is akinesia. It leads to the classic "masked face" (Fig. 18-4), paucity of trunk and limb movement (Figs. 18-5 and 18-6), and impairment of dressing, bathing, and other "activities of daily living." Akinesia usually begins many months before tremor. In "hemiparkinsonism" it frequently develops asymmetrically or unilaterally, so that despite having normal strength and coodination, patients have difficulty using one arm and leg.

Akinesia is usually accompanied by "cogwheel" rigidity (Fig. 18-7). It is an important sign of Parkinson's disease and other extrapyramidal disorders. Its presence is especially helpful in distinguishing a Parkinson tremor from other tremor varieties.

A Parkinson's disease tremor typically occurs when patients sit with their arms supported and thus it is called a *resting tremor* (Fig. 18-8). It too can be asymmetric or unilateral; if so, it is more pronounced on the side of akinesia. This tremor differs from cerebellar tremor (see Fig. 2-11) and essential tremor (see below) not only in being found at rest and being accompanied by akinesia, but by having a regular rate and primarily involving the hands and the feet.

A myriad of other signs, some of which require special examinations, develop in patients who have had Parkinson's disease for several years. Many are important in their own right and several may also be found in other illnesses.

Patients have impairment or loss of *postural reflexes,* which are the mechanisms that alter muscle tone in response to change in position. Their loss in combination with akinesia and rigidity leads to a gait impairment, called *marche à petit pas* or *festinating gait* that is characterized by short steps and a tendency to accelerate (Fig.

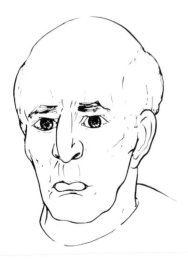

Fig. 18-4. Since Parkinson's patients have facial muscle akinesia and rigidity, they have remarkably infrequent blinking and facial expressions. In addition, widened palpebral fissures and lack of head motion give patients a "stare." Their facial appearance has been called a "masked facies," but this is a Latin term for "face" or "countenance," and the term *masked face* is becoming more widely used.

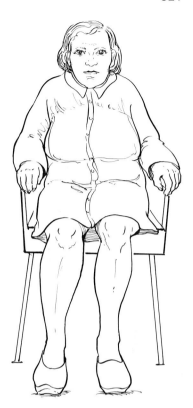

Fig. 18-5. When Parkinson's disease patients sit, they are typically immobile, with their legs uncrossed and their feet set flatly on the floor. Their arms remain on the chair or are held in their lap, but are rarely used for gesturing. In contrast to normal people and especially those with chorea, Parkinson's disease patients have virtually no repositioning movements in which they shift their weight from one hip to another, unnecessarily move their limbs, or perform other routine activities to make themselves comfortable.

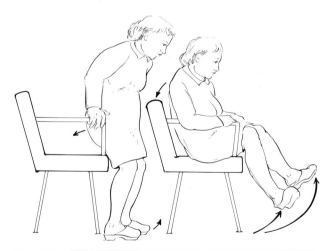

Fig. 18-6. Since Parkinson's disease patients have akinesia and rigidity, they cannot rapidly flex their spine, hips, or knees. When sitting, they tend to rock solidly backwards into a chair and their feet rise several inches off the floor. "Sitting *en bloc*" is an early, reliable manifestation of Parkinson's disease.

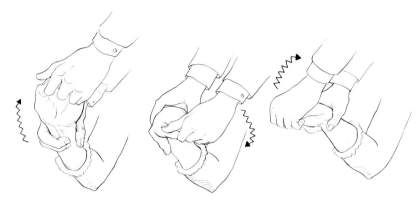

Fig. 18-7. In most cases of Parkinson's disease, "cogwheel rigidity" can be elicited by rotating the patient's wrist. It is characterized by firm resistance in all directions of movement and superimposed ratchetlike obstructions. In contrast, spasticity, which is the result of corticospinal tract damage, is sustained resistance up to a point, after which there is no resistance.

18-9). Of the several different characteristic gait abnormalities (see Table 2-4), the festinating gait is most similar to gait apraxia (see Fig. 7-7). Both disorders are characterized by small steps and slowed movements; however, gait apraxia is associated with impairment of voluntary leg motions and the presence of spasticity.

After patients have been ill for several years, their voice often becomes *hypophonic* (low in volume), and beset with a quavering or tremulous quality. Likewise, their handwriting becomes *micrographic* and shaky (Fig. 18-10).

More important, mental complications affect almost 50 percent of chronically ill Parkinson patients. Dementia, in which calculation ability and digit span recall are most severely affected, occurs in about 30 percent of patients. Although dementia practically never occurs as an initial symptom, it is found more frequently in older patients, when the illness has had a rapid onset, and when medications have had little effect (Lieberman). The dementia worsens with advancing age and increased physical impairments, especially greater akinesia. Although L-dopa and anticholinergic medications improve the physical aspects of the illness, they do not alleviate the dementia.

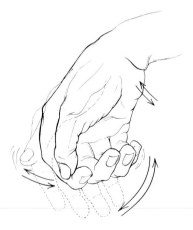

Fig. 18-8. The *resting tremor* is a relatively slow (4 to 6 cycles-per-second) to-and-fro flexion movement of the wrist, hand, thumb, and fingers. Since the cupped hand appears as though it were shaking pills, the movement is commonly known as a "pill-rolling" tremor. The tremor will be most apparent when patients sit comfortably. It is exaggerated or apparent only when patients are anxious. It will be momentarily reduced during the initial phase of many voluntary movements or by intense concentration. It is absent during sleep.

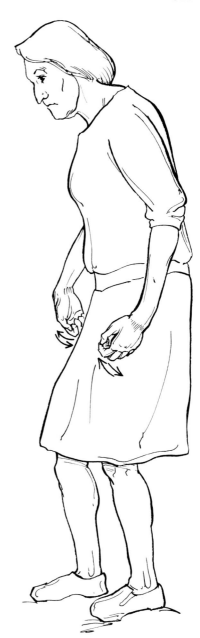

Fig. 18-9. When Parkinson's disease patients walk, they involuntarily tend to take short steps and accelerate their pace, i.e., they have a "festinating gait." In addition, they have a flexed posture and resting tremor. If they take several steps backwards, they usually are unable to stop, i.e., they have "retropulsion." They do not swing their arms, look about, or have other normal accessory movements. When turning, they simultaneously move their head, trunk, and legs without fluidity, i.e., they turn "en bloc."

Nevertheless, despite debilitating physical impairments, many patients, who must be carefully identified, have normal intelligence.

Late in the illness, about 10 percent of patients, especially those with dementia, develop psychotic episodes. These episodes are often precipitated by medications and are associated with the physical manifestations of excessive dopamine activity, such as dyskinesias. In treating such psychosis, the first step is to reduce the aniparkinson medication, especially the nighttime doses. Minor tranquilizers then might be given. Although neuroleptics are often necessary, the concurrent use of L-dopa and dopamine antagonist neuroleptics should be avoided.

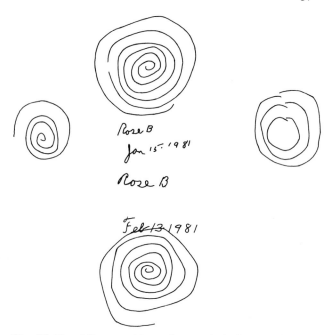

Fig. 18-10. *Micrographia,* a characteristic feature of Parkinson's disease, is shown in the patient's upper three spirals, date, and signature. In the lower examples, which were obtained after treatment was initiated, the excursions were larger, bolder, and relatively free of tremor.

Depression affects 25 to 50 percent of patients. It is also associated with dementia and increasing physical disability. Likewise, depression does not improve if medications improve the physical symptoms. Although depression may result in part from dopamine depletion, loss of other neurotransmitters, such as serotonin, may be responsible (Mayeux).

Treatment of depression in Parkinson's disease is often difficult because of coexistent physical and cognitive disabilities. Nevertheless, antidepressants are helpful, and their anticholinergic side-effects are at least theoretically beneficial to physical manifestations of Parkinson's disease. Electroconvulsive therapy has been suggested for patients who are unresponsive to antidepressants.

In contrast to the relatively high frequency of dementia and depression in Parkinson's disease, manic-depressive illness and schizophrenia rarely occur.

Pathology

Although in the past almost all cases of Parkinson's disease have been caused by encephalitis, now almost all cases are caused by an idiopathic degenerative illness. Contrary to a popular idea, however, Parkinson's disease does not result from cerebrovascular infarctions. Notably, the concordance rate in dizygotic twins is virtually zero.

The "pigmented nuclei" of the brain (the substantia nigra, locus ceruleus, and the tenth cranial dorsal motor nuclei) are all depigmented and their neurons contain *Lewy bodies,* which are eosinophilic, intracytoplasmic inclusions. As previously mentioned, nigrostriatal neurons are depleted of dopamine.

In many patients the cerebral cortex has changes indicative of Alzheimer's disease. Patients have an increased number of senile plaques, neurofibrillary tangles, and neuron loss. Also, demented patients have a decreased concentration of CAT in proportion to dementia (Chapter 7).

Differential Diagnosis

A Parkinson-like clinical state, or *parkinsonism,* can be caused by use of an illicit synthetic heroin methylphenyltetrahydropyridine (MPTP) or common phenothiazines, haloperidol, and other dopamine antagonist neuroleptics. Without a patient's history, the distinction between postencephalitic and medication-induced parkinsonism might be difficult; however, usually in Parkinson's disease, the onset is slow and the signs may be initially asymmetric. As a practical consideration, the coincidence of Parkinson's disease and schizophrenia is so low that whenever schizophrenic patients seem to have Parkinson's disease, they must be considered, in almost all cases, to have either medication-induced parkinsonism or a neurologic disorder other than Parkinson's disease.

The other neurologic conditions that cause parkinsonism are cerebral palsy, the juvenile form of Huntington's chorea, Wilson's disease, manganese intoxication, cerebral anoxia (especially from drug overdose), punch-drunk syndrome (dementia pugilistica, Chapter 7), and a group of rarely occurring degenerative neurologic conditions. Most affect young adults and cause mental impairment, and some may be correctable.

Therapy

Until the introduction of L-dopa, neurosurgery was the best available treatment. Small lesions were made in the thalamus or striatum. When patients had hemiparkinsonism, lesions were made in the basal ganglia contralateral to the affected limbs. In most cases, surgery was successful in relieving symptoms for several years. However, it was occasionally complicated by damage to the corticospinal tract in the adjacent internal capsule (Fig. 18-1), or, with bilateral procedures, corticobulbar tract damage that caused pseudobulbar palsy (Chaper 4).

Similar ablative surgical procedures have also been advocated for other movement disorders, including athetosis and dystonia. However, benefits are typically inconsistent or present for less than 1 year. Moreover, these procedures are also hazardous. Surgeons are now advocating spinal cord stimulation. This relatively harmless procedure has been said to have helped patients with tremor, dystonia, and other neurologic disorders.

Current medical treatment, which is usually satisfactory, attempts to maintain normal dopamine activity. Combinations of L-dopa and carbidopa (Sinemet) are the medical mainstay in the first five years of the illness, when sufficient (possibly 20 percent) nigrostriatal neurons are intact and can convert L-dopa to dopamine. The effect of dopamine can be enhanced by amantadine (Symmetrel) or mimicked by agonists, such as bromocriptine (Parlodel) (Fig. 18-2). Dopamine toxicity, manifested by dyskinesias and mental aberrations, limits dopamine replacement, especially late in the illness when dementia is often present.

Another standard medication, but one that is not as effective as L-dopa, are the anticholinergics (Table 18-1). They presumably are effective because dopamine depletion results in relatively excessive ACh activity, and anticholinergic medicines correct the imbalance (Fig. 18-11). In moderate doses, the side effects of anticholinergic medicine are usually dry mouth, constipation, and urinary retention. However, when larger doses are used, patients can develop confusion and agitation.

An experimental approach is to transplant adrenal cells, which are capable of synthesizing dopamine, into the brain. These cells may be able to provide sufficient dopamine to cure Parkinson's disease.

ATHETOSIS

Athetosis is a slow, regular, continual twisting of muscles. It is at one end of a spectrum, and chorea and hemiballismus at the other, where movements are of progressively greater amplitude and irregularity. Athetosis predominantly affects the distal parts of the limbs, and is almost always bilateral and symmetric (Fig. 18-12). It is often combined with chorea, in *choreoathetosis*.

Athetosis, which almost always becomes apparent in early childhood, results from perinatal hyperbilirubinemia (kernicterus), hypoxia, or prematurity, i.e., choreoathetotic cerebral palsy (Chapter 13). Although athetosis is closely associated with mental retardation, when the perinatal damage is confined to the basal ganglia, some patients have relatively normal intelligence despite having marked movement disorders and garbled voice.

For treatment of choreoathetotic cerebral palsy, neurosurgeons have created thalamic or basal ganglia lesions, and have installed spinal cord stimulators. Dopamine

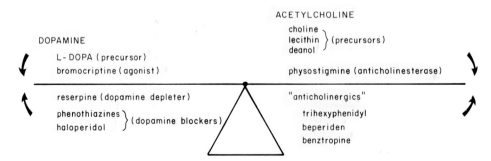

Fig. 18-11. The countervaling effects of dopamine and acetylcholine can be pictured as a balanced scale. In this model, the right side of the scale would be pushed downward when there is dopamine depletion, as in Parkinson's disease; however, it would be realigned by dopamine precursors, dopamine agonists, or anticholinergics. In cases where excessive dopamine activity is postulated, the left side would be pushed downward; however, it could be realigned by dopamine antagonists, dopamine depleters, or acetylcholine precursors.

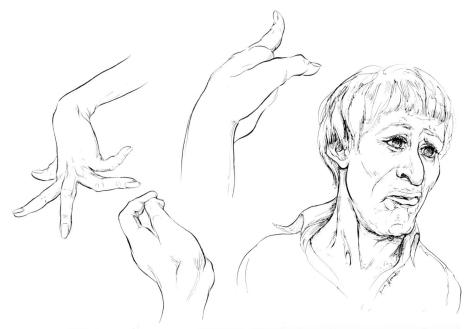

Fig. 18-12.   In athetosis, the face has incessant grimacing and fractions of smiles that alternate with frowns. Neck muscles contract and rotate the head. Laryngeal contraction and irregular chest and diaphragm muscle movements cause dysarthria that has an irregular cadence and nasal pitch. Fingers writhe constantly and tend to assume hyperextension postures, while the wrists rotate, flex, and extend. These movements prevent writing, buttoning, and other fine hand movements, but they usually permit gross shoulder, trunk, and hip movements.

antagonists suppress the movements, but their long-term use may lead to complications.

HUNTINGTON'S CHOREA

Huntington's chorea, which is genetically transmitted in an autosomal dominant pattern, is characterized by chorea and dementia. It becomes apparent, on the average, at age 35 years and causes death about 15 years later from aspiration and inanition. Between 2 and 6 per 100,000 persons suffer from Huntington's chorea, making it a relatively common disorder and one of the most frequent causes of dementia in middle-aged adults (Chapter 7). Although families of all races and ethnic backgrounds have been diagnosed as having Huntington's chorea, cases in the United States have been traced to several 17th century English immigrants.

Abnormalities in the basal ganglia and cerebral cortex are probably responsible for the major symptoms. The caudate nuclei are atrophied, and GABA and GAD concentrations in the striatum are reduced to less than 50 percent of normal. The cerebral cortex, especially in the frontal lobes, is also atrophied; however, there the GABA and GAD concentrations are normal. More important, in contrast to Parkinson's disease and Alzheimer's disease, cerebral cortex CAT concentrations are normal.

Clinical Features

In contrast to the continual writhing movements of athetosis, chorea consists of frequent discrete brisk movements, "jerks," of the pelvis, trunk, and limbs (Fig. 18-13). Also, the face has intermittent, rather than continual, frowns, grimaces, and smirks (Fig. 18-14). Abrupt pelvic movements when walking, superimposed on the normal pelvic tilting and rotation, give the gait of patients a characteristic "herky-jerky" pattern (Fig. 18-15) that served as the origin of the term *chorea,* which is Greek for "dance."

When Huntington's chorea is fully developed, the presence of an involuntary movement disorder, if not chorea itself, is easy to recognize. However, in its earliest stages, chorea is often so subtle that it mimics the nonspecific movements that result from anxiety, restlessness, discomfort, or clumsiness. At this stage, chorea may consist of only excessive face or hand gestures, frequent weight shifting, continual leg crossing, or twitching fingers (Fig. 18-16).

In 5 to 10 percent of Huntington's chorea cases, symptoms appear before patients are 20 years old. This variety, *juvenile Huntington's chorea,* is characterized not by chorea, but by rigidity and dystonic posturing (see below). Also in contrast to the common adult variety, the juvenile variety causes seizures, face and trunk akinesia, and a slow and short-stepped gait. Although these patients may appear to have Parkinson's disease, their invariable mental deterioration and the course of the illness are similar to Huntington's chorea.

The dementia may begin, typically, one year either before or after the chorea; however, some authors have claimed that mental symptoms can precede the chorea by a decade. Patients with frank chorea have impaired judgment, and later they develop profound dementia. In the beginning, irritability and depression may be present or, in some cases, may have been the first symptom of the illness. Many patients become

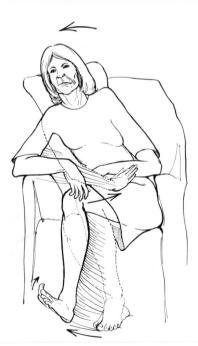

Fig. 18-13. Patients with chorea, such as this one who has Huntington's chorea, have intermittent and brisk pelvic, trunk, and limb movements that are most often a wrist flick, a jutting of the leg forward, or a shrugging of the shoulder.

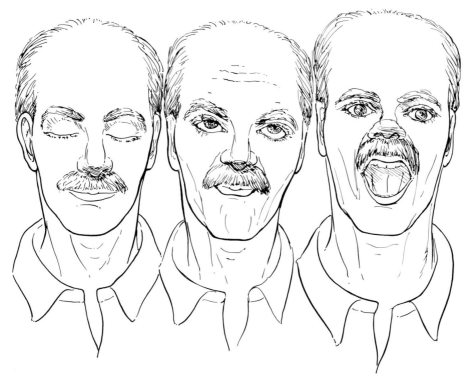

Fig. 18-14. Huntington's chorea patients have frequent, unexpected facial movements, including frowns, eyebrow raisings, smiles, and a variety of fractions of these expressions.

alcoholics or commit suicide. However, patients do not have intellectual or emotional changes that are sufficiently characteristic for diagnostic purposes.

In the future, the diagnosis will be made by analysis of genetic material, such as DNA. Now, the diagnosis rests on finding chorea and dementia and establishing that a parent had been afflicted with a similar disorder. Finding a low GABA concentration in the CSF will support the clinical diagnosis.

The electroencephalogram (EEG) shows only nonspecific, low voltage activity with a poorly organized background (Chapter 10). Computed tomography (CT) reveals atrophy of the cerebral cortex, absence of the caudate nuclei, and an outward expansion of the anterior horns of the third ventricle (see Fig. 20-12). Unfortunately, EEG and CT findings are found late in the illness and usually after the diagnosis can be achieved on clinical grounds.

Giving L-dopa as a diagnostic "provocative" agent usually precipitates a transient chorea when it is given to asymptomatic Huntington's chorea carriers, i.e., persons who carry the affected gene but are too young to have developed overt symptoms. The problems with this method of detecting affected persons, especially before they have children, are that sometimes the chorea does not recede and that some carriers may fail to develop it.

When chorea is mild, it may be suppressed by dopamine antagonists, e.g., haloperidol, which are sometimes supplemented by dopamine synthesis inhibitors, such as alpha-methyl-paratyrosine (Fig. 18-2). Attempts have also been made to

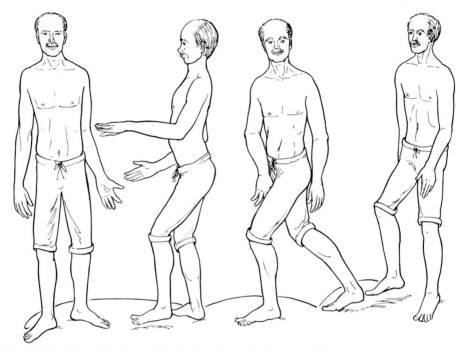

Fig. 18-15. The gait abnormality in Huntington's chorea, which is a characteristic feature, results from superimposed, intermittent trunk and pelvic motions. These movements along with those of the face and hands give the gait a dance-like appearance; however, the gait is not rhythmic or graceful, but lurching and contorted.

enhance GABA and ACh activity, but they resulted in little or no reduction in chorea. The dementia is unaffected by any of these treatments.

Other Varieties of Chorea

Sydenham's chorea (St. Vitus' dance or chorea minor) is a "major diagnostic criterion" of rheumatic fever that begins 1 to 6 months after the carditis and has an average duration of 2 months. It almost only affects children between the ages of 5

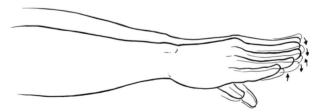

Fig. 18-16. The hands of Huntington's chorea patients make fidgety movements that could reasonably be mistaken for manifestations of anxiety or restlessness. Their true nature, however, can be demonstrated by having patients stretch out their hands and arms for 30 seconds. This maneuver precipitates characteristic, momentary flexion or extension finger movements and continuous hyperextension of the wrists.

and 15 years: Notably, of those children older than 10 years, girls are affected twice as frequently as boys. With the decreasing incidence of rheumatic fever, the incidence of Sydenham's chorea has fallen dramatically. Nevertheless, Sydenham's chorea remains an important condition because it is often the most prominent manifestation of an illness that can have life-long physical and mental consequences.

Children who develop Sydenham's chorea have an insidious onset of grimacing, limb movements, and other stigmata of chorea (Fig. 18-17). During the illness, patients have listlessness, irritability, apathy, and emotional lability. Although they do not develop cognitive impairment or major psychiatric disorders, about 50 percent of them have residual permanent minor psychologic disturbances. The brains of patients that have been inspected at postmortem examination, which were clearly from the worst cases, have had extensive microscopic hemorrhages.

Chorea recurs in about 20 percent of patients following another attack of rheumatic fever, the initiation of taking oral contraceptives (see below), or conception (see below). In addition, the close relatives of patients are liable to develop chorea under any of these same circumstances.

The etiology of Sydenham's chorea is probably a genetically induced susceptibility to a cerebrovascular inflammatory illness that can be triggered by streptococcal infections. The movements are thought to recur because of a permanent increased

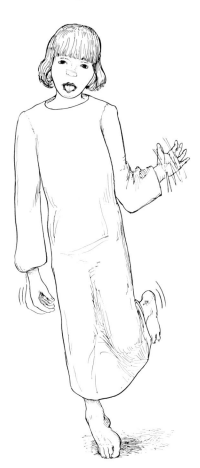

Fig. 18-17. Children with Sydenham's chorea may appear to have coy smiles and brief grimaces. They walk with a playful sashay. However, the chorea can be made obvious if the children attempt to hold a fixed position, such as standing at attention or standing on the ball of one foot.

dopamine sensitivity, when estrogen levels are elevated, as during female puberty, use of oral contraceptives, and pregnancy. The mental abnormalities during the illness are attributable to exhaustion or cerebral vascular inflammation; however, increased dopamine sensitivity has also been suggested to be the cause of the mental changes that occur both during and after episodes of Sydenham's chorea.

Treatment usually requires dopamine antagonists. They suppress the movements and also usually provide much needed sedation.

Oral contraceptive-induced chorea is a rare reaction to oral contraceptives. It occurs in women who are younger than 20 years old 1 or 2 months after starting a contraceptive containing estrogen and resolves after contraceptives are stopped. This variety of chorea is not associated with mental abnormalities.

Chorea gravidarum, another rarely occurring variety, almost always develops in young primigravidas during their first trimester of pregnancy. Many patients or their close relatives have had Sydenham's chorea, oral contraceptive-induced chorea, or chorea gravidarum. Patients with this condition often become so exhausted, frightened, and irrational that it frequently precipitates a spontaneous abortion or necessitates a therapeutic one. In either case, all symptoms resolve several days after the pregnancy is ended.

Withdrawal-emergent dyskinesia consists of choreoathetoid and other movements and also systemic symptoms, such as nausea and diaphoresis, immediately following a course of dopamine antagonist neuroleptic therapy. It especially affects children and usually lasts less than 6 weeks. Cases lasting longer than 6 months are probably ones of tardive dyskinesia.

Other causes of chorea have been described (Table 18-2). In many of these conditions, structural lesions or metabolic derangements injure the basal ganglia. In others, dopamine activity is selectively increased. Although chorea may occur without accompanying neurologic abnormality, in most disorders it is associated with dementia, delirium, or other mental impairment.

HEMIBALLISMUS

Hemiballismus is intermittent, gross movements of one side of the body that are similar to those found in chorea, except that they are unilateral and more of a flinging (ballistic) motion (Fig. 18-18). Since the lesion that causes hemiballismus is almost always a small, cerebrovascular infarction in the (contralateral) subthalamic nucleus, hemiballismus is not associated with mental abnormalities or accompanied by paresis or other signs of corticospinal tract injury.

Patients, who are almost always older than 65 years, have hemiballismus for several days to several weeks. Afterwards, the movements subside, but sometimes a residual hemichorea-like movement persists for years. When hemiballismus is severe, neuroleptics suppress it, possibly by blocking dopamine activity, providing sedation, or both.

The CSF concentration of the metabolite of dopamine, homovanillic acid (HVA), has been found to be increased. This finding is consistent with the observation that excessive dopamine activity is associated with dyskinesia. Although increased GABA activity should reduce the movements, GABA and its precursors and agonists have not been helpful.

Table 18-2

Causes of Chorea
_____

Basal ganglia lesions
   Perinatal injury, e.g., anoxia, kernicterus
   Cerebrovascular accidents
   Tumors
Genetic disorders
   Huntington's chorea
   Wilson's disease
Metabolic derangements
   Hypocalcemia
   Hypothyroidism
   Hepatic encephalopathy
Drugs
   Oral contraceptives*
   L-dopa compounds, precursors, and agonists
   Amphetamines, methylphenidate (Ritalin)
   Neuroleptics†
Vascular inflammatory conditions
   Sydenham's chorea
   Pertussis, diphtheria, and other encephalitides
   Systemic lupus erythematosus (SLE)
Miscellaneous
   Carbon monoxide poisoning
   Senile chorea
   Polycythemia
_____

*And chorea gravidarum.
†Withdrawal emergent and tardive dyskinesias.

WILSON'S DISEASE

Wilson's disease *(hepatolenticular degeneration)* is an autosomal recessive genetic illness characterized by dementia, a variety of involuntary movements, and hepatic insufficiency. It is caused by an abnormality of copper metabolism that leads to destructive deposits in many organs, including the brain. In advanced cases, the globus pallidus and putamen develop cavitary lesions that can be detected with CT.

Symptoms become evident between the ages of 10 and 40 years. The dementia, which may begin before the movements, can initially be overshadowed by personality changes, mood alterations, or thought disorders; however, no particular pattern or psychologic test is sufficiently reliable to distinguish it from the dementia caused by other neurologic illnesses.

Likewise, the appearance of the movements is highly variable. They may consist of rigidity, akinesia, chorea, a *wing-beating* tremor (Fig. 18-19), or dystonic posturing (see below). These movements tend to occur in combination and to be accompanied by signs of damage to the corticospinal and corticobulbar tract.

In addition, nonneurologic signs may be present and more obvious than neurologic ones. In particular, liver involvement leads to cirrhosis, and copper deposition in the cornea leads to a Kayser-Fleischer ring (Fig. 18-20).

The protean manifestations of Wilson's disease require that physicians test for this illness despite its infrequent occurrence (1 per 100,000 persons) in young adults who develop a wide variety of conditions, including tremor, other movement disor-

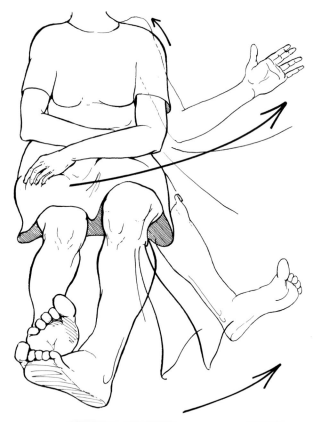

Fig. 18-18. Hemiballismus is large-scale movements of the limbs on one side of the body. Patients attempt to suppress the movements by pressing their body or unaffected limbs against the involuntarily moving ones. They also attempt to hide the involuntary movements by converting them into apparently purposeful movements. For example, if a patient's arm were to fly upward, he or she might incorporate the movement into a gesture, such as waving to someone.

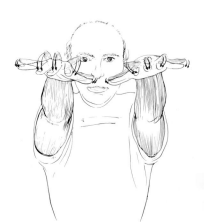

Fig. 18-19. Patients with Wilson's disease may have any of a variety of movement disorders; however, the *wing-beating tremor* is characteristic. Unlike most other tremors, it is coarse and involves the shoulders, and, as its name implies, patients move their arms as though they were attempting to fly. The bizarre appearance of such patients makes them especially liable to be misdiagnosed as having a psychogenic disturbance.

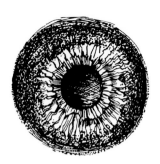

Fig. 18-20. The Kayser-Fleischer ring, which is pathognomonic of Wilson's disease affecting the brain, is a green-brown pigment in the periphery of the cornea. Typically, it is most obvious at the superior and inferior margins of the cornea where it obscures the fine structure of the iris. However, when the ring is forming, it can be seen only with an ophthalmologist's slit-lamp.

ders, atypical psychosis, dementia, dysarthria, or chronic hepatitis. Since the Kayser-Fleischer ring can be observed in virtually all cases in which neurologic symptoms are present, any suspected case should undergo a slit lamp examination. A test that is diagnostic, even when the illness does not affect the brain, is the determination of the concentration of serum ceruloplasmin (the serum protein to which copper adheres): In cases of Wilson's disease, its concentration is very low. Penicillamine, when given early enough, can usually reverse the mental deterioration, movement disorder, and nonneurologic manifestations.

DYSTONIA

Dystonia Musculorum Deformans

Dystonia musculorum deformans, or *torsion dystonia,* is a group of conditions that are characterized by *dystonia,* which is prolonged, powerful muscle contractions. Limb (appendicular) and neck, trunkal, and pelvic (axial) muscle contractions contort the body and create "dystonic postures." In addition, they act as isometric exercises and lead to muscle hypertrophy.

In about 30 percent of cases, the cause is an autosomal recessive genetic trait. In these cases, symptoms develop in children, who are predominantly Askenazi Jewish, between ages 8 and 14 years. The initial symptom of this "childhood onset" variety is usually appendicular dystonia, such as a slow, inward twisting (torsion) of one foot (Fig. 18-21). Over the next several years, affected children develop torsion of other limbs, the pelvis (tortipelvis), trunk, and neck (torticollis) (Fig. 18-22). Although these children become physically incapacitated, their mental abilities remain intact.

In an "adult-onset" variety, an equal proportion of patients who are mostly non-Jewish and have an autosomal dominant inheritance develop axial muscle involvement as young or middle-aged adults. Their dystonia subsequently spreads slowly or stops when involvement is limited to only one muscle group. These patients, like those with childhood onset, have no intellectual impairment.

The diagnosis of dystonia musculorum deformans is entirely clinical, since there is no diagnostic blood, EEG, CT, or anatomic abnormality. In experimental studies, CSF obtained from the ventricles shows decreased concentration of a norepinephrine metabolite, 3-methoxy-4-hydroxyphenylglycol (MHGP) in childhood onset cases, and decreased concentration of HVA in adult onset cases. Medications, which are inconsistently effective, have included carbamazepine (Tegretol) and anticholinergic

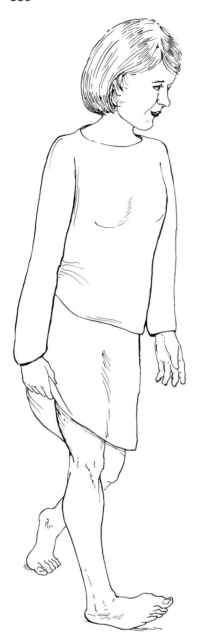

Fig. 18-21. Patients with dystonia musculorum deformans typically first have involuntary inturning (tortion) of one foot. In this case, because of torsion of the right ankle and hip, the girl's foot twists inward and onto its side.

medicines. Spinal cord stimulation has had its most impressive results with this movement disorder.

Other varieties of dystonia musculorum deformans include sporadic cases that do not fit either genetic pattern. In addition, dystonic posturing is a prominent manifestation of choreoathetosis, Wilson's disease, the juvenile form of Huntington's chorea, and several rare degenerative neurologic diseases.

Of this last group, *Lesch-Nyhan syndrome* is most notable. It is a sex-linked recessive genetic illness in which dystonia and other movements develop in children

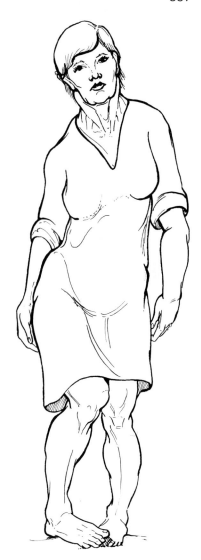

Fig. 18-22. As dystonia musculorum deformans progresses to encompass other portions of the appendicular and also the axial musculature, patients have writhing postures. Their muscles are hypertrophied and, because of the continuous exertion, patients have little subcutaneous fat.

aged 2 to 6 years. Patients also develop self-mutilation, other bizarre behavior, mental retardation, corticospinal tract signs, seizures, and hyperuricemia. Although brain concentrations of dopamine, HVA, and CAT are low, the basic abnormality is a deficiency in hypoxanthine-guanine phosphoribosyl transferase (HGPRT), which is an enzyme that is crucial to urea metabolism.

Focal Dystonia

Several conditions, called the *focal, segmental,* or *partial dystonias,* usually begin in adulthood and consist of dystonia of a single muscle group. As in dystonia musculorum deformans, focal dystonias are unaccompanied by mental impairment, no confirmatory laboratory test is available, and dopamine and ACh manipulations are rarely effective.

Spasmodic torticollis is a focal dystonia in which the sternocleidomastoid and other neck muscles undergo involuntary contractions and force the head to rotate to the opposite side for periods of several seconds to several minutes (Fig. 18-23). Although spasmodic torticollis is occasionally a component of dystonia musculorum deformans, it usually occurs alone. Neck muscle contractions can also develop as a side-effect of neuroleptics or L-dopa, or can be the result of cervical nerve root irritation ("wry neck").

Treatment by transection of the neck muscles or their nerves has resulted in unacceptable loss of head control without a reduction in the involuntary movements caused by remaining muscles. Although classic psychotherapy has produced no sustained benefit, biofeedback has been reported to be beneficial.

Occupational spasms are varieties of dystonia in which patients have painful hand muscle contractions (cramps) shortly after engaging in a particular activity that is often the basis of their livelihood. However, patients can use the same hand in performing similar functions. The most commonly occurring varieties are the writer's, pianist's, and violinist's cramp. For example, a patient with a writer's cramp would develop painful dystonic hand postures shortly after starting to write with a pen but would still be able, using the same hand, to type, eat, and button clothing.

Examination of these patients sometimes reveals subtle signs of extrapyramidal or corticospinal tract impairment, but in most cases the diagnosis rests entirely on the clinical situation. Biofeedback has also been reported to be helpful.

Spastic dysphonia is a poorly understood disorder that is considered to be a dystonia although it might actually be a manifestation of pseudobulbar palsy or buccofacial apraxia (Chapter 8). It is an involuntary contraction of the larynx that occurs only when patients attempt to speak and restricts them to speaking in a high-

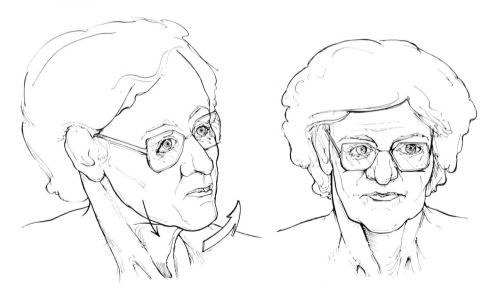

Fig. 18-23. In spasmodic torticollis, patients have a rotation of their head in a downward and contralateral sweep because of continuous contraction of the sternocleidomastoid muscle. The continuous contractions also lead to muscle hypertrophy. The involuntary rotation can be overcome with a great deal of voluntary effort, which induces a tremor, or a slight counter-rotational pressure exerted by a finger pushed against the opposite chin.

pitched whisper. Nevertheless, patients can sometimes shout or sing, and they can almost always use many of these same muscles when swallowing. Aside from crushing one of the recurrent laryngeal nerves to paralyze one side of the larynx, no therapy is available.

Meige's syndrome is a condition in which patients have eyelid and forehead muscle dystonia that forces their eyelids lightly shut (*blepharospasm*), accompanied by lower facial muscle grimacing and jaw closure (*oromandibular dystonia*) (Fig. 18-24). Since Meige's syndrome mimics buccolingual dyskinesia, even though it does not follow neuroleptic administration, it is considered in the differential diagnosis of tardive dyskinesia.

The following conditions are often included in discussions of involuntary movement disorders. However, their clinical characteristics are different from those of the conditions discussed so far. Moreover, investigations have failed to find structural abnormalities of the basal ganglia, neurotransmitter imbalances, or, with the exception of Tourette's syndrome, a beneficial response to dopamine or ACh manipulation.

ESSENTIAL TREMOR

Patients with essential tremor, which is sometimes called an "action" or "postural tremor," have a fine tremor of their wrists, hands, and fingers that is elicited by certain hand actions or positions. Patients with severe cases will also have to-and-fro head shaking (titubation) and a quavering voice. The hand tremor is fine and has a frequency that ranges from 4 to 12 Hz.

It usually develops in young and middle-aged adults and affects about 400 per 100,000 people who are older than 40 years. In some persons, who are said to have *benign familial tremor,* essential tremor is inherited in an autosomal dominant genetic pattern. Other cases may develop in elderly people, who are said to have *senile tremor.*

The most characteristic feature of the tremor is that it appears when patients hold their hands against gravity in fixed positions or perform delicate tasks. For example, the tremor is provoked when patients write, hold out their hands, or bring cups or cigarettes toward their mouth (Fig. 18-25).

Another important feature is that the amplitude of the tremor is suppressed, often

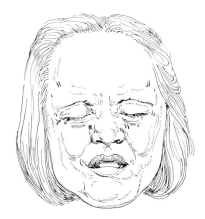

Fig. 18-24. Patients with Meige's syndrome have forced, dystonic eyelid closure (blepharospasm) and often also lower face and jaw contractions (oromandibular dystonia). These movements, which do not stem from neuroleptic use, differ from the buccolingual movements of tardive dyskinesia in their predominant involvement of the upper face, symmetry, and absence of tongue protrusions.

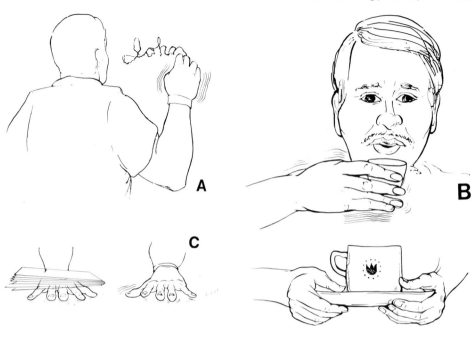

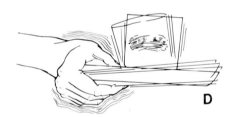

Fig. 18-25. An essential tremor may be demonstrated by having the patient (A) write his or her name, (C) support an envelope on his or her outstretched hands, (B) drink from a filled glass, or (D) transfer a cup and saucer from one hand to the other. The tremor that these movements elicit is not only diagnostically significant, when seen in public, it is often socially disastrous.

to the point of complete elimination, by beverages containing alcohol or the use of beta-adrenergic blockers, such as propranolol (Inderal). Its response to propranolol, which completes with catecholamines (including norepinephrine), indicates that essential tremor probably does not result from extrapyramidal dysfunction, but from excessive beta-adrenergic sympathetic nervous system activity.*

Several other tremor varieties share a similar appearance, origin in excessive adrenergic system activity, and suppression with propranolol. These tremors result from anxiety, hyperthyroidism, or use of steroids or beta-adrenergic stimulating agents, such as isoproterenol (Isuprel). Similarly appearing tremors are also found in patients who take amitriptyline (Elavil) or lithium (see below).

---

*Stimulation of alpha-adrenergic receptor sites leads to peripheral artery vasoconstriction. Stimulation of beta$_1$-adrenergic sites leads to cardiac acceleration and lipolysis. Stimulation of beta$_2$-adrenergic sites leads to bronchodilation and vasodilation of coronary, peripheral, and possibly meningeal arteries. Propranolol blocks both beta$_1$- and beta$_2$-adrenergic sites, and metoprolol (Lopressor), which also suppresses essential tremor is a relatively selective beta$_1$-adrenergic blocker.

In contrast, the parkinson "pill rolling tremor" occurs at rest and is diminished by the initiation of movements (Fig. 18-8). In addition, it is almost always accompanied by rigidity and akinesia. The "intention" tremor that results from cerebellar dysfunction is coarse, irregular, and elicited by gross actions (see Fig. 2-11). The wing-beating tremor of Wilson's disease remains difficult to categorize, but it appears to be a combination of a parkinson and cerebellar tremor.

TICS

Tics, which are sometimes referred to as habit spasms or mannerisms, are usually rapid, repetitive, stereotyped movements of muscle groups of the face, neck, or throat. Frequently observed tics are a "head toss," prolonged eye blink, shoulder jerk, throat clearing, and asymmetric smile. In general, tics move the affected part of the body away from the midline and occur with extraordinary rapidity and chronicity. Their frequency and intensity, as in the classic movement disorders, are increased by anxiety and fatigue and decreased by relaxation. They are also alleviated during sexual intercourse. In contrast, tics persist during sleep, when they are apt to be accompanied by night terrors and sleepwalking (Chapter 17). Also, after periods of years, single tics tend to subside spontaneously.

Tics develop in 2 to 20 percent of children between the ages of 5 and 10 years in most Western countries. A disproportionate number of these children have a close relative with one or more tics. Although tics are assumed to be a manifestation of anxiety, affected children have no consistent emotional, intellectual, or neurologic abnormalities, and their tics do not respond to psychotherapy or minor tranquilizers. Fortunately, by the end of adolescence, all but 6 percent of patients have a spontaneous remission.

Tics may also be found in some adults who have chorea, myoclonus, postencephalitic Parkinson's disease, and other illnesses that cause extensive brain damage. In addition, a small group of adults who have had no predisposing illness develop tics, usually between ages 40 and 60 years.

TOURETTE'S SYNDROME

Gilles de la Tourette's (Tourette's) syndrome is a disorder in which children develop vocal and *multiple* motor tics (Fig. 18-26). It affects boys three times more frequently than girls, and 90 percent of cases develop by age 10 years. Unlike most cases of single tics in childhood, Tourette's syndrome is a life-long illness in which, over periods of 2 to 6 months, tics change in distribution, vary in intensity, and undergo transient remissions. One third of patients have had a similarly affected parent, and an even greater proportion have a close relative with a single tic.

Although affected children appear to have attention deficits and hyperactivity as well as psychosocial disturbances induced by the illness, they have normal intelligence and no propensity to develop psychosis. About 50 percent have soft neurologic signs and 13 to 50 percent have minor, nonspecific EEG abnormalities.

The cardinal feature of Tourette's syndrome is vocal tics, which are repetitive, stereotyped vocalizations that are blurted out in a rapid, irresistible, and almost

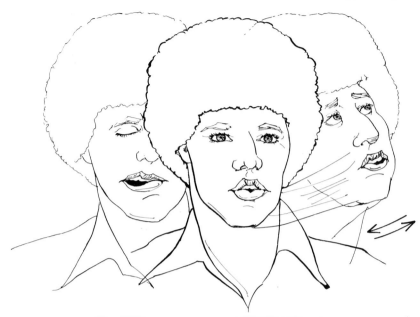

Fig. 18-26. In a typical Tourette's syndrome case, a young man has multiple motor tics, including leftward head jerking, grimacing of the right side of his mouth, and elevation of his forehead. The motor tics are accompanied by vocal tics, such as various noises. All tics continue throughout the day, being unaffected by conversation, eating, and social situations. After several months of a particular pattern, individual tics may recede or be replaced by others.

compulsive fashion. Initially and throughout the course of the illness, the vocal tics of most patients consist of inarticulate sounds, such as sniffing, throat clearing, or clicks; however, many patients begin to make increasingly louder and more disconcerting noises, such as grunting, snorting, or honking. This symptom can culminate in unprovoked outbursts of obscene words, *coprolalia*. Although most such explosions contain only fractions of obscene words, such as "shi," "fu," or "cun," some are well articulated, short series of obscenities.

The original description of the illness and many subsequent reports emphasize coprolalia. However, current studies have found that only 60 percent of patients have this symptom and, when it does occur, its onset is about 6 years after the onset of the tics. Therefore, despite its conspicuous and disturbing nature, coprolalia is not a diagnostic requirement for Tourette's syndrome.

Another symptom is repetition of the spoken words of others (*echolalia*), which is similar to perseveration but not to either aphasia or the language patterns of autistic children (Chapter 8). Still another one is an incessant tendency to touch other people in a compulsive, but furtive, and often sexual manner.

Treatment with haloperidol, in about 80 percent of cases, dramatically suppresses the vocalizations, most motor tics, and many of the other symptoms. In Tourette's syndrome patients, haloperidol rarely induces tardive dyskinesia. Although some other dopamine antagonists, such as fluphenazine (Prolixin) and pimozide (Orap), are reported to be effective, most others, including chlorpromazine, are ineffective. In occasional cases, clonidine (Catapres), which is an alpha-adrenergic agonist, has also been reported to be helpful.

These medications are not indicated for children with single tics, and guidelines are not established for adults with either single or multiple motor but no verbal tics. Although traditional psychotherapy and behavior modification plans have no significant or sustained effect, they can reduce the psychosocial burden of Tourette's syndrome.

Clinical and experimental data have provided interesting clues, but the etiology of Tourette's syndrome remains unexplained. Individual cases have developed in children who received methyphenidate (Ritalin). Family studies indicate that tics and Tourette's syndrome may both be manifestations of a single disorder inherited in an autosomal dominant pattern with variable degrees of penetrance (expression). Other studies have suggested abnormalities in brain ACh activity, dopamine receptor sensitivity, platelet monoamine oxidase concentration, and serotonin metabolism. Overall, despite its unknown etiology and extraordinary symptoms, Tourette's syndrome is now generally believed to be a neurologic illness.

MYOCLONUS

Myoclonus is asynchronous, irregular, brief, and usually generalized muscle contractions. Unlike the classic movement disorders, it persists when patients are asleep or comatose, and it can be elicited by either voluntarily movement on the part of the patient (action myoclonus) or the examiner stimulating the patient with noise, touch, or light (stimulus sensitive myoclonus). Also, myoclonus originates from abnormalities of the motor neurons in the cerebral cortex, brainstem, or spinal cord.

When myoclonus is generalized, it usually results from extensive damage to the cerebral cortex and is associated with dementia, delirium, or seizures. As mentioned in discussions of dementia and EEGs (Chapters 7 and 10), generalized myoclonus is the most prominent physical manifestation of both subacute sclerosing panencephalitis (SSPE) and Creutzfeldt-Jakob's disease—two conditions in which patients have myoclonus, dementia, and periodic EEG complexes (see Fig. 10-6). Myoclonus also results from cerebral anoxia, uremic encephalopathy, penicillin intoxication, excessive meperidine (Demerol) use, and, rarely, Alzheimer's disease. In most of these conditions, 5-hydroxytryptophan (5-HTP) or clonazepam (Clonopin) can suppress the myoclonus.

Palatal myoclonus is symmetric soft palate contractions that occur regularly 120 to 140 times-per-minute during sleep as well as wakefulness. Despite its name, palatal myoclonus has little relationship to generalized myoclonus. In particular, it usually results from small brainstem infarctions and it is not associated with dementia.

MEDICATION-INDUCED MOVEMENT DISORDERS

Dopamine Antagonist Neuroleptics

In addition to neuroleptics occasionally causing the neuroleptic-malignant syndrome (Chapter 6), seizure threshhold and EEG alterations (Chapter 10), and retinal abnormalities (Chapter 12), they induce a variety of striking movement disorders. These disorders, like classic ones, are usually intensified by anxiety, reduced by concentration, and abolished by sleep. They have also been postulated to result from dopamine activity abnormalities.

The most dramatic neuroleptic-induced movement disorder is *acute dystonia.* It consists of patients' suddenly developing limb or trunk dystonic postures, repetitive jaw and face contractions, torticollis, or *oculogyric crisis* (Fig. 18-27). Most cases develop within one week of the beginning of neuroleptic therapy or its being raised to a higher dose. Many cases occur when phenothiazines are used to treat nausea and other nonpsychiatric conditions. Acute dystonia is immediately reversed by an intravenous injection of an anticholinergic medicine (Table 18-1).

A related condition, *tardive dystonia,* can also complicate neuroleptic therapy; however, it develops long after neuroleptics are begun and becomes a chronic condition. Since tardive dystonia is often accompanied by tardive dyskinesia and responds, in many cases, to dopamine depletion using tetrabenazine, it is believed to originate from dopamine hypersensitivity (see below).

Akathisia is a continual leg movement that causes patients to shuffle their feet continuously while lying, sitting, or standing (Fig. 18-28). It often compels them to pace. Although the leg movements are similar to those in chorea and L-dopa excess, the patients' desire or need to move about is unique.

Akathisia recedes as neuroleptic treatment continues, but it can be alleviated more rapidly by reducing the dosage. Some studies claim that akathisia can also be alleviated by amantadine, anticholinergics, or reserpine; however, as in other neuroleptic-induced movement disorders, the reports are largely anecdotal. In any case, amantadine and anticholinergics, which directly or indirectly increase dopamine activity, are unlikely to produce the same effect as reserpine, which reduces it.

As introduced previously, the *withdrawal emergent syndrome,* which is characterized by choreoathetoid and myoclonic movements, occurs primarily in children and follows the abrupt withdrawal of a neuroleptic. It is a transient condition that may be reversed by reinstituting the neuroleptic and then slowly tapering it. Thus, the origin of the syndrome is also probably dopamine hypersensitivity.

In contrast to these disorders that involve excessive movement, neuroleptic-induced parkinsonism produces akinesia and related symptoms. The akinesia is the most important one because, even when still mild and subtle, it can create impediments to normal daily activities. Although the parkinsonism resolves spontaneously, it

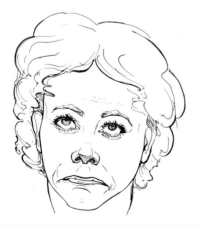

Fig. 18-27. During an oculogyric crisis, the patient's eyes roll upward or sideward, and grimacing and other facial movements often occur. Oculogyric crisis may be related to the impaired ocular movements in schizophrenic patients (Chapter 12) because both conditions may be caused by dopamine neurotransmission abnormalities in the basal ganglia.

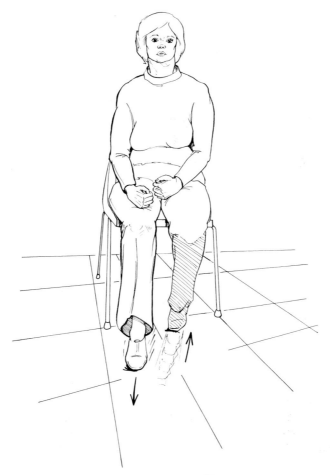

Fig. 18-28. Akathisia consists of continual to-and-fro leg movements accompanied by a feeling of intense restlessness. The leg movements are accented by neuroleptic-induced arm and face akinesia.

can be reduced by decreasing the dosage of the neuroleptic or administering anticholinergics or amantadine. L-dopa should not be given because it can stimulate cerebral cortex dopamine receptors and precipitate a toxic psychosis.

Tardive Dyskinesia

Tardive dyskinesia, or the *buccolinguomasticatory* or *orofacial syndrome* (Fig. 18-29), the most troublesome neuroleptic-induced movement disorder, has been repeatedly postulated to result from dopamine hypersensitivity (Fig. 18-30). Despite the limitations of this theory, it is consistent with several of major clinical features of tardive dyskinesia. For example, tardive dyskinesia begins only a relatively long time after neuroleptics are instituted, when denervation hypersensitivity would develop. It is worsened by reducing the dosage of the neuroleptic or adding L-dopa, presumably

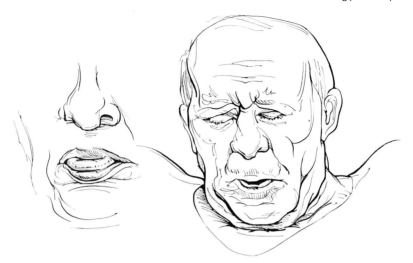

Fig. 18-29. The most prominent feature of tardive dyskinesia is darting tongue movements accompanied by continual jaw and facial muscle contractions. The blepharospasms, which are also an important part of this syndrome, are similar to that seen in Meige's syndrome. In addition to these movements, patients often have chorea or dystonia of the trunk and limbs.

since these changes expose the postsynaptic neuron to greater quantities of dopamine. Likewise, it is alleviated, to a certain degree, by increasing the dosage of the neuroleptic, which would reduce the stimulation of the postsynaptic neuron. Also, in many cases, it spontaneously remits, which is not only a clinically important observation but a possible explanation for some anecdotal reports of the effectiveness of particular medications.

The prominent or exclusive tongue, jaw, and facial movements, however, are not peculiar to tardive dyskinesia. They are observable in normal elderly people who are said to have "senile buccolingual dyskinesia" and in schizophrenic patients who have never received neuroleptics. They may also be found in patients who take L-dopa medications and in those who have chorea, Meige's syndrome, tics, and acute dystonia. In addition, edentulous persons may have an *orofacial dyskinesia,* with minimal tongue involvement, that is correctable with properly fitting dentures.

Treatment of tardive dyskinesia, based on the dopamine denervation hypersensitivity theory, attempts to reduce postsynaptic dopamine activity. Increasing the dosage of a neuroleptic or substituting a more potent one, which blocks dopamine postsynaptically, will temporarily relieve symptoms, but this plan creates a vicious cycle. Reserpine and tetrabenazine, which deplete presynaptic dopamine, or alpha-methyltyrosine, which is a false neurotransmitter, have been helpful in many cases, but none are consistently effective.

A similar strategy attempts to balance excessive dopamine activity by enhancing ACh activity. Physostigmine, which prolongs ACh activity, and ACh precursors, such as deanol (Deaner), lecithin, or choline (Fig. 18-11), have all been administered; however, except for brief periods, such treatments have not been significantly benefi-

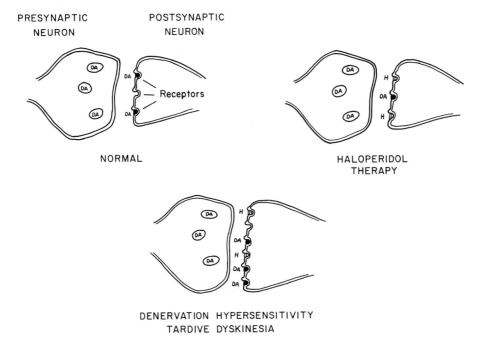

PRESYNAPTIC NEURON   POSTSYNAPTIC NEURON

— Receptors

NORMAL

HALOPERIDOL THERAPY

DENERVATION HYPERSENSITIVITY
TARDIVE DYSKINESIA

Fig. 18-30. The denervation hypersensitivity theory holds that when postsynaptic dopamine receptors are occupied by neuroleptics, such as haloperidol, a dopamine blockage denervates the receptors. As would occur in any denervated neuron, receptor sites become more numerous, increasingly sensitive, or both. Then, even minute quantities of dopamine (or other neurotransmitters), which continue to reach the postsynaptic neuron from the presynaptic neuron or ambient fluid, trigger the receptor.

cial. In several empiric or rationally based studies, GABA agonists, such as valproate (Depakene and Depakote) and baclofen (Lioresal), lithium, and clonazepam (Clonopin) have been administered, but none were consistently helpful.

Other Medications

Antidepressants, because of their anticholinergic properties, cause ocular accommodation impairment (see Fig. 12-4), rare cases of narrow angle glaucoma (see Fig. 12-7), and bladder dysfunction (see Fig. 15-4). In addition, about 10 percent of patients who are taking tricyclic antidepressants, even in the appropriate dosage, develop a fine tremor that appears similar to essential tremor and also responds to propranolol. Otherwise, although some antidepressants, such as amoxapine (Ascendin), have dopamine antagonist properties, they virtually never cause movement disorders or other signs of extrapyramidal dysfunction.

In contrast, lithium routinely causes extrapyramidal dysfunction. Even in slightly excessive concentrations, it causes a coarse, parkinsonlike tremor that is suppressed by propranolol. At greater concentrations, lithium causes akinesia, cogwheel rigidity, and dysarthria. In general, tremors and other extrapyramidal symptoms are signs of lithium toxicity.

Table 18-3
Commonly Cited Movement Disorders that
Begin in Childhood or Adolescence

Early Childhood
   Athetosis or choreoathetosis
   Lesch-Nyhan syndrome*
Childhood
   Dystonia musculorum deformans (childhood onset variety)*
   Myoclonus from subacute sclerosing panencephalitis (SSPE)
   Tourette's syndrome*
Adolescence
   Wilson's disease*
   Huntington's chorea (juvenile form)*
   Essential tremor*

    *Genetic transmission established.

SUMMARY

Many but not all involuntary movement disorders are believed to result from neurotransmitter abnormalities of the basal ganglia. Those illnesses that are characterized by dyskinesias are thought to result from increased dopamine activity. Similarly, medicines that either enhance or substitute for dopamine activity precipitate dyskinesias and also psychotic behavior. In contrast, when dopamine activity is reduced, whether by illness or dopamine antagonist neuroleptics, akinesia ensues.

The involuntary movement disorders are almost always diagnosed on the basis of the appearance of the movements. Other important diagnostic features are a family history indicative of genetic transmission, the patient's being a child or adolescent at the onset of the illness (Table 18-3), and the presence of mental abnormalities (Table 18-4). The illnesses for which confirmatory laboratory tests are available are Wilson's disease, SSPE, Lesch-Nyhan syndrome, and, in the near future, Huntington's chorea.

Table 18-4
Commonly Cited Movement Disorders that are
Associated with Mental Abnormalities*

Early childhood
   Athetosis or choreoathetosis†
   Lesch-Nyhan syndrome
Childhood and adolescence
   Myoclonus from SSPE
   Wilson's disease
   Huntington's chorea‡
Older adults
   Parkinson's disease§
   Myoclonus from Creutzfeldt-Jakob disease and rarely Alzheimer's disease

    *Dementia, depression, or psychotic behavior.
    †Despite severe movement disorders, many choreoathetosis patients will not have mental abnormalities (Chapter 13).
    ‡Sydenham's chorea may cause persistent, minor abnormalities.
    §About 50 percent of Parkinson's disease patients with chronic illness have mental abnormalities.

REFERENCES

Andersen J, Aabro E, Gulmann N, et al: Anti-depressive treatment in Parkinson's disease. Acta Neurol Scand 62:210, 1980

Asnis G: Parkinson's disease, depression, and ECT. Am J Psychiatry 132:191, 1977

Barabas G, Matthews WS, Ferrari M: Disorders of arousal in Gilles de la Tourette's syndrome. Neurology 34:815, 1984

Burke RE, Fahn S, Jankovic J, et al: Tardive dystonia: Late-onset and persistent dystonia caused by antipsychotic drugs. Neurology 32:1335, 1982

Folstein SE, Abbott MH, Chase GA, et al: The association of affective disorder with Huntington's Disease in a case series and in families. Psychol Med 13:537, 1983

Folstein SE, Franz ML, Jensen BA, et al: Conduct disorder and affective disorder among the offspring of patients with Huntington's Disease. Psychol Med 13:45, 1983

Friedhoff AJ, Chase TN (eds): Gilles de la Tourette's Syndrome. Advances in Neurology. New York, Raven Press, 1982

Golden GS: Psychologic and neuropsychologic aspects of Tourette's syndrome. In Symposium on the Borderland Between Neurology and Psychiatry. Neurol Clin 2:91, 1984

Gualtieri CT, Barnhill J, McGimsey J, et al: Tardive dyskinesia and other movement disorders in children treated with psychotropic drugs. J Am Acad Child Psychiatry 19:491, 1980

Jankovic J, Ford J: Blepharospasm and orofacial-cervical dystonia: Clinical and pharmacological findings in 100 patients. Ann Neurol 13:402, 1983

Klawans HL, Moses S, Nausieda PA, et al: Treatment and prognosis of hemiballismus. N Engl J Med 295:1348, 1976

Koller WC: Edentulous orodyskinesia. Ann Neurol 13:97, 1983

Koller WC: Propranolol therapy for essential tremor of the head. Neurology 34:1077, 1984

Korein J, Brundy J: Integrated EMG feedback in the management of spasmodic torticollis and focal dystonia: A prospective study of 80 patients. In Yahr MD (ed): The Basal Ganglia. New York, Raven Press, 1976

Lieberman A, Dziatolowski M, Kupersmith M, et al: Dementia in Parkinson's disease. Ann Neurol 6:355, 1979

Martin JB: Huntington's disease: New approaches to an old problem. Neurology 34:1959, 1984

Mayeux R: Emotional changes associated with basal ganglia disorders. In Heilman KM, Satz P (eds): Neuropsychology of Human Emotion. New York, The Guilford Press, 1983

Mayeux R, Stern Y, Cote L, et al: Altered serotonin metabolism in depressed patients with Parkinson's disease. Neurology 34:642, 1984

Mayeux R, Stern Y, Rosen J, et al: Depression, intellectual impairment, and Parkinson disease. Neurology 31:645, 1981

Nausieda PA, Bieliauskas LA, Bacon LD, et al: Chronic dopaminergic sensitivity after Sydenham's chorea. Neurology 33:750, 1983

Nausieda PA, Koller WC, Weiner WJ, et al: Chorea induced by oral contraceptives. Neurology 29:1605, 1979

Shapiro AK, Shapiro ES, Brun RD, et al (eds): Gilles de la Tourette's syndrome. New York, Raven Press, 1978

Sheehy MP, Marsden CD: Writer's cramp—A focal dystonia. Brain 105:461, 1982

Wolfson N, Sharpless NS, Thal LJ, et al: Decreased ventricular fluid norepinephrine metabolite in childhood-onset dystonia. Neurology 33:369, 1983

Young RR, Growdon JH, Shahani BT: Beta-adrenergic mechanisms in action tremor. N Engl J Med 293:950, 1975

QUESTIONS

1–5.   Pick the correct answer(s).

1.   In general, movement disorders:
   a.   Are present intermittently 24 hours a day
   b.   Are absent during sleep
   c.   May be suppressed for periods of up to 5 seconds by voluntary effort
   d.   Are made worse by anxiety

2.   Gilles de la Tourette's (Tourette's) syndrome is characterized by:
   a.   Multiple motor tics
   b.   Single motor tics
   c.   Vocal tics
   d.   Variation of the pattern of tics
   e.   Constant pattern of verbal and motor tics

3.   Obscenities in Tourette's syndrome are:
   a.   Present in all cases
   b.   Present in less than one half the cases
   c.   Usually develop as an initial symptom
   d.   A later manifestation when they occur
   e.   May be accompanied by echolalia

4.   Tourette's syndrome develops:
   a.   Usually before 5 years of age
   b.   Usually between 2 and 10 years of age
   c.   Predominantly in white Anglo-Saxon Protestants
   d.   In girls more than boys
   e.   After the age of 13 years

5.   Tourette's syndrome is associated with:
   a.   Soft neurologic signs
   b.   Nonspecific EEG abnormalities
   c.   Intellectual impairment
   d.   A tendency toward psychoses
   e.   Tics in close relatives

6–9.   Match the tremor with the examination that will elicit it:

6. Essential tremor	a. Finger–nose test
7. Cerebellar tremor	b. Causing psychologic stress
8. Parkinsonian tremor	c. Extending arms and hands
9. Anxiety-induced tremor	

10–15.   Match the tremor with the appropriate therapy.

10. Essential tremor	a. L-dopa
11. Cerebellar tremor	b. Propranolol (Inderal)
12. Parkinsonian tremor	c. Amantadine (Symmetrel)
13. Factitious tremor	d. Trihexyphenidyl (Artane)
14. Hyperthyroidism tremor	(for example)
15. Delirium tremens	e. None of the above

16–20.   Pick the correct answer(s).

16.   Spasmodic torticollis is:
   a.   Confined to the muscles of the neck and shoulders
   b.   May be the first manifestation of dystonia musculorum deformans
   c.   Often accompanied by retrocollis
   d.   May be resisted by slight pressure applied to the chin

17. In the recessively inherited form of dystonia musculorum deformans:
   a.   The illness progresses slowly
   b.   White Anglo-Saxon Protestants are affected most often
   c.   The symptoms first appear between ages 8 and 14 years
   d.   Mental abilities are preserved

18. In the dominantly inherited form of dystonia musculorum deformans:
   a.   Patients tend to have involvement of the trunk and neck muscles first
   b.   The symptoms begin in adult life
   c.   Patients may present with tortipelvis
   d.   Atrophy of the cerebellum has been seen on computed tomography

19. Dystonia musculorum deformans may be effectively treated with:
   a.   L-dopa
   b.   Neuroleptics
   c.   Spinal cord stimulation
   d.   Stereotactic ablation of portions of the thalamus

20. Dystonia of the head and neck muscles may result from:
   a.   L-dopa
   b.   Wilson's disease
   c.   Cerebral palsy
   d.   Neuroleptic medications

21–31. Match the movement disorder with its symptoms.

21. Unilateral involvement	a. Athetosis
22. Bilateral involvement	b. Chorea
23. Most often associated with dementia	c. Hemiballismus
24. Associated with mental retardation and seizures	
25. Continual movements	
26. Intermittent movements	
27. Greatest movement in distal portions of the extremities	
28. Prominent involvement of facial muscles	
29. Exacerbated by anxiety	
30. Dance-like quality to gait	
31. Patients suppress movements by pressure from the rest of their body.	

32–40. Match the illness with its description.

32. Recessive sex-linked inheritance	a. Huntington's chorea
33. Autosomal recessive inheritance	b. Sydenham's chorea
34. Autosomal dominant inheritance	c. Wilson's disease
35. May develop in children	d. None of the above
36. *Not* associated with progressive mental deterioration	
37. Mental changes may precede involuntary movements	
38. Movements may be ameliorated with neuroleptics	
39. Presence of Kayser-Fleischer ring	
40. Associated with rheumatic fever	

41–49. Match the illness with the underlying abnormality.

41. Cerebral cortical anoxia
42. Increased CSF antibodies to measles
43. Perinatal kernicterus
44. Low serum ceruloplasmin
45. Infarction of the subthalamic nucleus
46. Depigmentation of substantia nigra
47. Probably an infectious agent
48. Atrophy of the caudate heads
49. Cavitary lesions of the globus pallidus
    and putamen

a. Huntington's chorea
b. Wilson's disease
c. Hemiballismus
d. Creutzfeldt-Jakob disease
e. Choreoathetotic cerebral palsy
f. Parkinson's disease
g. Myoclonus
h. SSPE

50–53. Is the statement true or false?

50. Only one neuroleptic-induced movement disorder may occur at a time.

51. Neuroleptic-induced movement disorders develop independently of the antipsychotic strength of the medication.

52. Phenothiazines induce oculogyric crises and other acute dystonias only when used as an antipsychotic medication.

53. Tardive dyskinesia is rarely an adverse effect of use of haloperidol (Haldol) for Tourette's syndrome.

54–58. Match the description with the condition.

54. Akathisia
55. Oculogyic crisis
56. Acute dystonic reactions
57. Parkinsonism
58. Buccolinguomasticatory
    syndrome

a. Occurs early in course of treatment
b. Improves when the medication
   is reduced
c. Responds to anticholinergic
   medications, such as
   diphenhydramine (Benadryl)
d. May be briefly suppressed by
   voluntary effort
e. Improves as patient remains
   on medication

59. Which disorders, that may develop in adolescence, are associated with mental impairments and involuntary movements?

a. Creutzfeldt-Jakob disease
b. Wilson's disease
c. Choreoathetotic cerebral palsy
d. Huntington's chorea
e. SSPE
f. Essential tremor

60. In which ways does the childhood variety of Huntington's chorea differ from its adult variety?

a. Patients have marked rigidity.
b. Dementia does not develop.
c. The outcome is not fatal.
d. Patients appear to have
   Parkinson's disease.
e. Seizures are frequent.
f. Chorea is absent or minimal.

61–65. Match the disturbances, which are often felt to be psychogenic, with their neurologic description:

61. A 70-year-old man develops a
    high-pitched squeaky voice, forcing him
    to speak in a whisper

62. An actor begins to have a high-pitched
    voice and hand tremor while on stage

63. Continual forced eyelid closure

64. A middle-aged woman develops
    continual face, eyelid, and jaw
    contractions

a. Blespharospasm
b. Writer's cramp
c. Spasmodic dysphonia
d. Meige's syndrome
e. Oromandibular dystonia
f. Axiety-induced tremor

65. An author develops hand cramps when writing with a pen

66. Which of the following structures are usually considered to be portions of the corpus striatum?
   a. Substantia nigra
   b. Caudate nuclei
   c. Putamen
   d. Subthalamic nuclei
   e. Globus pallidus

67. What are the characteristics of the nigrostriatal tract?
   a. It links the substantia nigra to the corpus striatum
   b. The substantia nigra are normally black, but in Parkinson's disease one or both are discolored
   c. It governs about 80 percent of the dopamine regulation of the brain
   d. Its stimulation inhibits caudate activity
   e. It cannot be seen under the microscope

68. Sinemet is a combination of L-dopa and which other substance?
   a. Carbidopa, a dopa decarboxylase inhibitor
   b. Bromocriptine (Parlodel)
   c. Anticholinergics

69. About 50 percent of Parkinson's disease patients have depression, dementia, or both. In these patients, which clinical, histologic, or chemical abnormalities are present?
   a. Senile plaques, neurofibrillary tangles, and neuron loss
   b. Physical incapacity
   c. Long duration of illness
   d. A reduction in choline acetyltransferase in proportion to the dementia

70. Which of the following statements describe the Lesch-Nyhan syndrome?
   a. It is characterized by the onset of dystonia and other movements in children aged 2 to 6 years.
   b. It is an autosomal dominant transmitted genetic illness.
   c. Brain HVA and CAT concentrations are low.
   d. The basic deficit is a deficiency of HGPRT.
   e. Hyperuricemia is always present.

71. In which conditions is myoclonus found?
   a. Cerebral anoxia
   b. SSPE
   c. Creutzfeldt-Jakob disease
   d. Alzheimer's disease
   e. Meperidine (Demerol) use
   f. Psychogenic disturbances

72. Which of the following are characteristics of palatal myoclonus?
   a. A frequency of 1 to 3 Hz
   b. A frequency of 120 to 140 per minute
   c. Disappearance during sleep
   d. Underlying brainstem infarction
   e. Association with dementia

ANSWERS

1.	b, c, d	**5.**	a, b, e	**9.**	a, b, c
2.	a, c, d	**6.**	c	**10.**	b
3.	b, d, e	**7.**	a	**11.**	e
4.	b	**8.**	b	**12.**	c, d

13. e	**34.** a	**55.** a, c
14. b	**35.** a, b, c	**56.** a, c
15. e	**36.** b	**57.** b, c, d
16. a, b, c, d	**37.** a, c	**58.** d
17. c, d	**38.** a, b, c	**59.** b, d, e
18. a, b, c	**39.** c	**60.** a, d, e, f
19. c, d	**40.** b	**61.** c
20. a, b, c, d	**41.** g	**62.** f
21. c	**42.** h	**63.** a
22. a, b	**43.** e	**64.** d
23. b	**44.** b	**65.** b
24. a	**45.** c	**66.** b, c, e
25. a	**46.** f	**67.** a, b, c, d
26. b, c	**47.** d, h	**68.** a
27. a	**48.** a	**69.** a, b, c, d
28. a, b	**49.** b	**70.** a, d, e
29. a, b, c	**50.** False	**71.** a, b, c, d (rarely), e
30. b	**51.** False	**72.** b, d
31. a, b, c	**52.** False	
32. d	**53.** True	
33. c	**54.** a, b, d, e	

19

Brain Tumors

Brain tumors rarely occur in young and middle-aged adults. Even in older people, in whom their frequency is greatest, brain tumors occur less than 5 percent as often as CVAs (Chapter 11). Despite the association of brain tumors with headaches, for example, less than 1 out of 1,000 people with headaches suffer from such tumors.

Nevertheless, brain tumors do deserve careful attention. They often develop insidiously and may cause symptoms mistaken for Alzheimer's disease or for depression. They are the cause of considerable morbidity, mortality, and tragedy. In addition, for psychiatrists, brain tumors may be the epitome of "organicity."

This chapter will describe the major varieties of brain tumors and their frequently encountered clinical manifestations. It will discuss similar conditions, such as subdural hematomas, and review the appropriate diagnostic tests for these conditions.

VARIETIES

Tumors that arise within the brain or its covering, the meninges, are called primary brain tumors. This category includes the slowly growing *astrocytoma* and the highly malignant *glioblastoma multiforme.* Astrocytomas are relatively benign, affect children, and tend to develop in the cerebellum, brainstem, or optic nerve. Glioblastomas are highly invasive, occur almost only in adults, and develop in the cerebrum (Fig. 19-1; see also Fig. 20-6).

When these tumors grow within a part of the brain that does not regulate a vital function, surgical excision is feasible and sometimes curative. If the tumor is inoperable, use of radiotherapy, steroids, and chemotherapy reduces the size and subsequent rate of regrowth of the tumor; this therapy often provides a prolonged (1 to 2 years), useful, and relatively comfortable survival.

Meningiomas, tumors that arise in the meninges, are another frequently occurring primary brain tumor. They grow slowly and develop almost exclusively in adults. Often meningiomas are small, innocuous, incidental findings that need not be

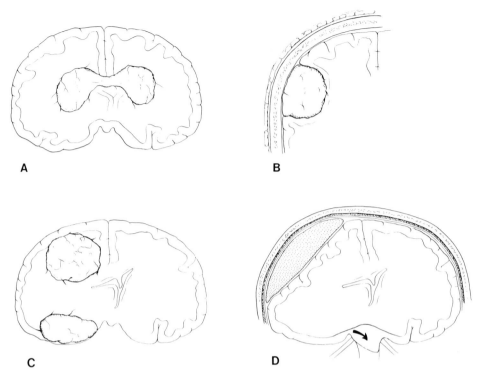

Fig. 19-1. (A) A *glioblastoma* typically infiltrates in a "butterfly pattern" from one cerebral hemisphere through the corpus callosum to the other, destroying both frontal lobes. (B) *Meningiomas* arise from the meninges on the surface of the brain. Since they grow slowly, meningiomas cause relatively little brain displacement or destruction (see Fig. 20-5). (C) *Metastatic tumors* are often multiple and surrounded by edema. Thus, large regions of brain are damaged (see Fig. 20-7). (D) A *subdural hematoma,* typically over the cerebral hemisphere (see Figs. 20-10 and 20-11), can compress the underlying brain and push it through the tentorial notch below, i.e., cause *transtentorial herniation.* In this usually fatal condition, the brainstem and ipsilateral oculomotor (third cranial) nerve are damaged.

removed. They are usually located over the surface of the brain, in surgically accessible locations (see Fig. 20-5).

In contrast to primary tumors, *metastatic* tumors are those that have spread to the brain from extracranial sites (see Fig. 20-7). Most metastatic tumors arise from lung or breast carcinomas. About 20 percent of cancer patients develop cerebral metastases and occasionally the discovery of a metastatic brain tumor is the first indication that the patient has cancer. Radiotherapy and steroids are palliative, but cure is rarely possible.

CLINICAL MANIFESTATIONS

The initial manifestations of a brain tumor are determined by *where* it is. Its variety, on the other hand, determines the *rapidity* with which clinical manifestations progress.

Depending upon the location, the most frequent manifestations are seizures, mental changes, headaches, and physical deficits. Seizures are the initial symptom of brain tumors in approximately one half of all cases. In people older than 50 years, seizures are caused about as often by brain tumors as by CVAs (Chapter 11). Since seizures from brain tumors are a manifestation of cerebral cortical involvement, they are usually the partial elementary or complex, including psychomotor, variety (Chapter 10). When a tumor-induced partial seizure occurs, it usually undergoes secondary generalization, causing tonic-clonic limb movements and loss of consciousness. The initial characteristics of a seizure, no matter how brief, are an important clue to the presence and location of a tumor. A tumor in the occipital lobe, for example, may cause visual hallucinations in the contralateral visual field; a tumor in the frontal lobe may cause clonic activity of the contralateral hand; and a tumor in the temporal lobe may cause psychomotor seizures.

The clinical diagnosis of brain tumor, or at least of a major neurologic problem, is easy when seizures or other physical signs are found; however, many patients during the initial phase of a brain tumor have no such findings. In particular, tumors in the nondominant hemisphere or either frontal lobe may attain considerable size and create substantial psychologic difficulties before physical impairments develop.

The mental changes that tumors produce usually are a mixture of various personality changes and intellectual impairment. Emotional dulling, lack of initiative, and disinterest are frequently the first symptoms of a brain tumor. Although aggressiveness is often cited, it is a rare manifestation. Unless the tumor involves both frontal lobes, dementia generally does not develop in the early stages of a brain tumor. More often, apathy retards intellectual function.

Brain tumor headaches occur frequently but are nonspecific. They are initially generalized, dull, not associated with nausea or vomiting, and responsive to aspirin. Like migraine headaches, they are worse in the early morning hours, often awakening a patient from sleep. Only in advanced cases are tumor headaches associated with nausea and vomiting.

Almost all of the effects of a tumor initially result from damage to the surrounding brain. Later, as the tumor grows and edema begins to surround it, symptoms result from the rise in intracranial pressure caused by the volume of the entire tumor mass. Increased intracranial pressure causes generalized cerebral dysfunction, severe headaches, and, as pressure is transmitted along the optic nerve to the optic disks, papilledema (Fig. 19-2). The physician must bear in mind that since papilledema occurs

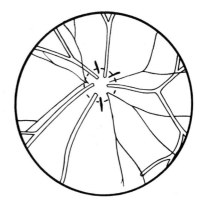

Fig. 19-2. Papilledema, which results from increased intracranial pressure, is characterized by reddening of the optic disk, which loses its distinct margin, and also by distention of the retinal veins. With acute papilledema, the disk is elevated (not pictured) and hemorrhages appear at its edge. (Compare with the normal disk in Fig. 4-3.)

relatively late in the course of brain tumors, it is present only in a minority of patients during initial examination.

While tumors of the cerebral hemisphere can cause contralateral hemiparesis, hemianopsia, or hemisensory loss, in the early stages of their growth most cause only mild physical impairments. Those tumors that arise from cranial nerves lead to readily recognizable deficits; optic nerve gliomas cause optic atrophy with blindness, and acoustic neuromas cause unilateral tinnitus and progressive hearing loss. Cerebellar tumors cause ipsilateral cerebellar signs and, if they compress the fourth ventricle, obstructive hydrocephalus.

DIAGNOSTIC TESTS

Computed tomography is the most readily available, cost-effective* diagnostic procedure (Chapter 20). It will reveal the size, location, and variety of a tumor and distinguish between CVAs, other lesions, and tumors. Equally important, a normal CT scan will virtually eliminate the possibility of brain tumors and other intracranial mass lesions.

In comparison, EEGs are simply not useful. Even with some large tumors, EEGs often show only minimal or nonspecific abnormalities. They can also be misleading because about 20 percent of normal people have abnormal studies.

Although arteriography and ventriculography are sometimes required, they should be performed only after a CT scan demonstrates an abnormality. Moreover, since they are hazardous, their use should always be restricted to specialists in neurologic disorders.

With rare exceptions, a lumbar puncture should not be performed when a brain tumor or other mass lesion is suspected. In cases of brain tumors, the CSF is usually either normal or only nonspecifically abnormal (Chapter 20). Moreover, following a lumbar puncture, mass lesions may cause transtentorial herniation (Fig. 19-3).

DISORDERS THAT MIMIC BRAIN TUMORS

Cerebrovascular accidents as well as tumors occur predominantly in older people and cause similar mental impairments, physical deficits, and seizures. The major clinical difference between these two illnesses is generally in their onset. Cerebrovascular accidents usually begin abruptly, especially on awakening in the morning, whereas brain tumors usually evolve over several weeks. However, some patients with brain tumors do have such an abrupt onset that their illness initially mimics a CVA.

Another difference is that following a CVA, even if patients have sustained extensive physical and intellectual deficits, they usually remain alert and free of headaches. For example, a patient with a CVA may be fully alert with a homonymous hemianopsia, hemiparesis, and hemisensory loss. To produce a comparable deficit, a

---

*The cost is about $300 in 1985.

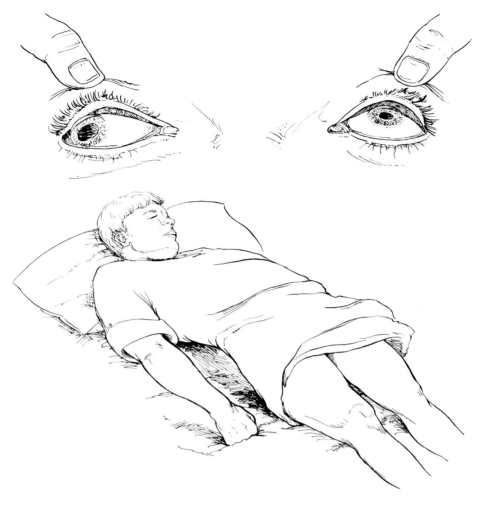

Fig. 19-3. A patient in *transtentorial herniation* from a right-sided subdural hematoma, as in Fig. 19-1 (D), has coma, decerebrate (extensor) posture, Babinski signs, and a dilated right pupil. This has resulted from the right temporal lobe compressing the right-sided oculomotor nerve and the brainstem.

tumor would have to extend through an entire cerebral hemisphere. It would then be so large that it would cause severe headache, stupor, and papilledema.

Finally, seizures from CVAs develop about 6 months after the CVA. In contrast, tumor seizures develop in the early phase of a tumor and are often its first symptom.

Subdural hematomas are another important disorder that mimics tumors. They begin when intracranial bleeding, usually triggered by head trauma, causes a hematoma in the potential space between the dura (a layer of the meninges) and the underlying brain (Fig. 19-1; see also Figs. 20-10, and 20-11). Over a period of several weeks, subdural hematomas, which may be either unilateral or bilateral, gather fluid and become progressively larger. As they grow they compress the cerebral hemispheres, causing generalized cerebral dysfunction.

Older people are especially prone to subdural hematomas because they develop intracranial bleeding after minor or even no apparent head injury. Also, once bleeding has started, it continues unchecked because atrophic brains do not press against the bleeding vessels.

Subdural hematomas probably occur as often as primary brain tumors. They cause headaches, seizures, and, most important, personality and intellectual impairments. Fortunately, subdural hematomas may be readily detected with CT and easily evacuated through small "twist-drill" holes. If promptly treated, cerebral function is fully restored. In other words, subdural hematomas are a relatively common form of correctable dementia.

Uncommon cerebral mass lesions—but ones that also begin with mental changes, physical deficits, or seizures—are brain abscesses and arteriovenous malformations (AVMs). Although life-threatening conditions, they need not be considered separately by the nonspecialist. Not only are they rare, they will be revealed by CT even if they are not specifically suggested by clinical evaluation.

Pseudotumor cerebri is an interesting metabolic disorder that is characterized by fluid retention in the brain. As its name suggests, pseudotumor can be confused with real tumor because the fluid retention causes intracranial pressure and thus leads to headaches and papilledema (Chapter 9). Although pseudotumor is found almost exclusively in obese young women who have menstrual irregularities, its etiology is unknown. A CT scan will indicate cerebral swelling and a lumbar puncture will show markedly elevated CSF pressure (300–600 mm H_2O).

Finally, some psychologic disorders may be confused with brain tumors. In depressive illness, for example, patients may complain of headache and perform poorly on mental status examinations (See Pseudodementia, Chapter 7). Physicians should not rely exclusively on any mental status examination to distinguish between psychologic disorders and brain tumors. Particularly in cases of possible pseudodementia, besides a CT scan, an EEG is often suggested because normal studies would indicate a psychologic disorder.

INDICATIONS FOR EVALUATION

Brain tumors and related conditions should be considered without waiting for florid physical deficits to appear. Initial and, if necessary, repeated neurologic examinations are easy to perform. A CT scan is accurate and readily available. It is especially inexpensive compared with the cost of a delayed diagnosis.

Besides looking specifically for brain tumors and subdural hematomas, neurologists generally order a CT scan, admittedly quite liberally, for patients who have intellectual decline and for those over 50 years who develop substantial emotional changes. They also often suggest a CT scan and other tests (Chapter 7) for patients who have an abrupt onset of any new mental illness severe enough to warrant hospitalization. Also, whenever the patient is worried about a brain tumor, no matter how groundlessly, a CT scan might be done to settle the issue and permit appropriate therapy to begin. Finally, neurologists often require a CT scan before depressed patients have electroshock therapy because if tumors or other mass lesions are present, besides being the cause of depression, they might either precipitate status epilepticus or enlarge and cause transtentorial herniation.

SUMMARY

The possibility of a brain tumor should be considered in patients who develop intellectual impairment, personality changes, or seizures even without overt physical impairments. Mental changes, which are usually an early manifestation, may result from tumors in the frontal lobe, increased intracranial pressure, or partial complex (e.g., psychomotor) seizures. Papilledema, severe headache, and extensive paresis are symptoms of advanced disease. Patients who are suspected of having a brain tumor should have a CT scan for diagnosis and be considered for alternative conditions, such as CVAs, subdural hematomas, and depression.

QUESTIONS

1. An 8-year-old boy who had a 6-week history of progressively greater difficulty with athletic activities, develops a severe headache, papilledema, and ataxia. Of the following, which is the most likely illness?
    a. Meningioma of the cerebellum
    b. Glioblastoma of the cerebrum
    c. Metastatic carcinoma
    d. Astrocytoma of the cerebellum

2. A 60-year-old man who has smoked two packs of cigarettes daily since age 20 develops psychomotor seizures. He has headaches, a left superior quadrantanopsia, and mild left hemiparesis. In addition, he has right-sided dysmetria and intention tremor. Of the following conditions, which is the most likely illness?
    a. Subdural hematomas
    b. Metastatic carcinoma: right temporal lobe and right cerebellar hemisphere
    c. Glioblastoma of the left temporal lobe
    d. Cerebrovascular accidents in the right temporal lobe and right cerebellar hemisphere

3. A 60-year-old woman has apathy and impaired ability to concentrate. Otherwise her history is unremarkable and neurologic examination is unrevealing. What should be the next step in her evaluation, from a medical point of view?
    a. CT scan
    b. EEG
    c. Lumbar puncture
    d. Additional preliminary assessment

4. A 30-year-old woman with neurofibromatosis has impaired ability to hear while listening with the telephone receiver next to her right ear. She also has tinnitus on the right. Aside from mild loss of auditory acuity on the right, her neurologic examination is normal. Of the following, which is the most likely illness?
    a. Left temporal lobe meningioma
    b. Hysteria
    c. Otitis media
    d. Right-sided acoustic neuroma

5. A 55-year-old woman developed mild paresis of the left leg, where hyperactive DTRs and a Babinski sign were found. She refused further evaluation until 11 months later, when she had a seizure that began with clonic movements of the left foot, then leg, and finally the arm. On examination, there is left hemiparesis, hyperactive DTRs, and a Babinski sign. Of the following, which is the most likely illness?

    a. Right cerebral glioblastoma
    b. Right cerebral meningioma
    c. Left cerebral glioblastoma
    d. Left cerebral meningioma

6. Which of the following are apt to cause headaches in the elderly?

    a. Subdural hematomas
    b. Open angle glaucoma
    c. Brain tumors
    d. Pseudotumor cerebri
    e. Temporal arteritis
    f. Nitroglycerine and other vasodilator medications

7. Brain tumor headaches often begin with headaches that are worse in the early morning, waking patients from sleep. Which of the following headaches typically also begin in the early morning?

    a. Muscle contraction (tension) headache
    b. Pseudotumor cerebri
    c. Migraine
    d. Trigeminal neuralgia
    e. Postconcussive syndrome

8. An obese 22-year-old woman with moderately severe, generalized headaches, has papilledema and a right sixth cranial nerve palsy. She is alert and otherwise her neurologic and general medical examination is normal. After routine blood and chemistry tests are found to be normal, a CT scan shows small ventricles, but no indication of an intracranial mass lesion. What would be the most appropriate next step?

    a. Arteriography to look for a brainstem glioma or cerebrovascular accident
    b. EEG
    c. Lumbar puncture to measure the pressure and withdraw CSF

9. A 45-year-old policeman with various emotional difficulties has become obsessed in thinking that he has a brain tumor. Careful medical and neurologic examinations are normal. What would most neurologists do next?

    a. Offer reassurance
    b. Suggest psychotherapy
    c. Give an antidepressant
    d. Treat him for tension headaches
    e. Other

10. A 60-year-old man with pulmonary carcinoma develops confusion and agitation. He refuses a full neurologic examination but physicians find that he has no obvious hemiparesis or nuchal rigidity. Which of the following are frequent causes of an alteration in mental state in such a patient?

    a. Seizures
    b. Pneumonia
    c. Metastasis to the brain
    d. Increased intracranial pressure

11. In the above case, a CT scan reveals two ring-shaped lesions with surrounding lucency. The patient becomes combative during the evaluation. Which medication should be given?

      a. Haloperidol or another neuroleptic
      b. Antidepressants
      c. Steroids
      d. Hypnotics

12. A 65-year-old woman with an onset of dementia has no physical or neurologic abnormalities, aside from frontal release reflexes and hyperactive DTRs. A full laboratory and EEG evaluation reveals no specific abnormality. A CT scan shows atrophy and a small meningioma in the right parietal convexity. What would be the most appropriate next step?

      a. Have the tumor removed
      b. Tentatively diagnose Alzheimer's disease and repeat the clinical evaluation and the CT scan in 6 to 12 months

ANSWERS

1. d. The lesion is in the cerebellum because of the ataxia. The papilledema indicates that there is hydrocephalus. Astrocytomas, the most common variety of brain tumors occurring in childhood, often develop in the cerebellum, and, in children, are curable.

2. b. The patient has psychomotor seizures, visual field loss, and hemiparesis from a right temporal lobe lesion. He also has right-sided coordination impairments from a right cerebellar lesion. These two lesions are probably manifestations of multiple metastatic tumors, but multiple cerebrovascular accidents are also possible. Subdural hematomas rarely cause seizures or cerebellar dysfunction, although they also often occur bilaterally. He is too old to have developed multiple sclerosis, and headaches are not a usual manifestation of multiple sclerosis.

3. d. Patients who may have either psychologic or medical (including neurologic) illness should have a *complete* physical examination. They usually should have routine medical tests that include CBC, SMA 6 and 12, thyroid function, and serology tests. Of those aimed at detecting a brain tumor, CT is the most efficient. An EEG is necessary because of the possibility of her having Creutzfeldt-Jakob disease and metabolic abnormalities associated with dementia. Of course, at the conclusion of the evaluation, the patient may be diagnosed as having pseudodementia.

4. d. Neurofibromatosis or von Recklinghausen's disease is associated with neuromas of the acoustic as well as other nerves. Acoustic neuromas typically cause speech discrimination impairment, tinnitus, and gradual loss of auditory acuity. Lesions of the cerebral hemispheres or the brainstem do not cause such auditory disturbances (Chapter 4).

5. b. The evolution of a hemiparesis over a relatively long (11-month) time, especially when it is accompanied by a partial (motor) seizure, suggests a cerebral tumor. In view of the chronicity, a meningioma is much more likely than a glioblastoma.

6. a, c, e, f. Open angle glaucoma (b) is not associated with headaches. Pseudotumor (d), although it causes headaches, occurs almost exclusively in young adults.

7. c. Migraine headaches characteristically develop during REM sleep, which occurs predominantly in the early morning.

8. c. A lumbar puncture for diagnostic and therapeutic reasons should be performed as soon as possible. The patient has pseudotumor cerebri with stretching of the sixth cranial nerves. (Sixth or third cranial nerve dysfunction because of increased intracranial pressure is called a "false localizing sign.") In pseudotumor, the CSF pressure will be above 300 mm— markedly elevated. Prolonged papilledema, because of the increased intracranial pressure, will lead to optic atrophy and then blindness. Pseudotumor is one of the rare exceptions where lumbar puncture is done in the presence of papilledema.

9. e. Even though brain tumors are rare in people at that age, most neurologists would, of course, order a CT scan. Almost 40 percent of the patients with tumors have no overt *physical* neurologic deficits referable to a tumor. Other structural lesions, such as an arteriovenous malformation or subdural hematoma, could be responsible for the patient's symptoms. Furthermore, from the perspective of a neurologist, with a normal CT scan the physician can give more secure reassurance and feel protected in the unlikely event of a medical-legal problem.

10. a, b, c, d.

11. a, c. A neuroleptic should be given at least until the patient's behavioral disturbances subside. Steroids, such as dexamethasone (Decadron®, Hexadrol® and others) will rapidly and effectively reduce the edema and thus the volume of the lesion. They will bring about a rapid improvement in most cases. Some neurologists would also give an anticonvulsant prophylactically because cerebral metastases often cause seizures.

12. b. The meningioma is probably irrelevant to the dementia. These tumors grow so slowly that they can be followed with periodic CT scans. They should be removed, of course, if they are large enough to compress brain tissue or become symptomatic.

20

Lumbar Puncture and Computed Tomography

Cerebrospinal fluid (CSF) is usually obtained by a lumbar puncture* or "spinal tap," which is performed at or below the second lumbar interspace to avoid striking the spinal cord. However, lumbar puncture can be prevented by degenerative spine disease, which creates a mechanical barrier, or counterindicated by an extensive sacral decubitus ulcer, which could lead to meningitis. In such cases, CSF can be obtained, although with some risk of damaging the spinal cord, by a puncture at the first cervical interspace.

The most common counterindication to a lumbar or cervical puncture is the presence of an intracranial lesion. This prohibition is based on the theory that the "mass effect" of an intracranial lesion tends to force the cerebrum downwards through the tentorial notch, and since these procedures suddenly reduce pressure in the spinal canal, the unopposed force of the lesion can precipitate transtentorial herniation (see Fig. 19-3).

Besides lumbar puncture being dangerous in the presence of an intracranial lesion, CSF analysis is not helpful in identifying the common lesions, such as cerebrovascular accidents, brain tumors, subdural hematomas, and brain abscesses. Therefore, unless physicians suspect acute bacterial meningitis, where rapid diagnosis is paramount, they usually postpone puncture until after computed tomography (CT) has been performed to exclude an intracranial lesion.

The CSF examination is helpful in evaluating several specific symptoms and illnesses, of which some are potentially fatal but readily diagnosable by CSF examination. In acute care hospitals, lumbar puncture is performed most commonly in evaluating patients who have a toxic-metabolic encephalopathy or "delirium." In these patients, lumbar puncture may reveal evidence of bacterial meningitis, other central nervous system (CNS) infections, or subarachnoid hemorrhage (Table 20-1).

The next most frequent indication for lumbar puncture is in the evaluation of patients who have suddenly developed an unusually severe headache, because this

---

*The cost of lumbar puncture in 1985 is about $250.

Table 20-1
Cerebrospinal Fluid (CSF) Profiles

	Color	WBC/mm^3	Protein/ mg/100 ml	Glucose/ mg/100 ml	Miscellaneous
Normal	Clear	0–4*	30–45	60–100	
Bacterial meningitis	Turbid	100–500	75–200	0–40	Gram-stain may reveal organisms
Viral meningitis	Turbid	50–100*	50–100	40–60	
Fungal meningitis†	Turbid	100–500*	100–500	40–60	Cryptococcal antigen titer should be determined
Neurosyphilis	Clear	5–200*	45–100	40–80	VDRL is often negative‡
Subarachnoid hemorrhage	Bloody	§	45–80	60–100	Supernatant may be xanthochromic

*Mostly lymphocytes.
†In tuberculous meningitis the CSF profile is similar except that the glucose concentration is lower. In carcinomatous meningitis the CSF has similar profile but malignant cells may be detected.
‡See Chapter 7.
§In normal proportion (1:1,000) to red cells.

symptom could be a manifestation of bacterial meningitis or subarachnoid hemorrhage. As a general practice, neurologists often perform lumbar puncture on patients who complain of the "worst headache" of their life to exclude these conditions, which are potentially fatal.

Another common indication for lumbar puncture is to diagnose tuberculous or fungal, particularly cryptococcal, meningitis. These forms of chronic meningitis typically cause fever, malaise, dementia, and headache. They are apt to develop in patients who have conditions that impair their immunologic capacity, such as steroid or other immunosuppressive treatment for systemic lupus erythematosus, chemotherapy for cancer and renal transplantation, leukemia, and acquired immune deficiency syndrome (AIDS).

A lumbar puncture is not a screening test in the evaluation of patients who have dementia, but the CSF should be inspected when neurosyphilis is suspected. However, although a positive CSF VDRL test is virtually diagnostic of neurosyphilis, about 40 percent of patients with neurosyphilis have a negative CSF VDRL test (Chapter 7). In multiple sclerosis, the CSF may contain myelin basic protein, oligoclonal bands, and an increased percentage of gamma globulin (Chapter 15). In subacute sclerosing panencephalitis (SSPE), the CSF often contains measles antibodies (Chapter 7).

COMPUTED TOMOGRAPHY

In CT, normal brain tissue is arbitrarily portrayed as gray. Structures that are increasingly more radiodense than brain tissue, such as tumors, blood, and calcifications, are portrayed as being progressively closer to white. The ventricles are portrayed as being black because they are filled with CSF, which is radiolucent. Since

CSF also accumulates in cerebral infarctions, chronic subdural hematomas, and in brain edema surrounding tumors, these areas are darker than normal brain.

When "contrast" solutions containing iodine are administered, blood-filled structures become more radiodense. This phenomenon, "contrast enhancement," highlights vascular structures, such as arteriovenous malformations, glioblastomas, and chronic subdural hematomas.

In several situations CT should be avoided or, at least, the procedure should be modified. The radiation is slightly greater than in a conventional x-ray skull series. Thus, even though the radiation dose is still relatively small and is confined to the head, examinations must be limited in frequency. Also, the contrast solution can provoke an allergic reaction and, especially in patients with diabetes or dehydration, renal failure.

Neurologists and other physicians are accused of indiscriminately ordering CT scans. However, it is quite cost-effective,* much more reliable than the electroencephalogram (EEG) and isotopic brain scan, and indicated for most of the conditions discussed in this book, including dementia and delirium, aphasia and other specific neuropsychologic deficits, headaches in elderly people, partial seizures, and structural lesions, such as subdural hematomas, brain tumors, and cerebrovascular infarctions (Figs. 20-1 to 20-12). It is also performed in most cases of cerebral palsy, multiple sclerosis, and classic movement disorders. Although criteria are not yet established for ordering CT scans for patients who appear to have psychiatric illness, their use has become commonplace in the evaluation of patients who have developed psychosis, profound depression, or episodic behavioral disturbances.

On the other hand, CT is rarely indicated in cases of chronic pain, sleep disturbances, absence (petit mal) seizures, cluster and migraine headaches, Parkinson's disease, tics, and essential tremor. It is not indicated, of course, in muscle and peripheral nerve diseases, including myasthenia gravis, amyotrophic lateral sclerosis (ALS), polyneuropathy, and muscular dystrophy.

The CT scan in about 20 percent of chronic schizophrenic patients shows a pattern of large ventricles and small brain volume, which is called "hydrocephalus ex vacuo" or "increased ventricular-brain ratio." Also, some of these patients lack the normal cerebral asymmetry, in which the cortex of the dominant (usually left) hemisphere is more convoluted than that of the nondominant hemisphere (Chapter 8). These CT abnormalities are not attributable to age, medications, or electroshock therapy. Moreover, since people with marked cerebral atrophy can have normal or high intelligence, the atrophy itself does not necessarily reflect generalized cerebral dysfunction.

Overall, chronic schizophrenic patients with CT abnormalities, compared with those without these abnormalities, have more severe illness. They have more resistance to medications, greater cognitive impairments, and worse prognosis.

Loss of cerebral asymmetry and other dominant hemisphere CT abnormalities have also been described in autistic children. However, the abnormalities have been found inconsistently and were present mostly in children who also had mental retardation or congenital physical neurologic impairments.

---

*The cost of a CT scan in 1985 is about $300.

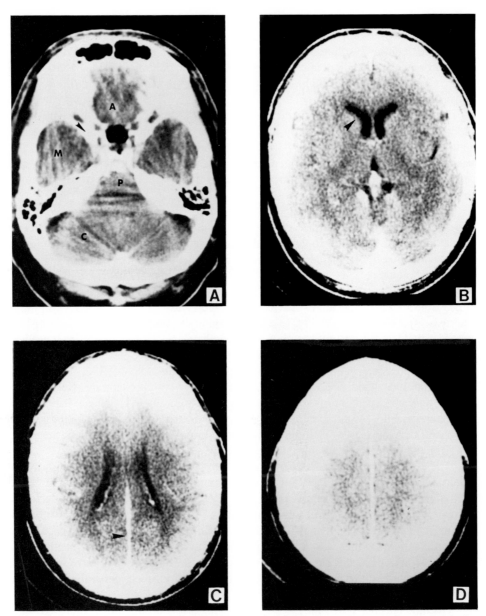

Fig. 20-1. Four representative, progressively higher axial view CT scans of a normal brain. (A) The anterior fossae **(A)** contain the anterior frontal lobes and the olfactory nerves. The middle fossae **(M)** contain the anterior temporal lobes, which are situated behind the sphenoid wing (arrow). The posterior fossae contain the cerebellum **(C)** and the medulla and pons **(P)**, which are called the *bulb*. (B) The anterior horns of the lateral ventricles are concave because of indentation by the heads of the caudate nuclei (arrow). A calcified pineal gland is the small white structure in the center. The third ventricle is the thin elongated black area anterior to the pineal gland. (C) The lateral ventricles spread lengthwise in the hemispheres, which are separated by the white, straight sagittal sinus (open arrow). (D) The cerebral cortex is adjacent to the skull. Thus, individual gyri and sulci are not discernible.

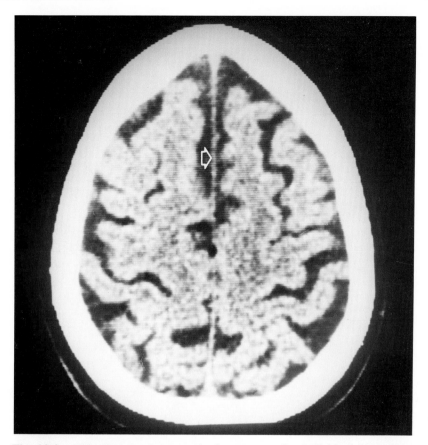

Fig. 20-2. This CT scan shows cerebral cortex atrophy: Individual thin gyri are distinct and wide sulci are prominent. The cerebral hemispheres are retracted from the inner table of the skull and from the sagittal sinus (open arrow). Although cerebral atrophy is associated with Alzheimer's disease, Down's syndrome, other illnesses that cause dementia, and some varieties of schizophrenia, it is a normal concomitant of old age and it is not necessarily associated with intellectual deterioration. For example, many elderly individuals with normal or high intelligence have marked cerebral atrophy.

Magnetic Resonance Imaging

When nuclei are exposed to a magnetic field, they tend to vibrate (resonate). As the nuclei return to their natural alignments, they emit energy. Hydrogen nuclei (protons) produce a characteristic pattern that permits a tomographic portrayal of tissues containing water.

Unlike CT, magnetic resonance imaging (MRI) imaging does not use ionizing radiation or contrast solutions. Also, although MRI is expensive,* it has no known risks and can be used repeatedly to evaluate large regions of patients' bodies.

---

*The cost of NMR in 1985 is about $850.

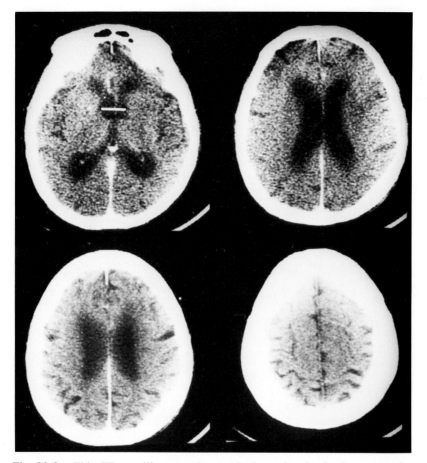

Fig. 20-3. This CT scan illustrates that cerebral atrophy also leads to expansion of the lateral ventricle, "hydrocephalus ex vacuo" or an "increased ventricular-brain ratio," and widening of the third ventricle (line).

Magnetic resonance imaging reveals the brain and other intracranial contents in exquisite detail. (Fig. 20-13). It can contrast gray and white matter because gray matter has a water content that is 20 percent greater. It can portray structures, such as the spinal cord, that are normally obscured by bone. It can highlight areas of the brain where the chemical composition of the tissues, but not gross anatomy, have been altered. This capability is especially useful in the diagnosis of multiple sclerosis, where plaques of demyelination can be detected by MRI but not CT. Unfortunately, MRI has not been significantly more helpful than CT in diagnosing psychiatric conditions or Alzheimer's disease.

Positron Emission Tomography

While the role of CT is to delineate the anatomy of the brain, and that of MRI is to display its chemical abnormalities as well as gross anatomy, the unique role of positron emission tomography (PET) is to reveal the metabolic activity of the brain

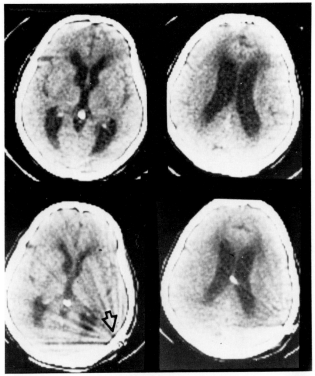

Fig. 20-4. (Top) In normal pressure hydrocephalus (NPH), the CT scan shows ventricular dilatation, including widening of the temporal horns of the lateral ventricles (not pictured), but no cerebral cortex atrophy. (Bottom) Following instillation of a shunt (open arrow), the size of the ventricles decreases. Unfortunately, distinction, based on CT, between NPH and hydrocephalus ex vacuo is unreliable.

during normal and abnormal conditions. The technique is based on detecting energy, in the form of positrons, produced during metabolism of fluorine-18-labeled fluorodeoxyglucose (FDG). Since FDG is metabolized as though it were common glucose, a greater positron emission rate indicates a higher metabolic rate and more voracious glucose utilization. In the future, metabolism of other substrates, such as phosphate, can be studied. However, FDG and other substrates must be produced in a cyclotron.

Positron emission tomography has been used to study cerebral metabolism in a variety of normal activities, such as speaking. One of its most clinically useful applications is to study metabolism during seizures and to identify the foci of partial complex seizures. Positron emission tomography has also been used to study cerebrovascular accidents, Huntington's chorea, and other neurologic illnesses. However, its resolution is so low that metabolic activity can be correlated with only relatively large structures, such as the basal ganglia.

Nevertheless, in Alzheimer's disease, PET has shown decreased glucose metabolism in the cerebral cortex (Chapter 7). In studies of schizophrenic patients, preliminary results indicate that there is glucose hypometabolism in the frontal lobe cortex.

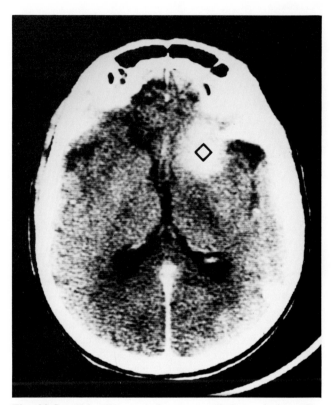

Fig. 20-5. This CT scan shows a radiodense lesion (diamond), typical of a meningioma, arising from the right sphenoid wing. These lesions can irritate the temporal lobe posteriorly, triggering partial complex seizures, or they can grow anteriorly and compress the frontal lobe and the olfactory (first cranial) nerve, i.e., cause the Foster-Kennedy syndrome (Chapter 4). In contrast to glioblastomas (Fig. 20-6), large infarctions (Fig. 20-8), and subdural hematomas (Fig. 20-10), meningiomas are slowly developing and exert little mass effect. Moreover, small meningiomas are commonplace and do not produce mental changes.

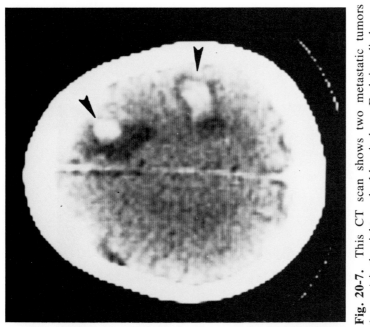

Fig. 20-7. This CT scan shows two metastatic tumors (arrows) in the right cerebral hemisphere. Each is radiodense, relatively solid, and surrounded by edema.

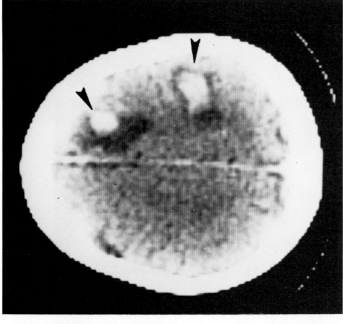

Fig. 20-6. This CT scan illustrates a glioblastoma. It has a white contrast-enhancing ring (R) and surrounding black brain edema. The mass effect of the lesion (open arrows) compresses the adjacent brain and shifts midline structures, such as the sagittal sinus, contralaterally.

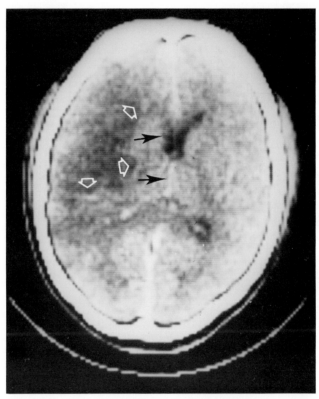

Fig. 20-8. This left middle cerebral artery infarction (open arrows) is typically radiolucent and, since it is large, has a mass effect that compresses the adjacent lateral ventricle and shifts midline structures contralaterally (solid arrows).

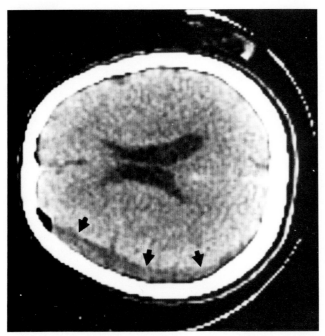

Fig. 20-10. This CT scan of a left-sided chronic subdural hematoma (arrows) illustrates its typical radiolucent interior, faint surrounding membranes, and compression of the adjacent lateral ventricle. Chronic subdural hematomas not only cause headaches and dementia, but they can also lead to transtentorial herniation (see Figs. 19-1 and 19-3).

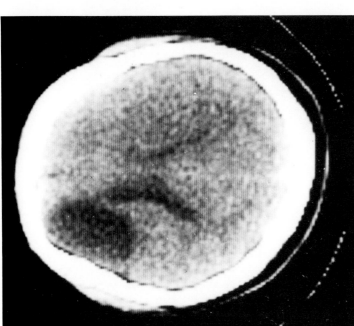

Fig. 20-9. A porencephaly, or "brain cyst," is a common congenital cerebral injury that is often responsible for seizures, spastic contralateral hemiparesis, and mental retardation. It is radiolucent and, unlike lesions with mass effect, enlarges the adjacent ventricle and tends to draw midline structures ipsilaterally.

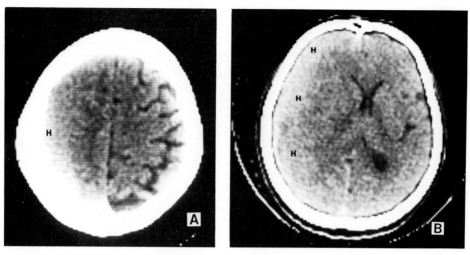

Fig. 20-11. As these CT scans illustrate, occasionally the interior of a subdural hematoma (H) is virtually isodense to brain. Such isodense subdural hematomas, which are life-threatening, are notoriously difficult to identify; however, their presence can be suggested by (A) a mass effect and (B) unilateral "loss," by compression, of the gyri-sulci pattern.

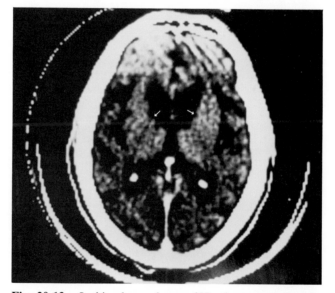

Fig. 20-12. In this advanced case of Huntington's chorea, the CT scan shows that the anterior horns of the lateral ventricles are convex (arrows) because of atrophy of the caudate nuclei. (Contrast their shape to the normal concave shape of the ventricles, Fig. 20-1, Top Right.) Also, the CT scan shows prominent gyri and sulci, which indicate cerebral atrophy. Although these CT findings are characteristic of Huntington's chorea, they have usually not yet appeared when dementia or chorea is first detected.

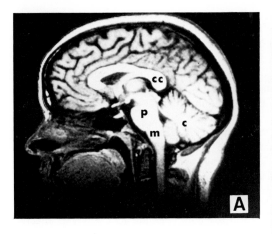
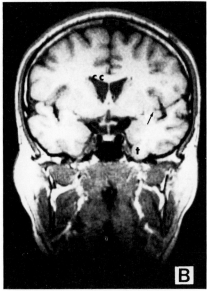

Fig. 20-13. (A) A magnetic resonance imaging (MRI) sagittal view of a normal brain reveals exquisitely detailed cerebral gyri and sulci, the corpus callosum (**cc**), and the pons (**p**), medulla (**m**), and cerebellum (**c**) of the posterior fossa. In addition, the cervicomedullary junction and various nonneurologic soft tissue structures are easily visualized. (B) This MRI coronal view illustrates the corpus callosum (**cc**) joining the cerebral hemispheres. The white matter of the corpus callosum and cerebral hemispheres is distinct from the superficial gray matter of the cortex. The anterior horns of the lateral ventricles, with their concave lateral borders, are beneath the corpus callosum and lateral to the caudate nuclei and internal capsule (see Figs. 7-6 and 18-1). The cerebral cortex around the left sylvian fissure (arrow) is more convoluted than that around the right. The frontal lobe is above the fissure and the temporal lobe is below. The mesial-inferior surface of the temporal lobe, which is the origin of most partial complex seizures, is sequestered by the bulk of the temporal lobe and the sphenoid wing, far from where scalp EEG electrodes are applied.

After treatment, although brain metabolism is generally increased, frontal lobe cortex hypometabolism persists. Similar results have been found in patients with affective disorders.

REFERENCES

Ackerman RH, Alpert NM, Correia JA, et al: Positron imaging in ischemic stroke disease. Ann Neurol 15(suppl):S126, 1984

Brodie JD, Christman DR, Corona JF, et al: Patterns of metabolic activity in the treatment of schizophrenia. Ann Neurol 15(suppl):S166, 1984

Buchsbaum MS, Cappelletti J, Ball R, et al: Positron emission tomographic image measurement in schizophrenia and affective disorders. Ann Neurol 15(suppl):S157, 1984

Chase TN, Foster NL, Fedio P, et al: Regional cortical dysfunction in Alzheimer's disease as determined by positron emission tomography. Ann Neurol 15(suppl):S170, 1984

Damasio H, Maurer RG, Damasio AR, et al: Computerized tomographic scan findings in
    patients with autistic behavior. Arch Neurol 37:504, 1980
Engel J: The use of positron emission tomographic scanning in epilepsy. Ann Neurol
    15(suppl):S180, 1984
Farkas T, Wolf AP, Jaeger J, et al: Regional brain glucose metabolism in chronic schizophre-
    nia: A positron emission transaxial tomographic study. Arch Gen Psychiatry 41:293, 1984
Gonzalez CF, Grossman CB, Masdeu JC: Head and Spine Imaging. New York, Wiley Medi-
    cal, 1984
Kuhl DE, Metter EJ, Riege WH, et al: Patterns of cerebral glucose utilization in Parkinson's
    disease and Huntington's disease. Ann Neurol 15(suppl):S119, 1984
Luchins DJ, Weinberger DR, Wyatt RJ: Schizophrenia and cerebral asymmetry detected by
    computed tomography. Am J Psychiatry 136:753, 1982
Partain CL, James AE, Rollo FD, et al: Nuclear Magnetic Resonance (NMR) Imaging.
    Philadelphia, W.B. Saunders, 1983
Phelps ME, Mazziotta JC, Baxter L, et al: Positron emission tomographic study of affective
    disorders: Problems and strategies. Ann Neurol 15(suppl):S149, 1984
Prior MR, Tress B, Hoffman WL, et al: Computed tomography study of children with classic
    autism. Arch Neurol 41:482, 1984
Weinberger DR, Delisi LE, Perman GP, et al: Computed tomography in schizophreniform
    disorder and other acute psychiatric disorders. Arch Gen Psychiatry 39:778, 1982

Additional Review Questions

Q1: Match the side effect with the anticonvulsant medication most likely to produce it:

1.	Stevens-Johnson syndrome	a.	Primidone (Mysoline)
2.	Granulocytopenia	b.	Carbamazepine (Tegretol)
3.	Hypertrichosis (hirsutism)	c.	Phenobarbital
4.	Gum (gingival) hyperplasia	d.	Phenytoin, diphenylhydantoin,
5.	More sedation than anticonvulsant activity compared with other medications		DPH (Dilantin)
6.	Status epilepticus with abrupt cessation		
7.	Paradoxical hyperkinesis in children		
8.	Liver toxicity		
9.	Lethargy at blood levels above the therapeutic range		
10.	Ataxia		
11.	Fetal-hydantoin syndrome		

A1:
1. d, occasionally c
2. b
3. d
4. d
5. a
6. a, b, c, d
7. c
8. b
9. a, b, c, d
10. d
11. d

Q2: A 22-year-old man with tonic-clonic seizures has about one seizure a week. Which of the following are likely causes of this high frequency of seizure activity?

a. Noncompliance with medication(s)
b. Presence of hysteric as well as genuine seizures
c. He suffers from neurofibromatosis
d. He suffers from Jakob-Creutzfeldt disease
e. He suffers from tuberous sclerosis
f. He takes drugs, alcohol, or medications other than anticonvulsants
g. The wrong anticonvulsant or the incorrect dose has been prescribed

A2: a, b, e, f, g
a. Noncompliance is a frequently occurring cause of "uncontrollable" or refractory seizures.
b. Hysteric seizures are often found in patients with genuine seizure disorders.
e. Tuberous sclerosis is a neurocutaneous disorder characterized by facial adenomata, dementia, and refractory seizures.

   f.   Use of many medications interferes with anticonvulsant activity, although most
        often they potentiate anticonvulsant activity, precipitating toxicity.
   g.   The physician should always consider the possibility that he erred in the
        diagnosis or treatment plan.

Q3:   The patient is found to have a phenytoin (Dilantin) level of 8 mg/dL (the therapeutic
level is 10 to 20 mg/dL). Of the possibilities listed above, which is the single most likely
possibility?

A3:   a

Q4:   When therapeutic concentrations of phenytoin (Dilantin) are achieved, genuine
seizures persist. Which of the plans should the physician follow?
   a.   Increase the phenytoin dose
   b.   Stop the phenytoin
   c.   Add a second anticonvulsant, such as phenobarbital, to phenytoin
   d.   Reconsider the diagnosis and treatment

A4:   c, d
   c.   Adding a second anticonvulsant, now that therapeutic levels of one
        anticonvulsant are achieved, is the best plan.
   d.   Reconsideration should always be performed when therapies do not achieve the
        expected result, but often two anticonvulsants are necessary.
   a.   Little additional benefit will result and toxicity will ensue at greater than
        therapeutic levels.
   b.   Abrupt cessation of any anticonvulsant may precipitate status epilepticus.

Q5:   A 19-year-old Marine recruit has status epilepticus, fever, stupor, and nuchal rigidity. Which therapies or diagnostic tests should be performed as soon as possible?
   a.   Parenteral anticonvulsants
   b.   Oral anticonvulsants
   c.   Thiamine (50 mg. I.V.)
   d.   Lumbar puncture
   e.   Penicillin or penicillin in combination with chloramphenicol

A5:   a, d, e
The presumptive diagnosis is meningitis-induced seizures.

Q6:   A 30-year-old man with a long history of aggressive behavior and other antisocial
actions has an EEG that shows an isolated, phase-reversed spike focus intermittently over the
left frontal lobe. Which statements are appropriate?
   a.   In retrospect, the behavioral disturbances were the result of partial complex
        (psychomotor) seizures.
   b.   The EEG has absolutely no bearing on the case.
   c.   Certain EEG abnormalities are characteristically found in antisocial people.
   d.   Both the EEG and the behavior may reflect cerebral damage.

A6:   d.   The EEG indicates the presence of a structural lesion in the left frontal lobe that
could be a source of seizures. Lesions in the frontal lobe as well as those in the temporal lobe
can cause the partial complex seizures. However, while this patient may be a seizure suspect,
since there are no stereotyped behavioral disturbances and the EEG shows no paroxysmal
activity, most neurologists would not make the diagnosis of seizures with the information at
hand.

Q7:   A 16-year-old woman who has had both absence (petit mal) and generalized tonic-
clonic seizures, which require high doses of two anticonvulsants, has confusion, disorientation,
agitation, and dysarthria. Otherwise her medical and neurologic examination reveals no abnormality. Which conditions may be the cause of her mental abnormalities?
   a.   Anticonvulsant intoxication
   b.   Postictal psychosis following an absence (petit mal)
   c.   Postictal psychosis following a tonic-clonic seizure

     d. Petit mal status

     e. Oral contraceptive-induced seizures

A7: a, c, d

     a. Anticonvulsant intoxication is common and it is the most likely cause.

     c. Postictal confusion is often accompanied by agitation and behavior abnormalities.

     d. Petit mal status is rare but possible.

Incorrect answers:

     b. There are no postictal symptoms with petit mal seizures.

     e. There is no such thing.

Q8: In the case just described, what would be the best therapeutic plan after routine evaluation reveals no other abnormalities?

     a. Obtain blood for anticonvulsant determination

     b. Stop the anticonvulsant administration for the present

     c. Give diazepam intravenously

     d. Obtain an EEG

A8: a, b, d

Q9: An 8-year-old boy begins to have 10- to 20-second episodes of repetitive lip smacking, eyelid fluttering, and finger rubbing. During these episodes he is incoherent. Afterwards he is confused and sleepy. What is the most likely diagnosis?

     a. Absence (petit mal) seizures

     b. Partial complex (psychomotor) seizures

     c. Attention deficit disorder

     d. Psychologic aberrations

A9: b   This child is having typical partial complex seizures; he has incoherence, not loss of consciousness; stereotyped, simple, repetitive movements and sounds; and subsequent (postictal) confusion and somnolence.

Q10: If the EEG in the case just described shows an intraictal pattern that supports the diagnosis, which medicine would be the most appropriate?

     a. Valproate (Depakene)

     b. Carbamazepine (Tegretol)

     c. Phenytoin (Dilantin)

     d. Ethosuximide (Zarontin)

A10: b   Carbamazepine (Tegretol), although some authors might suggest phenytoin (Dilantin) or primidone (Mysoline).

Q11: During the course of evaluation for dementia, a patient's CT scan reveals a small, dense lesion without surrounding edema arising from the right parietal convexity. The brain is not compressed by the lesion, which is felt to be a meningioma. What symptoms might such a lesion likely cause?

     a. Dementia

     b. Partial complex seizures

     c. Absence seizures

     d. Partial seizures without secondary generalization

     e. Partial seizures with secondary generalization

A11: d, e   Small meningiomas that do not have edema and do not compress the underlying brain are commonplace and are rarely of medical consequence. Although they are considered "brain tumors," such meningiomas are usually innocuous, incidental findings. They might, however, cause seizures by irritating the underlying cortex. In this case, partial seizures might arise from the underlying parietal cortex, causing sensory symptoms on the left side of the body. While the seizure activity might remain limited to sensory phenomena, it also might undergo generalization to cause generalized tonic-clonic activity. Such a small meningioma, however, would not cause dementia because its small size and lack of cerebral compression would not damage enough cerebral tissue to interfere with intellectual function.

Q12: An 18-year-old woman has had 2 years of premenstrual episodes, lasting one to three days, consisting of malaise, "depression," nausea, and a dull, throbbing headache behind her left eye. An EEG during an episode reveals some theta (slow) activity diffusely and intermittently. What is the single most likely diagnosis?

    a. Partial complex seizure(s)
    b. Cyclic depression
    c. Premenstrual tension
    d. An arteriovenous malformation (AVM)
    e. None of the above

A12: e. Most likely, the young lady has premenstrual common migraine headaches. Partial complex seizures are not usually accompanied by a headache, usually do not last more than 20 minutes, and do not have merely scattered theta activity on an intraictal EEG. An AVM would not cause multiple headaches, autonomic symptoms, or mood changes.

Q13: Which of the following patients is most likely to have a seizure?

    a. A 65-year-old man with left Bell's palsy
    b. A 70-year-old woman with a right third cranial nerve palsy and left hemiparesis
    c. A 55-year-old woman with rapidly progressive paresis and sensory loss of her left arm and more so her left leg, which have hyperactive DTRs and a Babinski sign
    d. A 40-year-old man who, following an upper respiratory tract infection, develops ascending flaccid, areflexic weakness of the legs

A13: c. This patient probably has a right parasagittal (parafalcine) meningioma, a right frontal glioblastoma, or another mass lesion in this location. Whatever its nature, any cerebral mass lesion routinely causes seizures. Only lesions of the cerebral cortex itself or ones of the meninges that press on the cortex are likely to cause seizures. Thus, the patient with the left seventh cranial nerve palsy (a), right midbrain (b), or Guillain-Barré syndrome (d), would not be expected to have seizures.

Q14: Many phenomena, conditions, tests, and illnesses have been named after two neurologists, i.e., paired eponyms. Match the eponyms with one or more of the associated findings:

1. Kayser-Fleischer	a. None of the ones below
2. Brown-Sequard	b. Peripheral neuropathy and mental
3. Watson-Schwartz	changes
4. Wernicke-Korsakoff	c. An opacity in the cornea indicative
5. Creutzfeldt-Jakob	of an illness characterized by
6. Niemann-Pick	dementia and involuntary
7. Niemann-Marcus	movement
	d. Disassociation of pain and
	temperature in the legs
	e. Disassociation of paresis and
	position sense loss in the legs
	f. Disassociation of paresis and
	hypalgesia in the legs
	g. Dementia with myoclonus in an
	elderly man
	h. Fatal illness of infancy
	i. Detectable in utero or prenatally

A14: Correct answers: 1c Wilson's disease; 2f spinal cord transsection; 3b acute intermittent porphyria; 4b; 5g; 6h, i; 7a.

Q15: Changes in deep tendon, plantar, and gag reflexes are a salient feature of many neurologic illnesses. Match the illnesses with one or more of the expected reflex alterations.

1.	Guillain-Barré syndrome	a.	Hyperactive deep tendon reflexes
2.	Multiple sclerosis	b.	Hypoactive deep tendon reflexes
3.	Acute intermittent porphyria	c.	Extensor plantar reflexes (Babinski signs)
4.	Myasthenia gravis		
5.	Wernicke-Korsakoff syndrome	d.	Unresponsive or flexor plantar reflexes
6.	Amyotrophic lateral sclerosis		
7.	Brachial plexus injury	e.	Hyperactive gag reflex
8.	Herniated lumbar intervertebral disc	f.	Hypoactive gag reflex

9. Parasagittal meningioma
10. Multiple cerebral infarctions
11. Spastic hemiparesis
12. Brainstem infarctions
13. Myotonic dystrophy
14. Duchenne's muscular dystrophy
15. Chronic nitrous oxide abuse
16. Diabetes mellitus neuropathy
17. Cauda equina syndrome
18. Lupus cerebritis
19. Lupus neuropathy
20. Ascending polyneuropathy
21. Poliomyelitis
22. Pseudobulbar palsy
23. Bulbar palsy
24. "Sciatica"
25. Brown-Sequard syndrome
26. Tabes dorsalis
27. Optic neuritis
28. Combined system disease
29. Anxiety
30. Multi-infarction dementia

A15:

1.	b, d, f	**16.**	b, d	
2.	a, c, e	**17.**	b, d	
3.	b, d, f	**18.**	a, c, e	
4.	f, d	**19.**	b, d	
5.	b, d	**20.**	b, d (i.e., Guillain-Barré)	
6.	a, c, e	**21.**	b, d, f (in bulbar form)	
7.	b, d	**22.**	e (reflexes variable)	
8.	b, d	**23.**	f (reflexes variable)	
9.	a, c	**24.**	b, d	
10.	a, c, e	**25.**	a, c	
11.	a, c	**26.**	b, d	
12.	a, c, e or f (depending on site of lesion)	**27.**	d	
13.	b, d	**28.**	a, c	
14.	b, d	**29.**	a, e	
15.	b, d	**30.**	a, c, e	

Q16: Which conditions in question 15 involve upper motor neuron injury?
A16: 2, 6, 9, 10, 11, 12, 18, 22, 25, 28, 30.

Q17: Which conditions in question 15 involve lower motor neuron injury?
A17: 1, 3, 4 (neuromuscular junction), 5, 6, 7, 8, 15, 16, 17, 19, 20, 21, 23, 24.

Q18: Match the most appropriate diagnostic or confirmatory procedure with the condition:

1. Multiple sclerosis	a. Computed tomography (CT)
2. Cerebellar infarction	b. Electroencephalography
3. Subdural hematoma	(EEG)
4. Bacterial meningitis	c. Electromyography (EMG) and
5. Hydrocephalus	nerve conduction velocity
6. Myotonic dystrophy	(NCV)
7. Myasthenia gravis	d. Lumbar puncture (LP)
8. Muscular dystrophy	e. Myelography
9. Diabetic neuropathy	f. Pneumoencephalography
10. Alzheimer's disease	g. Slit lamp examination
11. Wilson's disease	h. Tensilon test
12. Spinal cord compression	i. None of the above

13. Absence (petit mal) seizures
14. Combined system disease (pernicious anemia)
15. Hepatic encephalopathy
16. Radial nerve palsy
17. Meningioma of sphenoid ridge
18. Subacute sclerosing panencephalitis (SSPE)
19. Down's syndrome
20. Brain abscess
21. Creutzfeldt-Jakob disease
22. Meningioma of spinal cord
23. Partial complex seizures
24. Carpal tunnel syndrome
25. Mental retardation
26. Cerebral arteriovenous malformation
27. "Cerebral palsy"
28. Cryptococcal meningitis
29. Optic neuritis
30. Lumbar herniated intervertebral disk
31. Huntington's chorea
32. Wernicke's encephalopathy
33. Amaurosis fugax
34. Frontal lobe tumor
35. Lithium toxicity
36. Parkinsonism
37. Postictal *v* functional seizures
38. Herpes encephalitis
39. Normal pressure hydrocephalus
40. Porphyria with mental changes
41. Pseudotumor cerebri
42. Postconcussive syndrome
43. Wallenberg's syndrome
44. Sydenham's chorea

A18: **1.** i. The diagnosis of multiple sclerosis is predominantly a clinical one, although the CSF might be helpful if it reveals myelin basic protein or oligoclonal bands. Visual evoked responses (VER) are helpful but not diagnostic.

2. a.
3. a.
4. d.
5. a.
6. c. (EMG)
7. h.
8. i. Muscular dystrophy is predominantly a clinical diagnosis, but CPK and other serum enzymes determinations and a muscle biopsy would be helpful confirmatory information.
9. c (NCV)
10. i. Both the CT and EEG may be normal in early Alzheimer's disease.
11. g. Alternatively a serum ceruloplasmin determination would be an appropriate test.
12. e.
13. b.
14. i. A serum B_{12} determination or a Schilling test would be the appropriate tests.
15. b.
16. c (EMG and NCV)
17. a.
18. b.
19. i. A chromosome test would reveal trisomy or translocation of chromosome 21.
20. a.
21. b. A brain biopsy, however, would be definitive.
22. e. In the future, a CT scan of the spinal cord will be the procedure of choice.
23. b.
24. c.
25. i.
26. a.
27. i.
28. d. The CSF must be analyzed for cryptococcal antigen, an India ink preparation must be made, and fluid should be cultured for fungus.
29. i. VER would be abnormal.
30. e. In the near future, a CT scan of the spine will be the procedure of choice.
31. i. Although a CT scan might show atrophy of the caudate nuclei, such a finding would be present only in advanced cases.
32. i. Mamillary body hemorrhages and other pathologic changes are too small to be seen on CT.
33. i. Carotid arteriography might reveal atherosclerotic stenosis and ulcerations, which might form a nidus for platelet emboli.
34. a.
35. i. A test of the blood level would be the most appropriate, but the EEG would be clearly abnormal early in toxicity.
36. i.
37. b. Postictally, EEGs are depressed and serum prolactins elevated.
38. a, b, d.
39. a. A CT scan would be helpful but there is no one specific diagnostic test.
40. i. When porphyria is associated with mental changes, it is of the "acute intermittent" variety. During an attack, examination of the urine will show excessive porphyrins. A Watson-Schwartz test will be positive.

41. d and a. A lumbar puncture will reveal abnormal pressures (usually in excess of 300 mm). Since the differential diagnosis of pseudotumor is tumor, a CT scan must be performed. Besides showing absence of a tumor or other mass lesions, the CT scan will show small ventricles.

42. i. Minor, inconsistent EEG abnormalities are often but not necessarily found in this admittedly nebulous condition.

43. i. Infarctions of the lateral medulla (Wallenberg syndrome) cannot be detected with any of these tests.

44. i. The CT scan is normal in cases of Sydenham's chorea. It is abnormal in Huntington's chorea and Wilson's disease.

Q19–21: A 67-year-old man has had 3 weeks of progressively more severe, dull, bifrontal headaches, which are worse in the morning and relieved partially by aspirin. The patient is apathetic and inattentive, but allowing for his age, there is no cognitive impairment. He is unsteady, but the housestaff find no other physical deficit.

Q19: Which of the following causes of headaches might be seriously considered in this case?

    a.   Glioblastoma or metastatic carcinoma
    b.   Migraine headaches
    c.   Carbon dioxide retention
    d.   Cryptococcal meningitis
    e.   Subdural hematoma, despite lack of trauma
    f.   Meningococcal meningitis
    g.   Cluster headaches
    h.   Trigeminal neuralgia
    i.   Brain abscess

A19: a, c, d, e, i

Q20: What should the order be of the immediate diagnostic steps?

    a.   EEG
    b.   Lumbar puncture
    c.   Routine laboratory evaluation, including a chest x-ray
    d.   Arterial blood gas analysis
    e.   Complete history and physical
    f.   Computed tomography

A20: e, c, f. If these are normal, a, b, and possibly d

Q21: Before any tests could be performed, the attending neurologist finds that the patient does have papilledema, paresis of the left leg, and a left Babinski sign. Where would he or she expect that the CT scan would show a lesion?

    a.   Left side of the spinal cord
    b.   Right side of the brainstem
    c.   Right internal capsule
    d.   Right frontal lobe

A21: d

Q22–23: A 29-year-old woman has a 19-year history of monthly, almost exclusively left frontal and periorbital dull, throbbing, aching headaches. They begin in the early morning and are associated with slight nausea, photophobia, and hunger, despite the nausea. Her mother has had similar headaches. The patient's physical examination and routine laboratory tests are normal.

Q22: Which would be the best initial management plan?

    a.   Obtain a CT scan
    b.   Obtain an EEG
    c.   Give a therapeutic trial of a vasoconstrictor medication, e.g. Cafergot

    d.   Give a therapeutic trial of a mild analgesic/sedative combination, e.g., Fiorinal, including trials of medication at bedtime

    e.   If possible, eliminate skipped meals, excessive as well as insufficient sleep, and all food and beverages containing alcohol.

A22: e and either c or d (this author suggests d). If the patient responds to simple measures, no further evaluation is indicated. With a typical case of common migraine headache such as this, further evaluation is not warranted if the patient responds. In any case, an EEG would not be very helpful and CT scan should be avoided in young people, especially women in their child-bearing years.

Q23: The woman, however, begins to have more frequent, intense, and incapacitating headaches. Plans c, d, and e do not help. A CT scan is done and shows no abnormalities. What should the next therapeutic plan be?

    a.   Prophylactic treatment with beta blockers, e.g., propranolol (Inderal)

    b.   Prophylactic treatment with methysergide (Sansert)

    c.   Daily use of vasoconstrictor medications

A23: a

When common or classic migraine headaches occur more than once a week, prophylactic therapy is indicated. In this case, a beta blocker medication would probably be effective and not subject the patient to the risks of retroperitoneal fibrosis, which may be a complication of (improper) use of methysergide (Sansert).

Q24–29: Match the clinical features of the headache with the diagnosis:

Q24:	Severe, prostrating headache occurring during coitus	a.	Pseudotumor cerebri
		b.	Subarachnoid hemorrhage
Q25:	Generalized dull headache in an obese young woman with papilledema and sixth cranial nerve palsy	c.	Trigeminal neuralia
		d.	Temporal arteritis
		e.	Open-angle glaucoma
Q26:	Frontal headaches in a 70-year-old man	f.	Closed angle glaucoma
		g.	Cluster

Q27: A series of 30-minute periorbital headaches in a 30-year-old man that are often precipitated by wine

Q28: If untreated, may be complicated by blindness

Q29: Brief periods (less than 5 seconds) of sharp pains in the right lower jaw that may be precipitated by brushing teeth

A24–29:

24:	b	**27:**	g
25:	a	**28:**	a, d, e, f
26:	d, f	**29:**	c

Q30–36: Match the medication(s) that are effective in the treatment of these various headaches:

30:	Furosemide (Lasix)	a.	Cluster
31:	Cafergot	b.	Pseudotumor cerebri
32:	Propranolol (Inderal)	c.	Trigeminal neuralgia
33:	Prednisone	d.	Temporal arteritis
34:	Carbamazepine (Tegretol)	e.	Common migraine
35:	Lithium		
36:	Methysergide (Sansert)		

A30–36:

30:	b	**34:**	c
31:	e	**35:**	a
32:	a, e	**36:**	a, e
33:	a, b, d		

Q37–49: Match the headaches with precipitating causes:

37:	Menses	a.	Common or classic migraine
38:	Red wine	b.	Cluster headache
39:	REM sleep	c.	Tic douloureux
40:	Touching affected area	d.	None of the above
41:	Too much sleep		
42:	Cool breeze		
43:	Genetic factors		
44:	A vascular loop pressing on the trigeminal nerve		
45:	Histamine		
46:	Type A personality		
47:	Exclusively high socioeconomic background		
48:	(May occur in) childhood		
49:	Almost only above age 55		

A37–49:

37:	a	**41:**	a	**45:**	d
38:	a, b	**42:**	c	**46:**	d
39:	a, b	**43:**	a	**47:**	d
40:	c	**44:**	c	**48:**	a
				49:	c

Q50: A 29-year-old woman has had several headaches every week for 10 years. They are usually present on awakening in the morning, although she may develop them if she misses her 10:00 AM coffee break. Her headaches also occur in the afternoon, while driving her car for several hours, or during psychologically stressful episodes. Most headaches are bitemporal, more on the left than the right. After several hours, her headaches become generalized and dull. Sometimes, however, they begin as a dull ache in the upper neck and then seem to gravitate to behind the left eye. Rest, aspirin compound products, and coffee often relieve the headaches. She rarely has to leave work early because of the pain. Afternoon naps relieve most headaches completely. The patient's mother, maternal grandmother, and 11-year-old daughter have had headaches, but she is unaware of the details of their headaches. The remaining medical history, physical and neurologic examinations, and routine laboratory work are unremarkable. Formulate a diagnosis and suggest initial management.

A50: This patient probably has the most frequently occurring headache problem that neurologists encounter: a combination of muscle contraction (tension) and common migraine headaches. There is no indication that the patient suffers from a structural lesion in view of the chronicity of the headaches and lack of accompanying neurologic physical signs.

The components of the headaches that suggest that they are partly migrainous are the following: The headaches begin in the early morning and may be averted by taking coffee (caffeine). They are often located unilaterally, especially in the periorbital or retro-orbital area. They are relieved by sleep, not merely resting, and they are alleviated by aspirin-caffeine compounds. Finally, although muscle contraction headaches may have a familial occurrence (on a psychogenic basis), a female-family incidence, as in this case, is indicative of genetically inherited susceptibility.

The headaches are also partly the result of muscle contractions. Those headaches located in the neck and dull bitemporal headaches are from muscle contracting as are those that occur after difficult work, long drives, and psychologically stressful episodes.

An important, typical feature of this case is that the two types of headaches alternate, vary, and blend because prolonged muscle contraction headaches lead to migraine headaches and mild, prolonged common migraine leads to muscle contraction headaches. Either or both, of course, cause anxiety, which exacerbates the pain and discomfort.

Opinion might differ over the appropriate initial management. Some physicians would perform computed tomography (CT) to alleviate their own as well as the patient's concern about a structural lesion, such as a brain tumor or arteriovenous malformation. Other physicians, including the author, would postpone CT while attempting to eliminate the headaches by simple medical means.

Therapy would start by having the patient record the various headaches and potential precipitating factors on a calendar. Menses, excessive work days, vacations, use of wine, and other factors would be considered as possible provoking factors that then could be avoided.

Meanwhile therapy would be directed first toward the common migraine headache, by this author at least, because these headaches are more readily treated. When they occur once a week or less, a mild analgesic-sedative compound, such as Fiorinal, might be given. When they occur more frequently, prophylactic therapy with a beta-blocker might be given. Depending on the psychologic circumstances, treatment of the muscle contraction headaches might begin with aspirin. Then a mild sedative or even an antidepressant, which would provide analgesic as well as psychologic benefit, could be added.

Q51–56: Below are six sketches of spinal cords stained such that normal myelin is stained black, gray areas are crosshatched, and demyelinated areas are white (unstained). Match the sketches (Q51–56) with the descriptions of the clinical associations (A–F).

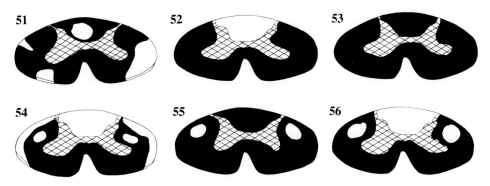

51   52   53

54   55   56

A. A 45-year-old man with progressively severe intellectual and personality impairment for 4 years has loss of vibration and position sensation, absent reflexes in the legs, and a floppy-foot gait. His pupils are miotic and unreactive.

B. A 65-year-old man, who had a complete gastrectomy 4 years ago, now has dementia, hyperactive DTRs, bilateral Babinski signs, and loss of vibration sensation in the legs.

C. A 70-year-old lady has weakness of the left leg, right arm, and neck muscles. She has atrophy of many limb muscles and fasciculations of the tongue and most of the atrophic muscles.

D. A 35-year-old man has optic neuritis, internuclear ophthalmoplegia, and gait impairment because of ataxia, weakness, and spasticity.

E. A 40-year-old woman and her sister have pes cavus, intention tremor of the limbs, and loss of position and vibration sensation.

F. A 70-year-old man who has schizophrenia, sustains a frontal lobe gunshot wound. He takes Dilantin, which leads to cerebellar dysfunction. He becomes so distraught, he becomes an alcoholic and suffers an episode of severe confusion, nystagmus, and bilateral abducens nerve palsy.

A51–56:

51 D. The spinal cord shows multiple areas (plaques) of demyelination (sclerosis). The patient has signs of optic nerve, brainstem, and spinal cord dysfunction. Both the clinical and pathologic material indicate multiple sclerosis.

52 A. The spinal cord shows demyelination of the posterior columns. Loss of these tracts causes loss of position sensation, which makes patients walk with high, uncertain, and awkward steps. This patient also has a suggestion of Argyll-Robertson pupils as well as mental abnormalities. This is a case of syphilis of the brain and spinal cord (tabes dorsalis).

53 F. The spinal cord remains normal despite the cerebral injury, drug-induced cerebellar dysfunction, and Wernicke's encephalopathy.

54 E. There is degeneration of the spinocerebellar, posterior column, and corticospinal tracts. Loss of the spinocerebellar and posterior column tracts, which indicates a spinocerebellar degenerative illness, such as Friedreick's ataxia, causes intention tremor, position and vibration sense loss, and a foot deformity (pes cavus).

55 C. The spinal cord shows demyelination of the corticospinal tracts and loss of the anterior horns, which contain the motor neurons. This is the picture of motor neuron disease when, typically, both the upper and lower motor neuron systems degenerate. The patient has the clinical features of amyotrophic lateral sclerosis (ALS), the most common form of motor neuron disease.

56 B. The spinal cord shows demyelination of the posterior columns and the corticospinal tracts. This combination, termed "combined system disease," is associated with B_{12} deficiency from pernicious anemia or surgical removal of the stomach. It is associated with dementia, paraparesis, hyperactive DTRs, and position and vibration sense loss. These findings are similar to those of tabes dorsalis with dementia; however, combined system disease causes hyperactive DTRs and Babinski signs, while tabes dorsalis causes hypoactive DTRs and Argyll-Robertson pupils, but neither paraparesis nor Babinski signs.

Q57–61: Match the disease with the associated abnormality:

57. Idiopathic Parkinson's disease	a. Dopamine depletion
58. Hemiballismus	b. Dopamine block
59. Wilson's disease	c. Contralateral subthalamic nucleus
60. Huntington's chorea	infarction
61. Haloperidol-induced bradykinesia	d. Caudate atrophy
	e. Copper metabolism abnormality

A57–61:
    57. a   **58.** c   **59.** e   **60.** d   **61.** b

Q62–66: Match the medication with its potential side effects:

62. L-DOPA	a. Constipation
63. Anti cholinergics	b. Anhidrosis
64. Sinemet	c. Buccolingual dyskinesias
65. Oral contraceptives	d. Agitation
66. Choline	e. Fishy smell
	f. Sexual hyperactivity
	g. Chorea
	h. Somnolence
	i. Hallucinations
	j. Dry mouth
	k. May hasten development of tardive dyskinesia
	l. Pupillary dilatation

A62–66:
    62. c, d, f, g, i
    63. a, b, d (unusual), h (unusual), j, k, and l (minimal)
    64. same as 62
    65. g (Oral-contraceptive–induced chorea is a rare complication, found in young nulliparous women who usually themselves or their relatives have had Sydenham's chorea.)
    66. e

Q67–72: How does the tremor of parkinsonism differ from that of essential tremor? (True/False)

67. Only Parkinson's tremor is absent during sleep.
68. Only Parkinson's tremor is sometimes found in many family members.
69. Only essential tremor often begins in the third or fourth decade of life.
70. Only essential tremor is fine and rapid.
71. Only Parkinson's tremor is associated with rigidity or bradykinesia.
72. Only essential tremor may be reduced by alcoholic drinks and propranolol.

A67–72:
67. False: both are absent during sleep
68. False: a common variety of essential tremor is called "benign familial tremor."
69. True, with rare exceptions
70. True
71. True
72. True

Q73–79: Which conditions induce tremor? (Yes/No)
73. Excessive coffee consumption
74. Lithium usage
75. Amantadine (Symmetrel)
76. Steroids
77. Amitriptyline (Elavil)
78. Hypothyroidism
79. Hyperthyroidism

A73–79:
73. Yes.
74. Yes. Fine tremor is often associated with mild lithium intoxication. Gross tremor is a clear sign of intoxication.
75. No. This antiviral medication suppresses Parkinson's tremor.
76. Yes, although high doses are required.
77. Yes, but unlike lithium use, mild tremor with amitriptyline use is not clearly a sign of toxicity.
78. No.
79. Yes.

Q80: A 71-year-old man has been receiving numerous psychotropic medications for many years. Fundoscopy reveals flecks of dark pigment scattered about the retina. Which of the following medications is (are) most likely responsible?

a.	Chlorpromazine (Thorazine)	c.	Thioridazine (Mellaril)
b.	Imipramine (Tofranil)	d.	Amitriptyline (Elavil)

A80: a, c

Q81–86: Match the visual field loss associated with each condition:

81.	Left homonymous hemianopsia with macular sparing	a.	Retinal injury, e.g., embolus or detachment
82.	Fortification scotoma	b.	Hysteria
83.	Central scotoma, lasting for two weeks	c.	Migraine
		d.	Diabetes insipidus
84.	Bitemporal hemianopsia	e.	Loss of libido
85.	Unilateral superior quadrantanopsia	f.	Optic atrophy
86.	Enlarged blind spot	g.	Amaurosis fujax
		h.	Internal capsule infarction
		i.	Aphasia
		j.	Occipital infarction
		k.	Optic or retrobulbar neuritis
		l.	Pseudotumor cerebri

A81–86:
    81. j   **84.** d, e, f (all associated with pituitary
    82. c   tumors)
    83. k   **85.** a
                            86. l

Q87–89: A 29-year-old woman awakens one morning with pain in and around her right eye. She can see only large objects using the right eye, but the vision in the left eye remains 20/30 corrected (using glasses). The pain in the right eye increases on any movement, but there is no diplopia. The pupils are round and equal. The optic discs and fundi appear normal. The condition lasts for at least 48 hours.

Q87: What is the most likely condition that has caused this problem?
    a.   Hysteria   d.   Multiple sclerosis
    b.   Left occipital infarction   e.   Classic migraine
    c.   Optic or retrobulbar neuritis   f.   None of the above

A87: c. Inflammation of the optic nerve (optic neuritis), typically in its portion behind the eyeball (retrobulbar neuritis), is the single most likely cause. While this condition is often a harbinger or complication of multiple sclerosis, in about two thirds of cases, patients never develop other indications of multiple sclerosis.

Q88: A skeptical physician believes that this patient has a conversion reaction. Which observations or positive tests would probably be present that would indicate that the patient does have optic neuritis?
    a.   Constriction of the right pupil as light is shown into it.
    b.   Dilatation of the right pupil as light is rapidly moved from the left to the right eye.
    c.   Finding abnormal visual evoked responses (VERs) in the right eye.
    d.   Abnormal CT scan.
    e.   Abnormal electroencephalogram (EEG).
    f.   Oligoclonal bands and myelin basic protein in the CSF.

A88: b, c, f

Q89: Which of the following medications or techniques have been said to be effective treatment for multiple sclerosis?
    a.   ACTH   c.   Plasmaphoresis
    b.   Phenytoin (Dilantin)   d.   Cyclophosphamide

A89: a, d

Q90: An 80-year-old man, who is being treated for depression, complains of right-sided frontotemporal headaches. His vision in the right eye is impaired. Temporal arteries are prominent, but not especially tender. There is no papilledema, hemiparesis, or other neurologic sign. Which conditions must be considered immediately?
    a.   Open angle glaucoma   d.   Optic neuritis
    b.   Metastases to the skull   e.   Temporal arteritis
    c.   Meningioma   f.   Narrow angle glaucoma

A90: e, f

Q91–102: Differences between Horner's syndrome and oculomotor (third cranial nerve) palsy are important. Indicate which features are associated with either one, both, or neither:
    91. Pupillary dilatation   a.   Horner's syndrome
    92. Ptosis   b.   Oculomotor nerve palsy
    93. Miosis (pupillary constriction)   c.   Migraine
    94. Associated with diabetes   d.   Neither
    95. Found in cluster headache
    96. Found with Pancoast's tumors
    97. Associated with medullary lesions

   98. Associated with pontine lesions
   99. Associated with midbrain lesions
   100. Causes diplopia
   101. Associated with syringomyelia
   102. Found rarely in migraine

A91–102:

91.	b	**95.**	a	**99.**	b
92.	c	**96.**	a	**100.**	b
93.	a	**97.**	a	**101.**	a
94.	b	**98.**	d	**102.**	b

Q103:   Which factors may precipitate angle closure glaucoma? (Yes/No)

   a.   Topically applied agents that cause pupillary dilatation, e.g., phenylephrine (Neosynephrine).
   b.   Atropine, scopolamine, and other atropine-like medications.
   c.   Sympathomimetic drugs.
   d.   Drugs that interfere with parasympathetic activity.
   e.   Tricyclic antidepressants because of their atropine-like effects.
   f.   Anticholinergic medications.
   g.   Propanolol and topically applied beta-blockers.
   h.   Ephedrine and neosynephrine.
   i.   Any medication that retards reuptake or metabolism of norepinephrine.
   j.   Any drug that acts like norepinephrine.

A103:

   a.   Yes. Such medications, which are often instilled during fundoscopy, sometimes precipitate angle closure glaucoma.
   b.   Yes.
   c.   Yes. Topically administered sympathomimetics, but not (for practical purposes) systemically administered sympathomimetics may precipitate glaucoma.
   d.   Yes. Only predisposed people, however, are at risk.
   e.   Yes. Phenothiazines too may cause glaucoma, although such a complication occurs very rarely.
   f.   Yes. Only predisposed people are at risk.
   g.   No. In fact, topically applied beta-blockers are used in treatment of glaucoma.
   h.   Yes.
   i.   Yes.
   j.   Yes.

Q104:   A 40-year-old alcoholic man who has mild, chronic cirrhosis is brought to the Emergency Room because he suddenly became confused. Examination reveals disorientation, slurred speech, and asterixis. There is no nystagmus, extraocular paresis, or pupillary abnormality. Laboratory data include the following: mildly abnormal liver function tests, 26% hematocrit, and blood in the stool. Which conditions ought to be considered?

   a.   Wernicke's encephalopathy   d.   Subdural hematoma
   b.   Alcohol-induced hypoglycemia   e.   Delirium tremens (DTs)
   c.   Hepatic encephalopathy

A104:   c. Hepatic encephalopathy is the most likely cause. People with cirrhosis or other causes of hepatic insufficiency will develop encephalopathy typically when gastrointestinal bleeding occurs from esophageal varices or gastric ulceration.

In this case, the anemia and bloody stool indicate gastrointestinal bleeding. Sometimes encephalopathy will occur merely following a meal of high protein content. Most important, mental changes and asterixis often occur, as in this case, before liver function test abnormalities become pronounced.

Wernicke's encephalopathy (a), alcohol-induced hypoglycemia (b), and subdural hematoma (d) should always be considered in alcoholics with mental changes. Although no neurologic signs indicate any of these diagnoses, all such patients routinely should receive intravenous thiamine and, after blood is drawn for tests, intravenous glucose.

Q105–113:   Match the ocular abnormality with the most probable site of lesion:

105. Right third cranial nerve paresis and left hemiparesis	a. Myasthenia gravis
	b. Scopolamine intoxication
106. Left sixth cranial nerve paresis and right hemiparesis	c. Right pontine lesion
	d. Left midbrain lesion
107. Right Horner's syndrome, right facial hypalgesia, right limb ataxis, and left limb and trunk hypalgesia	e. Left pontine lesion
	f. Right midbrain lesion
	g. Midline brainstem lesion
	h. Left lateral medullary lesion
108. Internuclear ophthalmoplegia	i. Right lateral medullary lesion
	j. Syphilis
	k. Heroin or methadone overdose

109. Right sixth and seventh cranial nerve paresis and left hemiparesis
110. Ophthalmoplegia with normally reactive pupils, ptosis, and facial paresis
111. Small, irregular pupils that accommodate but do not react
112. Fever, agitated confusion, and dilated pupils
113. Stupor, miosis, and pulmonary edema

A105–113:

105. f	107. i	109. c	111. j	113. k
106. e	108. g	110. a	112. b	

Q114:   Which of the following are found in the brains of people with Alzheimer's disease but not in brains of normal elderly persons?

a. Loss of weight
b. Increase in sulci width
c. Expansion of the lateral ventricles
d. Major loss of large cortical neurons
e. *Marked* reduction of choline acetyltransferase in the hippocampus
f. Mild memory impairment
g. *Multiple* neurofibrillary tangles
h. Similarity to brains of Down's syndrome patients and retired boxers
i. Presence of senile plaques

A114:   d, e, g, h

Cerebral atrophy (a, b, c) and the presence of some plaques (i), neurofibrillary tangles, and granulovacuolar degeneration are found in normal brains but are only quantitatively more pronounced in the brain with Alzheimer's disease. Likewise, mild memory impairment in people with early Alzheimer's disease is similar to that found in the normal elderly.

Q115-122:   Mental changes are often accompanied by physical abnormalities. Match the associated signs:

115. Parkinson's disease patient with agitation, hallucinations, and ____	a. Seventh cranial nerve palsy
	b. Incontinence
	c. Tremor and/or rigidity and bradykinesia
116. Dementia, gait apraxia, and ____	
117. Delirium, sixth cranial nerve palsy, ataxia, peripheral neuropathy, and ____	d. Nystagmus
	e. Myoclonus
	f. Pupils that do not react
118. Dementia, chronic hepatic insufficiency, corneal discoloration, and ____	g. Pupils that do not accommodate
	h. Seizures
	i. Dyskinesias

119. Dementia, position sense loss, positive VDRL, and miotic _____
120. Seizure patient with lethargy, confusion, dysarthria, ataxia, and, _____
121. Child with rapidly progressive mental and personality impairment, high measles antibody titre in the CSF, and _____
122. Elderly man with rapid development of dementia, periodic EEG, and _____

A15–122:

115. i	**117.** d	**119.** f	**121.** e
116. b	**118.** c	**120.** d	**122.** e

Q123–132: Match the illness with the findings in Q115–122 or note "none of the above":

123. Wernicke-Korsakoff syndrome	129. Subacute sclerosing panencephalitis (SSPE)
124. Normal pressure hydrocephalus	
125. Wilson's disease	130. Alzheimer's disease
126. Creutzfeldt-Jakob disease	131. Multiple sclerosis
127. Tertiary syphilis	132. Parkinson's disease with L-Dopa intoxication
128. Anticonvulsant intoxication	

A123–132:

123. 117	**128.** 120
124. 116	**129.** 121
125. 118	**130.** None of the above, but rarely 122
126. 122	**131.** None of the above
127. 119	**132.** 115

Q133: If a patient uses topical pilocarpine because he has narrow angle glaucoma, can he use tricyclic antidepressants and phenothiazine medications with impunity?

A133: Yes.

Q134: Which features indicate amyotrophic lateral sclerosis (ALS), peripheral neuropathy, both, or neither?

a. Muscle atrophy	d. Hypoactive DTR's
b. Fasciculations	e. Atrophy of tongue muscles
c. Babinski signs	f. Stocking-glove hypalgesia

A134:

a. both	c. ALS	e. ALS
b. ALS	d. Peripheral neuropathy	f. Peripheral neuropathy

Q135: Which of the following illnesses may cause peripheral neuropathy and mental changes?

a. Cervical spondylosis	e. Heavy metal intoxication
b. Wernicke-Korsakoff syndrome	f. Syphilis
c. Porphyria (Acute intermittent)	g. Uremia
d. ALS	h. Nitrous oxide abuse

A135: b, c, e, f, g, h

Q136: A 17-year-old woman complains of 10 days of progressively increasing weakness of the ankles and toes. On examination she has weakness in the hands and wrists as well as the ankles and toes, and also unreactive ankle DTRs and plantar reflexes. Which illness might explain her symptoms and signs?

a. Myasthenia gravis	d. Guillain-Barré syndrome
b. Toxic polyneuropathy	e. Thoracic spinal cord tumor
c. Polymyositis	f. Alcoholism

A136: b, d, f

Q137: A 6-year-old boy, who has begun to have difficulty standing, pushes himself up upon his legs. The boy is seemingly well-built, but has paresis of the pelvic-girdle muscles and areflexia of the quadriceps. A 7-year-old cousin has a similar problem.

Which illness is the patient most likely to have?

a. Peripheral neuropathy   d. Hysteria
b. Myasthenia   e. Childhood form of ALS
c. Duchenne's muscular dystrophy

A137: c

Q138: What is the sex of the cousin? Who are the carriers?

A138: Probably, the cousin is also a boy and the carriers are the boys' mothers, who are sisters.

Q139: In which illnesses will the Romberg test be positive?

a. Diabetic neuropathy   d. Cerebral infarction
b. Tabes dorsalis   e. Spinocerebellar (Friedreich's)
c. Cerebellar tumor   degeneration

A139: a (because of peripheral neuropathy) and b and e (because of posterior column injury)

Q140: Which of the following substances cause cerebellar dysfunction?

a. Ethanol   d. Elavil
b. Dilantin   e. Mercury
c. INH

A140: a, b, e (Elavil causes tremor, but not because of cerebellar damage).

Q141: A 35-year-old man staggers into the emergency room. He is lethargic and disoriented. There is nystagmus, gait ataxia and finger-to-nose dysmetria. Which illness is he most likely to have? What is the *specific* therapy?

a. Subdural hematoma   c. Wernicke-Korsakoff syndrome
b. Cerebral infarction   d. Hysteria

A141: c. Thiamine 50 mg IV

Q142: An 11-year-old boy is admitted because of headache, nausea, and vomiting. He has had clumsiness for the 2 weeks before admission. His optic disks are edematous. He has ataxia, hyperactive DTRs bilaterally, and Babinski signs bilaterally. Which is the most likely diagnosis?

a. Multiple sclerosis   c. Cerebellar tumor
b. Drug abuse   d. Spinocerebellar degeneration

A142: c. Cerebellar astrocytomas, which are relatively common in youngsters, block the aqueduct of Sylvius, creating hydrocephalus (manifested by headaches, nausea, vomiting, and papilledema).

Q143: An 18-year-old soldier sustained a mild head injury in basic training. Examination revealed striking tremors and ataxia of gait (although no falls occurred), but no dysarthria, nystagmus, or dysmetria. The best course to pursue would be:

a. Immediate CT   c. Lumbar puncture
b. Give thiamine IV   d. Observe

A143: The signs of cerebellar disease are incomplete and inconsistent. Failing to fall when apparently severely ataxic is *astasia abasia* and usually a sign of psychogenic difficulty. The best course would be to observe (d) or, for reassurance, obtain a CT scan (a), although this need not be performed immediately.

Q144: A 30-year-old man is brought to the Emergency Room of Elsewhere Hospital describing his new digital watch as a "timer for destruction of the world." He speaks in circumlocutions and tangents and he often repeats phrases and sentences, but he does not use jargon, neologisms, or paraphasias. Physicians are not able to obtain any additional history or to perform any physical or neurologic examinations.

What conditions must be given immediate consideration?

a. Aphasia   c. Psychiatric disturbances
b. Acute organic mental   d. The impending destruction of
    syndrome (delerium)   the world, i.e., the man is correct

A144: a, b, c

Q145: With calming and urging a small dose of phenothiazine, the man is able to cooperate. He then carefully describes the "powers" of his new watch. The physicians demonstrate that the man is oriented, has good memory, and his judgment is otherwise intact. Nevertheless, one physician insists that the patient is aphasic.

Which tests of language function must the skeptical physician perform?

A145: Metaphor is a linguistic phenomenon used by orators, poets, humorists, and sportscasters among other people. Psychotic patients may actually believe that objects have been transformed, but these people, when calm, will be able to identify the object. Even schizophrenics with true jargon speech, as well as this man, *will be able to follow the three routine tests of language function:*

- Following requests
- Naming common objects
- Repeating phrases

Q146: Which of the following symptoms might constitute a "narcoleptic tetrad?"
- a. Inability to move on awakening (sleep paralysis)
- b. Hunger or anorexia
- c. Vivid dreams when falling asleep (hypnogogic hallucinations)
- d. Daytime sleepiness (narcolepsy)
- e. Night terrors (pavor nocturnus)
- f. Episodic loss of muscle tone (cataplexy)

A146: a, c, d, f

Q147: Which of the following are characteristic of an attack of narcolepsy?
- a. Preceding boring situation
- b. Preceding feeling of fatigue
- c. Duration of 15 minutes or less
- d. Sleep onset REM
- e. Absent deep tendon reflexes (DTRs)
- f. Average age of onset before 25 years of age
- g. About a dozen episodes weekly
- h. Usually accompanied by total paralysis (cataplexy)
- i. Narcoleptic attacks begin several years before attacks of cataplexy

A147: a, b, c, d, e, f, g, i

("h" is incorrect because patients more often have loss of tone in a limited area of musculature, such as the legs or jaw, than of their entire body).

Q148: Which of the following conditions are associated with excessive daytime sleepiness?

- a. Night terrors
- b. Obstructive sleep apnea
- c. Jactatio capitis nocturnus (nightime head banging)
- d. Use of "sleeping pills" at bedtime
- e. Enuresis
- f. Narcolepsy
- g. Nonobstructive sleep apnea

A148: b, d, f, g

Q149: Besides excessive daytime sleepiness, which of the following are complications of obstructive sleep apnea?
- a. Systemic hypertension
- b. Pulmonary hypertension
- c. Cardiac arrhythmias

A149: a, b, c

Q150: How do night terrors differ from nightmares? (True/False)
- a. Night terrors, one of the "parasomnias," occur in stage three or four of NREM sleep, but nightmares occur in REM sleep.

b.   Both night terrors and nightmares are vivid, frightening dreams that might be analyzed.

c.   Night terrors usually occur early in the night, during the long stretches of stage 3 and 4 NREM sleep, often occurring when the child is abruptly stimulated. Nightmares occur mixed with other dreams, all of which the child may recall.

d.   The child with a nightmare typically awakens fully from the dream and may be able to recount many vivid details, but the child with a night terror usually returns to sleep.

e.   Frequent night terrors or nightmares are both indications for diazepam (Valium) or imipramine (Tofranil) at bedtime.

A150: a, true; b, false (night terrors are brief episodes of fear similar to a startle response); c, true; d, true; e, false (these and similar medications are indicated only for night terrors and then only when under certain circumstances).

Q151: Which of the following sleep-related phenomena occur during REM sleep, stage 3 or 4 of NREM sleep, or either?

a.	Sleepwalking somnambulism	h.	Teeth mashing (bruxism)
b.	Bedwetting (enuresis)	i.	1–3 Hz EEG activity
c.	Night terrors	j.	High frequency, asynchronous EEG activity
d.	Nightmares		
e.	Penile erections	k.	Flaccid muscles and absent DTRs.
f.	Cluster headaches		
g.	Dreams	l.	Increase in cerebral blood flow

A151:

a.	NREM	g.	REM
b.	NREM	h.	Either
c.	NREM	i.	NREM
d.	REM	j.	REM
e.	REM	k.	REM
f.	REM	l.	REM

Q152: As close as possible, match the developmental milestone with the month/year in which 50 percent of infants or children achieve it, according to the Denver Developmental Screening Test:

1. Stands alone well		a.	1 month
2. Pedals tricycle		b.	2 months
3. Smiles responsively		c.	4 months
4. Plays ball with examiner		d.	6 months
5. Walks well		e.	8 months
6. Stacks two blocks		f.	10 months
7. Separates from mother easily		g.	12 months
8. Draws a man in three parts		h.	14 months
9. Sits without support		i.	18 months
10. Three words other than mama, dada		j.	24 months
		k.	30 months
11. Pulls self to stand		l.	3 years
12. Laughs		m.	4 years

A152:

1. g	4. g	7. l	10. h
2. j	5. g	8. m	11. e
3. a	6. h	9. d	12. b

Q153: What is the sequence in which a child learns to copy the cross, circle, diamond, and square?

A153: circle, cross (or x), square, diamond

Q154: Children may have an acute confusional state. In children, which groups of substances are well-known causes of mental changes?

    a.   Phenytoin (Dilantin), phenothiazines, haloperidol, oral hypoglycemics

    b.   Sedatives, e.g. phenobarbitol

    c.   "Cold" medications, especially those containing antihistamine

    d.   Bronchodilators for treatment of asthma, especially those containing sympathomimetics

    e.   Alcohol or drug intoxication

A154: All of the above. Most notable is the paradoxical reaction in which a sedating substance causes agitation, hyperactivity, and insomnia in children. Other relatively common causes of acute confusional state would include (viral) encephalitis, head trauma, postictal confusion, and any bacterial infection e.g. pneumonia, otitis media.

Q155: Two days after an 11-year-old boy seems to have recovered from an upper respiratory tract viral illness, he has a series of seizures followed by coma. His temperature is 101°F and his liver is enlarged, but otherwise there are no abnormal physical abnormalities. Laboratory tests show an elevated serum transaminase (SGOT) and prolonged prothrombin time (PT).

Which conditions are likely to be the cause of the rapid onset of fever, coma with seizures, and such laboratory abnormalities following an upper respiratory tract infection?

    a.   Gullain-Barré syndrome   e.   Wernicke-Korsakoff

    b.   Multiple sclerosis   syndrome

    c.   Mononucleosis   f.   Reye's syndrome

    d.   Wilson's disease

A155: c, f

Q156: An adolescent with a chronic, major psychiatric disorder begins to drink excessive quantities of tap water and other fluids and to urinate large volumes. After 1 week, he develops a seizure and then coma. Which of the following conditions might have caused such voluminous fluid intake and excretion?

    a.   The psychiatric condition

    b.   Diabetes insipidus

    c.   Diabetes mellitus

    d.   Excessive salt intake

A156: a, b, c, d. Polyuria and polydipsia may be caused by psychogenic factors; an excessive serum solute load such as from glucose or sodium; or absence of antidiuretic hormone, such as found in pituitary tumors.

Q157: In the previous question, assuming the patient did not have excessive salt intake, what might be the cause of the seizure?

    a.   A hypothalamic or pituitary tumor that compresses the hypothalamus or grows into the temporal lobe.

    b.   Hyperglycemia/hyperosmolarity from diabetes mellitus.

    c.   Hyponatremia (serum sodium of 120 or below) from compulsive water ingestion.

A157: a, b, c

Q158: Which conditions can amniocentesis detect?

    a.   Down's syndrome   e.   Tay-Sach's disease

    b.   Cerebral palsy   f.   Mental retardation

    c.   Galactosemia   g.   Phenylkentonuria (PKU)

    d.   Wilson's disease   h.   Midline closure defects e.g. meningomyelocele

A158:   a, c, e, g, h

Q159:   Which conditions can fetal prenatal ultrasound scanning determine?
a.   Twins
b.   Placental placement
c.   Fetal sex
d.   Limb size
e.   Hydrocephalus
f.   Urinary tract abnormalities
g.   Fetal uterine placement
h.   Midline closure defects

A159:   a, b, c, d, e, f, g, h

Q160:   What side effects of antipsychotic drugs are caused by blockade of the tuberoin-fundibular dopamine tract?

A160:   Blockade of the tuberoinfundibular or hypothalamic-pituitary dopamine tract leads to an increase in prolactin, leading in some patients to gain weight, and in women sometimes to lactation and amenorrhea.

Q161:   Sinemet (L-dopa plus carbidopa) will potentially increase levels of which biogenic amines?

A161:   Since L-dopa is a precursor of dopamine, norepinephrine, and epinephrine, it will potentially increase levels of all three of these catecholamines.

Q162:   While both trihexyphenidyl (Artane) and amantadine (Symmetrel) treat drug-induced extrapyramidal side effects, they are believed to act at different sites. Explain. In what clinical situation might you choose amantadine over trihexyphenidyl?

A162:   Artane works primarily as an anticholinergic, whereas Symmetrel acts mainly as a direct dopamine agonist at postsynaptic nigrostriatal dopamine receptors. Amantadine would be the drug of choice for treating extrapyramidal symptoms in a patient who could not tolerate anticholinergic treatment, e.g. a patient who already had dry mouth, blurry vision, constipation, or urinary retention.

Q163:   Tardive dyskinesia is believed to reflect too much dopamine activity in the nigrostriatal system. Explain how antipsychotics, dopamine blockers, can possibly cause too much dopamine activity.

A163:   Postsynaptic dopamine receptor blockade is believed to lead to denervation super-sensitivity, i.e., the nigrostriatal dopamine receptors become more numerous or more sensitive or both.

Q164:   While still in the research phase, how might lecithin or Sinemet treat tardive dyskinesia?

A164:   Lecithin, phosphatidylcholine, is an acetylcholine precursor, and is believed by some to treat tardive dyskinesia by increasing the activity of the cholinergic system. Sinemet is postulated by some to treat tardive dyskinesia by desensitizing or down-regulating the hypothe-sized supersensitive dopamine receptors.

Q165:   In terms of the prevailing biogenic amine models of major psychiatric disorders, how might a compound that inhibited dopamine β-hydroxylase affect a schizophrenic subject? A patient with a severe endogenomorphic depression?

A165:   A compound that blocked dopamine β-hydroxylase activity would inhibit the conversion of dopamine to norepinephrine. This will theoretically exacerbate psychotic symptoms in a schizophrenic patient by increasing dopamine levels. It should also exacerbate depression by decreasing norepinephrine.

Q166:   Imipramine may be better than amitriptyline for depressed patients with low urinary MHPG. Explain why this may be so.

A166:   Low MHPG may reflect abnormally low norepinephrine activity. Imipramine (Tofranil) appears to affect the norepinephrine system preferentially, while amitryptiline (Elavil) appears to affect the serotonin system preferentially. Thus, imipramine theoretically is more effective on depressives with low MHPG.

Q167:   A 25-year-old man, who had had 2 weeks of premature ejaculation, develops spastic paresis and paresthesias below his waist. Otherwise, routine history and physical examinations are unremarkable. A myelogram and CT scan of the head shows no abnormalities. Of the following tests, which will be diagnostically helpful?

    a.   Visual evoked responses (VERs)
    b.   CSF oligoclonal band studies
    c.   CSF myelin basic protein
    d.   Antistriational antibody studies
    e.   Anti-ACh receptor antibodies
    f.   EEG

A167: a, b, c. These tests can indicate multiple sclerosis (MS), and VERs, in particular, can indicate optic nerve involvement (optic or retrobulbar neuritis). Antistriational antibodies indicate that a thymoma is present in a patient with myasthenia gravis. Anti-ACh receptor antibodies indicate general myasthenia gravis. An EEG is not diagnostically helpful for MS, myasthenia, or related conditions.

Q168: Which of the tests, listed in the above question, is generally positive in MS in exacerbation but negative in MS in remission?

A68: c. Myelin basic protein is found in exacerbation of MS but not when it is in remission. CSF oligoclonal bands are found in all stages of multiple sclerosis. When the optic nerves are involved even asymptomatically, the VERs are abnormal. However, each of these studies may be abnormal in conditions other than multiple sclerosis. Both CSF studies may be positive in chronic CNS inflammatory conditions, such as neurosyphilis and chronic fungal meningitis. VERS may be positive in optic nerve gliomas or other conditions affecting the optic pathways.

Q169: Which of the following results have *not* been shown by epidemiologic studies of MS patients?

    a.   The incidence of MS is roughly proportional to the distance from the equator in the Southern as well as in the Northern Hemisphere.
    b.   The incidence of MS is remarkably low in Orientals, black Africans, native Israelis, and Latin Americans.
    c.   Spouses have an increased incidence.
    d.   Blood relatives have an increased incidence.

A169: c

Q170: Which findings accompany MS-induced sexual impairment?

    a.   Optic neuritis
    b.   Urinary impairment
    c.   Internuclear ophthalmoplegia
    d.   Leg spasticity

A170: b, d. These are symptoms of spinal cord involvement, which is the cause of MS sexual impairment.

Q171: What do prolonged VER latencies indicate?

    a.   Optic or retrobulbar neuritis
    b.   Optic or retrobulbar neuritis, despite no clinically demonstrable visual impairment
    c.   Internuclear ophthalmoplegia (INO)
    d.   Psychogenic blindness rather than Anton's syndrome
    e.   Optic neuritis that is not a manifestation of multiple sclerosis

A171: a, b, e. Prolonged VER latencies are abnormal. They suggest a lesion of the visual system including the eye, optic nerve, and cerebral cortex. Only about one third of optic neuritis cases later develop multiple sclerosis.

Q172: Following surgery on the anterior communicating artery, a patient is found to be apathetic, mute, and paraparetic. The patient is also incontinent. Which of the following complications probably has developed?

    a.   The spinal cord and brain have been damaged
    b.   Depression has developed
    c.   Both anterior cerebral arteries were occluded
    d.   The patient developed normal pressure hydrocephalus (NPH), i.e., dementia, gait apraxia, and incontinence

A172: c. The anterior communicating arteries supply a large portion of the frontal lobes, including the medial surface of the motor strips. These regions control the voluntary function of the legs and bladder. Infarction of these arteries creates marked personality impairments along with weakness of both legs and loss of bladder control. NPH sometimes develops following subarachnoid hemorrhages, but NPH patients have gait apraxia rather than paraparesis.

Q173: Which of the following conditions might lead to a patient's having "putrid smells" that the physician cannot detect?
    a.   Seizures that originate in the uncus
    b.   Sinusitis
    c.   Migraine aura
    d.   Seizures that originate in the parietal lobe
    e.   Phenytoin

A173: a, b. Migraine headaches curiously, often have visual but rarely olfactory auras.

Q174: Which of the following conditions cause Horner's syndrome?
    a.   Lateral medullary infarctions
    b.   Cluster headaches
    c.   Lung carcinoma
    d.   Migraine headaches
    e.   Occlusion of the posterior inferior cerebellar artery
    f.   Cervical spinal cord lesions
    g.   Cerebral infarctions
    h.   Injury to C_8 and T_1 nerve roots

A174: a, b, c, e, f, h

Q175: An elderly man falls down a flight of stairs, fracturing his right femoral neck (hip) and right humerus (arm). After the hip is "pinned" and the arm is set, he is noted to be confused, agitated, and unintelligible. Which of the following possibilities must be considered?
    a.   Fat emboli
    b.   Neurologic illness precipitating the fall
    c.   A left cerebral infarction
    d.   The fall was complicated by development of a subdural hematoma
    e.   An electrolyte disturbance
    f.   A medication causing an adverse reaction
    g.   Aspiration pneumonia
    h.   Alcohol or other substance withdrawal

A175. a, b, c, d, e, f, g, h

Q176: Which of the following would be helpful in the case described in the preceding question?
    a.   CBC, electrolytes, BUN determinations
    b.   EEG
    c.   CT scan
    d.   Review of medications
    e.   Chest x-ray
    f.   Review of history
    g.   Lumbar puncture
    h.   Urine for fat analysis

     i.   Sedating the patient until the situation is clarified

     j.   Echoencephalogram

A176: a, c, d, e, f, h, i

Q177: In which conditions might lumbar puncture be indicated?

     a.   Subdural hematoma

     b.   Brain abscess

     c.   Brain tumor

     d.   Unruptured arteriovenous malformation

     e.   Pseudotumor cerebri

     f.   Multiple sclerosis

     g.   Bacterial meningitis

     h.   Subacute sclerosing panencephalitis (SSPE)

     i.   Viral encephalitis

     j.   Sexual impairment

A177: e, f, g, h, i. Lumbar punctures should not be done when intracranial mass lesions are suspected because CSF analysis will not be helpful and the procedure might precipitate transtentorial herniation.

Q178: Which of the following are complications of alcoholism?

     a.   Mamillary body hemorrhage

     b.   Peripheral neuropathy

     c.   Neurofibrillary tangles

     d.   Central pontine myelinolysis

     e.   Corpus callosum degeneration (Marchiafava-Bignami syndrome)

     f.   Cerebellar degeneration

     g.   Granulovacuolar changes

     h.   Sclerotic plaques

A178: a, b, d, e, f

Q179: Which of the following illness(es) is (are) characterized by a normal mental state despite quadriparesis and respiratory distress?

     a.   Guillain-Barré syndrome

     b.   Locked-in syndrome

     c.   Amyotrophic lateral sclerosis (ALS)

     d.   Myasthenia gravis

     e.   Porphyria

A179: a, b, c, d

Q180: An emaciated 13-year-old girl has weakness, sensory loss, and areflexia of her distal lower extremities. She then develops eversion and dorsiflexion weakness of her left ankle. How can both a peripheral neuropathy and a left superficial peroneal nerve injury be explained?

     a.   Her polyneuropathy is nutritional

     b.   The mononeuropathy is a compression injury

     c.   She has a vasculitis, e.g., lupus, which causes both polyneuropathy and mono-neuropathy multiplex

     d.   They cannot be explained

A180: c or a and b. A systemic illness, such as lupus, is possible, but patients rarely present with neurologic signs. Anorexia nervosa can lead to a nutritional neuropathy when the patients fail to take vitamins or high protein, fat-soluble foods. Whatever the cause of the weight loss, nerves lose their overlying subcutaneous fatty tissue. The nerves' protection then is lost and they are vulnerable to compression, even as slight as crossing one leg over the other.

Q181: An adolescent girl has twitchy, restless movements. Aside from irritability, her mental and emotional status is normal. Which tests would be most appropriate?

    a.   VDRL
    b.   Inquiries about oral contraceptives
    c.   Antistreptolysin O titer (ALSO)
    d.   Pregnancy test
    e.   Lupus preparation

A181: b, c, d, e. Chorea in adolescence can be a manifestation of pregnancy (chorea gravidarum), an idiosyncratic reaction to oral contraceptives, rheumatic fever (Sydenham's chorea), lupus, or various metabolic derangements. In adolescence, it may be indistinguishable from myoclonus (as seen in SSPE) or tremors (as seen in Wilson's disease). Curiously, in adolescents Huntington's chorea does not usually cause chorea, but rigidity that appears like parkinsonism.

Q182:   Which area of the brain is larger on one side than the other?
    a.   The uncus
    b.   The motor strip
    c.   The planum temporale
    d.   The basal ganglia
    e.   The cerebral hemispheres damaged by in utero vascular accident
    f.   The frontal lobe

A182: c, e. The planum temorale, the superior surface of the temporal lobe which contains Heschl's and Wernicke's areas, is almost always larger in the dominant than the nondominant hemisphere. This normal asymmetry is lost in brain damage, some schizophrenic patients, and many autistic children. When a cerebral hemisphere is damaged in utero, that hemisphere fails to grow fully. The contralateral limbs, in such cases, will be foreshortened. Also, focal seizures may originate from the damaged hemisphere.

Q183:   A 70-year-old man has the abrupt onset of confusion, amnesia, and personality changes. A neurologist makes a diagnosis of transient global amnesia (TGA). Most neurologists believe TGA is the result of ischemia of both posterior cerebral arteries. While that theory may be true, which test might be performed to diagnose other conditions that might mimic TGA?
    a.   Serum phenobarbital concentrations
    b.   EEG
    c.   Serum potassium
    d.   Blood glucose
    e.   Blood alcohol level

A183: a, b, d, e. Patients, especially those who are elderly, may develop mental aberrations, "a paradoxical reaction," if they take hypnotic medications including phenobarbital and alcohol. Partial complex seizures and hypoglycemia should always be considered in acute confusional states. However, although low serum potassium (hypokalemia) causes weakness, it does not cause mental disturbances.

Q184:   A 30-year-old man is admitted for psychotic behavior. "Organic" causes are excluded and he is treated with high doses of haloperidol. He becomes rigid and, although alert, unresponsive. His temperature rises to 106°F and he becomes diaphoretic and tremulous. What should be done?
    a.   Change to another antipsychotic medication
    b.   Treat for delirium tremens (DTs)
    c.   Search for an underlying infection, e.g., meningitis
    d.   Check fluid and electrolyte concentrations
    e.   Obtain electroencephalogram
    f.   Check CPK concentration

A184: b, c, d, f. (Depending on the circumstances, DTs (b) should be considered even though patients are rarely rigid.)

Q185: In the above question, before therapy can be instituted, the patient develops hypotension and renal failure. What is the source of the renal impairment?

    a.   Haloperidol (Haldol) is nephrotoxic

    b.   DTs

    c.   Hypotension causes renal insufficiency

    d.   Rhabdomyolysis

    e.   An inherited succinylcholine abnormality

A185: c, d

Q186: In which conditions are fever, muscle necrosis, and renal impairment possible complications?

a.	Malignant hyperthermia	d.	Hallucinogen intoxication
b.	DTs	e.	Duchenne's dystrophy
c.	Catatonia	f.	Neuroleptic-malignant syndrome

A186: a, b, c, d, f

Q187: In the above question, how does neuroleptic-malignant syndrome differ from the other choices?

A187: Neuroleptic-malignant syndrome follows use of neuroleptic medications that block dopamine transmission. Malignant hyperthermia, which is usually an inherited condition, follows administration of general anesthesia. Neuroleptic-malignant syndrome causes much more muscle rigidity and fever than catatonia, DTs, or hallucinogens.

Q188: What is the purpose of combining carbidopa with L-dopa, as in Sinemet?

    a.   Carbidopa is a peripheral dopamine decarboxylase inhibitor, which raises CNS levels of L-dopa

    b.   Carbidopa is a dopamine antagonist

    c.   Carbidopa is a dopamine agonist

    d.   Carbidopa is anticholinergic

    e.   Carbidopa acts on the postsynaptic neuron

A188: a

Q189: What is the purpose of using bromocriptine (Parlodel) in the treatment of Parkinson's disease?

    a.   It is a dopamine precursor

    b.   It is a dopamine agonist

    c.   It has anticholinergic properties

    d.   It affects the presynaptic neuron

    e.   It affects the postsynaptic neuron

A189: b, e

Q190: A 32-year-old man who suffers from partial complex epilepsy has developed increasing confusion, irritability, and lethargy. His current regimen is phenytoin (Dilantin) (300 mg/day) and primidone (Mysoline) (750 mg/day). Blood anticonvulsant levels, CT scan, lumbar puncture, EEG, and routine tests disclose no significant abnormality. Of the following, which would be the best management plan?

    a.   Increase both anticonvulsants

    b.   Substitute carbamazepine (Tegretol) for the primidone (Mysoline)

    c.   Stop both anticonvulsants

    d.   Add carbamazepine (Tegretol) to the two current anticonvulsants

A190: b. Primidone is the most likely offender. Although the patient may be anticonvulsant-toxic despite normal levels, anticonvulsants should not be abruptly withdrawn because it might precipitate status epilepticus.

Q191: Which anticonvulsant is metabolized into phenobarbital?

    a.   Primidone (Mysoline)

    b.   Phenytoin (Dilantin)
    c.   Carbamazepine (Tegretol)
    d.   Valproic acid (Depakene)

A191: a

Q192: Which procedures might be helpful in determining which hemisphere is dominant?

    a.   Positron emission tomography (PET)
    b.   CT scan
    c.   EEG with sphenoidal electrodes
    d.   Nuclear magnetic resonance (NMR) imaging
    e.   Intracarotid sodium amobarbital injection
    f.   Wada test
    g.   Visual evoked responses (VER)
    h.   Brainstem auditory evoked responses (BAER)

A192: a, e, f. The Wada test involves intracarotid amobarbital injections. (In the future, NMR (d) will be helpful.)

Q193: Which of the following may be found in a right-handed patient who undergoes a complete commissurotomy?

    a.   Stimulation of either hemisphere can provoke various emotions
    b.   The patient will not be able to describe what the right hand is doing
    c.   Seizures will be confined to a single hemisphere
    d.   The left hand will be able to copy a figure seen in the left visual field, but the patient will not be able either to write or say the name of the figure
    e.   The patient will be able to copy with the right hand what he or she sees in the right visual field, but will not be able to say or write the name of that figure
    f.   The patient will not be able to execute written commands with her right hand

A193: a, c, d, f

Q194: What is false about serotonin?

    a.   It is an indoleamine
    b.   5-hydroxyindoleacetic acid is its metabolic product
    c.   It is found in high concentrations in the dorsal raphe nucleus
    d.   It is an endogenous opiate
    e.   When it or its precursors are injected into the ventricles, sleep is induced

A194: d

Q195: Which analgesics does naloxone antagonize?

    a.   Heroin
    b.   Morphine
    c.   Stimulation-produced analgesia
    d.   Hypnosis

A195: a, b, c

Q196: When nonsteroidal anti-inflammatory agents are given for menstrual cramps, with which substances do they interfere?

    a.   Enkephalins
    b.   Endorphins
    c.   Prostaglandins
    d.   Serotonin
    e.   Dopamine

A196: c

Q197: Which statements are true regarding the dorsal raphe nucleus?

    a.   It contains high concentrations of endorphins

    b.   Stimulating it causes pain
    c.   Stimulating it produces analgesia
    d.   Stimulating it produces behavioral changes
    e.   Its destruction causes analgesia
    f.   It contains high serotonin concentrations
    g.   Microinjections of procaine (Novacaine) cause analgesia
    h.   Microinjections of morphine cause analgesia
  A197:   c, f

  Q198:   A 14-year-old boy is brought to the Emergency Room in stupor. He is apneic and his pupils are miotic. Which one of the following conditions is most likely to be the cause of this constellation of findings?
    a.   Brainstem stroke
    b.   Heroin or other narcotic overdose
    c.   Hypoglycemia
    d.   Postictal stupor
    e.   Psychogenic disturbance
  A198:   b. Pontine strokes may cause this constellation, but they rarely occur in this age group. The other conditions generally cause dilated pupils and do not cause apnea.

  A199:   Which of the following are complications of intravenous heroin use?
    a.   Pulmonary edema
    b.   Cerebrovascular accidents
    c.   Tetanus
    d.   Malaria
    e.   Acquired immune deficiency syndrome (AIDS)
  A199:   a, b, c, d, e

  Q200:   What are the effects that are common to endogenous opiates and morphine?
    a.   Euphoria
    b.   Addiction
    c.   Respiratory depression
    d.   Reversal with naloxone
  A200:   a, b, c, d

  Q201:   In which CNS areas are opiate receptors located?
    a.   The basal ganglia
    b.   A delta fibers
    c.   The spinal dorsal horn
    d.   The amygdala
    e.   Unmyelinated C fibers
  A201:   a, c, and d. The A delta and C fibers are parts of the peripheral nervous system. Although they carry pain sensation, but they do not use endogenous opiates for neurotransmission.

  Q202:   Which of the following roles have been ascribed to serotonin?
    a.   It is concentrated in the raphe nuclei where it modulates the sleep cycle
    b.   It is found in the dorsal horn of the spinal cord where it has a role in analgesia
    c.   It is found in the periaqueductal gray matter where it has a role in pain perception and modification
    d.   It is found in the nucleus raphe magnus, where it has a role in pain interpretation and reduction
    e.   Serotonin itself is an endogenous opiate
    f.   Some tricyclic antidepressants inhibit the uptake of serotonin
  A202:   a, b, c, d, f

  Q203:   Three family members brought to the Emergency Room are each suffering from respiratory distress and weakness of the head, neck, and shoulders. They also have dilated and poorly reactive pupils. Ocular motility impairments, that seem like internuclear ophthalmoplegia, are present. One patient, as a young woman, had had optic neuritis. Which of the following conditions is the most likely diagnosis?

  a. Multiple sclerosis
  b. Atropine intoxication
  c. Insecticide poisoning
  d. Botulism
  e. Myasthenia gravis

  A203: d. Botulism can produce bulbar palsy and ocular motility impairments that mimic internuclear ophthalmoplegia. Insecticide poisoning also produces respiratory distress, but in such cases the pupils are almost always miotic and fasciculations are prominent.

  Q204–206: This 29-year-old woman has developed a tremor that is most pronounced when she writes, drinks coffee, and lights a cigarette.

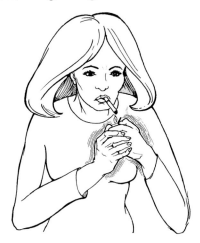

  Q204: Which of the following conditions can lead to such a tremor?

  a. Essential tremor   d. Huntington's chorea
  b. Wilson's disease   e. Athetosis
  c. Anxiety   f. Benign familial tremor

  A204: a, b, c, and f. Essential tremor and benign familial tremor are probably varieties of the same condition. Wilson's disease is a rare but important condition that is always to be considered in young adults who develop tremor. Anxiety can produce a tremor that is indistinguishable from essential tremor and that may have a similar etiology and response to beta-adrenergic blockers.

  Q205: Which tests should be performed to exclude Wilson's disease when only mild tremor were evident?

  a. CT scan   d. Serum ceruloplasmin
  b. EEG   e. Serum copper concentration
  c. Lumbar puncture   f. Slit-lamp examination

  A205: d, f

  Q206: If the patient did have an essential tremor, which group of medications are most often effective?

  a. Anticholinergics   d. Beta-adrenergic blockers
  b. Dopamine agonists   e. Antiviral agents
  c. Neuroleptics   f. Alpha-adrenergic blockers

  A206: d

Q207–213: Match the EEG pattern with the associated conditions.

Q207: Periodic complexes

Q208: Triphasic waves

Q209: Movement artifact

Q210: Excessive beta activity

Q211: 3-Hz spike-and-slow wave

Q212: Focal, phase-reversed delta activity

Q213: Postictal EEG depression

a. Absences

b. Brain tumor

c. Use of sedatives or tranquilizers

d. Psychogenic seizures

e. Electroshock therapy

f. Tonic-clonic seizure

g. Creutzfeldt-Jakob disease

h. Subacute sclerosing panencephalitis (SSPE)

i. Uremia

j. Hepatic encephalopathy

A207: g, h

A208: i, j

A209: d

A210: c

A211: a

A212: b

A213: e, f

Q214: What is the consequence of a deficiency in choline acetyltransferase?

    a. Decreased acetylcholine

    b. Increased cholinesterases

    c. Parkinson's disease

    d. Possibly dementia

A214: a, d

Q215: Which of the following analgesic systems do *not* use the endogenous opiate system?

    a. Narcotics

    b. Aspirin

    c. TENS

    d. Periventricular gray matter stimulation

    e. Hypnosis

    f. Tricyclic antidepressants

    g. Nonsteroidal anti-inflammatory agents

A215: b, e, f, g

Q216: How do neurotransmitters differ from classic endocrine hormones, such as T_4?

    a. They or their byproducts circulate in detectable quantities in the blood

    b. They are produced and stored at a site adjacent to the target organ

    c. They or their byproducts are present in significant quantity in the cerebrospinal fluid but not in the blood

    d. They are steroids

A216: b, c

Q217: Metachromatic leukodystrophy is a rare illness of adults, ages 19 to 46 years, although it affects children and adolescents more commonly. It may be diagnosed by finding decrease arylsulfatase activity in serum, white blood cells, fibroblasts, urine, and amniotic fluid cells. Unlike most other degenerative neurologic conditions, this illness affects both the peripheral and the central nervous systems. What are the clinical manifestations of this illness?

    a. Autosomal recessive inheritance

    b. Myopathy

    c. Peripheral neuropathy

    d. Seizures

    e. Cerebellar dysfunction

    f. Intellectual impairments

A217: a, c, d, e, f

Q218: In what way does Huntington's chorea in adolescents differ from that in adults?

a. Rigidity is prominent
b. No dementia
c. Akinesia prominent

d. Seizures frequent
e. Different course
f. Mimicks Parkinson's disease

A218: a, c, d, f

Q219: In which conditions might a lumbar puncture precipitate transtentorial herniation?
a. Acute subdural hematoma
b. Pseudotumor cerebri
c. Chronic subdural hematoma
d. Glioblastoma

A219: a, c, d

Q220: With which findings are the concentration of senile plaques associated?
a. Older age
b. Schizophrenia
c. Poor performance on the Blessed test

d. Depression
e. Trisomy 21
f. Nonviral infectious particles, "prions"

A220: a, c, e, f

Q221: In depressed people, which of the following neuroendocrine changes are routinely found?
a. Advance in MHPG excretion
b. Delay in body temperature nadir
c. Advanced shift of REM sleep
d. Delay in peak cortisol excretion
e. Advanced shift of body temperature nadir

A221: a, c, e

Q222: Which conditions frequently increase REM latency?
a. Depression
b. Drug withdrawal
c. Excessive alcohol use
d. Narcolepsy

A222: c

Q223: In Huntington's chorea, what is the change in CSF GABA concentration?
a. GABA is increased
b. GABA is decreased
c. GABA is unchanged

A223: b. Determination of a lowered GABA concentration in the CSF sometimes confirms the clinical impression of Huntington's chorea.

Q224–230: How are the following medications thought to treat or prevent pain?
224. Aspirin
225. Nonsteroidal anti-inflammatory agents
226. Tricyclic antidepressants
227. Methysergide
228. Cafergot
229. Inderal
230. Narcotics

a. Vasoconstriction
b. Activates the endogenous opiate system
c. Beta-adrenergic blocking
d. Inhibits prostaglandin synthesis
e. Interferes with platelet serotonin
f. Increases serotonin levels

A224. d
225. d
226. f
227. e
228. a
229. c
230. b

Q231: A 28-year-old woman complains of gait impairment. She has a history of vigorous exercise, taking large quantities of vitamins, and avoiding red meat and alcohol. On examination, she has marked sensory loss in all limbs and absent DTRs, but her strength is normal. Which of the following conditions are most likely to be responsible for her complaints?

    a.   Cervical spondylosis
    b.   Myopathy
    c.   Vitamin toxicity
    d.   Iron deficiency anemia

A231: c. Pyridoxine (vitamin B_6) in large daily doses creates a neuropathy that impairs sensation and is reversible after the vitamins are withdrawn. Although iron deficiency does not create a neuropathy, thiamine and folate deficiency, often a consequence of alcoholism, can produce a neuropathy.

Q232: A 68-year-old house painter has weakness, atrophy, and areflexic DTRs in his upper extremities. In addition, he has sensory loss in his right hand, brisk DTRs in his legs, and a right Babinski sign. Which of the features suggest that he has cervical spondylosis rather than ALS?

    a.   Hand atrophy
    b.   Hyperactive DTRs in the legs
    c.   Sensory loss
    d.   The Babinski sign

A232: c. House painting, which involves prolonged neck hyperextension, leads to cervical spondylosis as an occupational hazard. Whatever the cause, cervical spondylosis leads to sensory and lower motor neuron loss in the upper extremities and upper motor neuron signs in the lower extremities. Cervical spondylosis is a much more frequently occurring condition than ALS.

Q233: What are the potential neurologic side effects of oral contraceptives?

    a.   Dementia
    b.   Chorea
    c.   Multiple sclerosis
    d.   Increase in migraine headaches
    e.   Peripheral neuropathy
    f.   Cerebrovascular accidents in certain women

A233: b, d, f. The tendency towards cerebrovascular accidents, which is associated with high dose estrogen, is probably restricted to older women who are hypertensive or who smoke.

Q234: In which conditions might a contrast CT scan produce serious complications?

    a.   Asthma
    b.   Iodine allergy
    c.   Encephalitis
    d.   Diabetic nephropathy
    e.   Dehydration
    f.   Seizure disorder

A234: b, d, e. The contrast solution contains iodine, which might precipitate the Stevens-Johnson syndrome, laryngeal edema, or other manifestations of allergy. Patients with diabetes or dehydration might develop acute tubular necrosis.

Q235: What is the most characteristic finding in standard intelligence tests in people with early dementia?

    a.   Decreased performance, decreased verbal scales
    b.   Decreased performance, relatively normal verbal scales
    c.   Decreased verbal, relatively normal performance scales
    d.   Neither

A235: b

Q236: In contrast to patients with early dementia, what will standard intelligence tests show in patients with depression-induced cognitive changes?

    a.   Decreased performance, decreased verbal scales
    b.   Decreased performance, relatively normal verbal scales

     c.   Decreased verbal, relatively normal performance scales

     d.   Neither

A236: a. Verbal and performance scales are both lowered; however, performance scales, because of psychomotor retardation, might be profoundly low and the patient might have different results as his attention and mood fluctuate.

Q237: As people age, what is the most common EEG finding?

     a.   Loss of amplitude

     b.   Slowing of the background activity

     c.   Presence of beta activity

     d.   Fragmentation of background

A237: b

Q238: What are the consequences of alcohol withdrawal?

     a.   Increased REM activity

     b.   Insomnia

     c.   Increased dreaming

     d.   Tendency to have seizures

A238: a, b, c, d

Q239: Which test is the most likely to reveal asymptomatic frontal lobe multiple sclerosis plaques?

     a.   EEG

     b.   CT scan

     c.   Nuclear magnetic resonance imaging

     d.   Lumbar puncture

     e.   Visual-evoked responses

A239: c. Magnetic resonance imaging (MRI) is superior to the CT scan for detecting changes in the chemical composition of myelin, as occurs in multiple sclerosis. Moreover, it has better anatomic resolution.

Q240: Which findings are more closely associated with aphasia than dementia?

     a.   Right homonymous hemianopsia

     b.   Focal EEG slowing

     c.   Paraphasic errors

     d.   Seizures

     e.   Circumducted or hemiparetic gait

A240: a, b, c, d, e

Q241: Does use of phenytoin (Dilantin), phenobarbital, and carbamazepine (Tegretol) tend to give to false-positive, false-negative, or no different results in the dexamethasone suppression test?

A241: False-positive

Q242: In what ways do hypnogogic hallucinations *differ* from partial complex seizures?

     a.   They are associated with flaccid, areflexic musculature

     b.   They often have an auditory component

     c.   They are associated with EEG spikes

     d.   They have visual, auditory, and emotional aspects

     e.   They are varied

A242: a, e

Q243: Which analgesic properties are found with narcotics that are *not* found with nonsteroidal anti-inflammatory agents?

     a.   Antipyretic activity   e.   Euphoria

     b.   Dependence   f.   Withdrawal symptoms

     c.   Respiratory depression   g.   Prostaglandins synthesis inhibition

     d.   Tolerance

A243: b, c, d, e, f

Q244: Which structure contains 80 percent of the brain's dopamine content?
    a.   Third ventricle
    b.   Thalamus
    c.   Cerebral cortex
    d.   Corpus striatum
A244: d

Q245: Which structures will "enhance" during a contrast CT scan?
    a.   Glioblastoma
    b.   Cerebral infarct
    c.   Arteriovenous malformation (AVM)
    d.   Cerebral hemorrhage
    e.   The contents of a subdural hematoma
    f.   The membrane of a subdural hematoma
A245: a, c, f, rarely b

Q246: A 50-year-old man who has developed a slowly progressive dementia is suspected of having neurosyphilis. The CSF shows protein concentration of 100 mg/100 ml, 10 lymphocytes/mm, and a negative VDRL. Which of the following plans are appropriate?
    a.   Repeat the lumbar puncture to determine the CSF cryptococcal antigen titer, culture CSF for TB, and obtain CSF cytology
    b.   Disregard the negative VDRL and treat the patient for neurosyphilis
    c.   Perform a brain biopsy
    d.   Base the diagnosis on a CSF FTA-ABS test
A246: a, b. A CSF FTA-ABS test on spinal fluid is unreliable. This patient should be treated for neurosyphilis as further evaluation is undertaken. Notably, as many as 40 percent of neurosyphilis patients may have negative CSF VDRL tests because of natural resolution of the serologic variables or partial, possibly inadequate antibiotic treatment.

Q247: Which of the following conditions cause dementia that tends to occur in families?
    a.   Pick's disease
    b.   SSPE
    c.   Alzheimer's disease
    d.   Creutzfeldt-Jakob disease
A247: a, c. About one third of the patients with Alzheimer's disease have had a similarly affected parent or sibling. In rare families Alzheimer's disease appears to be transmitted as an autosomal dominant trait. In them, Alzheimer's disease appears at a younger age and follows a fulminant course. Pick's disease, which is rare in the United States, has a familial tendency, but genetic transmission has not been established.

Q248: Which condition is *not* associated with shortened REM latency?
    a.   Night terrors
    b.   Narcolepsy
    c.   Depression
    d.   Withdrawal from sedatives
    e.   Withdrawal from neuroleptics
    f.   Cataplexy
A248: a

Q249: A person complains of developing a recurrent, vivid dream. His bed partner has noted that after mumbling, the patient falls deeply asleep and, on two occasions, has had enuresis. What preliminary tests should be done?
    a.   He should be monitored in a sleep laboratory
    b.   He should have an EEG with hyperventilation and photic stimulation
    c.   He should undergo a sodium amytal interview
    d.   He should have an EEG following sleep deprivation
A249: b, d

Q250: The patient in the question 249 has an EEG following sleep deprivation that shows a paroxysm of a variety of spike and spike-and-wave activity, but further evaluation is unremarkable. What medication is indicated?

a. Sedatives
b. Hypnotics
c. Antidepressants

d. Neuroleptics
e. Anticonvulsants
f. Antabuse

A250: e

Q251: Which one of the following illnesses is the most likely cause of rapidly progressive intellectual impairment in an 8-year-old girl?

a. Mental retardation
b. A glycogen storage disease
c. SSPE
d. Duchenne's muscular dystrophy

A251: c. SSPE is probably the most common degenerative neurologic condition that affects children. Glycogen storage diseases are indolent and not necessarily associated with intellectual impairment. Duchenne's muscular dystrophy does not affect females. In males, it causes intellectual impairments that are subtle and slowly progressive.

Q252: Sometimes high-dose steroid treatment is complicated by "steroid psychosis," hypokalemic myopathy, or fungal meningitis—all conditions that initially may be misdiagnosed as psychogenic. Nevertheless, steroids are commonly used in a variety of neurologic illnesses. Which of the following illnesses are commonly treated with steroids?

a. Metastatic brain tumor
b. Multiple sclerosis
c. Lupus cerebritis

d. Bell's palsy
e. Uremic encephalopathy
f. Myasthenia gravis

A252: a, b, c, d, f

Q253: One week after a right cerebral infarction, a 60-year-old man develops burning pain in the left face, arm, leg, and trunk. There is marked sensory loss to all modalities in these regions and a mild left hemiparesis. What is the origin of the patient's pain?

a. Parietal lobe injury
b. Psychogenic impairment
c. Lateral spinothalamic damage
d. Thalamic injury

A253: d. The patient has "thalamic pain." This characteristically disturbing manifestation of a cerebrovascular accident can persist for years, but it is usually limited to about 6 months and often responsive to treatment with either phenytoin (Dilantin) or carbamazepam (Tegretol).

Q254: Which structures are usually considered to be parts of the basal ganglia?

a. The corpus striatum
b. The cerebellum
c. The putamen
d. The caudate nuclei

e. Meynert's nuclei
f. The globus pallidus
g. The substantia nigra
h. The subthalamic nucleus

A254: a, c, d, f, g, h

Q255: Which of the structures in question 254 are usually considered to be part of the corpus striatum?

A255: c, d, f

Q256: Which of the following tests *do not* rely on ionizing radiation?

a. CT
b. MRI
c. Isotopic brain scan
d. EEG

A256: b, d

Q257: What will the cisternogram show in classic cases of normal pressure hydrocephalus?

a. Radioactivity over the cerebral hemispheres
b. Persistent intraventricular radioactivity

      c.   Radioactivity lingering in the spinal canal
      d.   None of the above

A257: b

Q258: In cisternograms of patients with Alzheimer's disease with cerebral atrophy, what will the cisternogram show?
      a.   Radioactivity over the cerebral hemispheres
      b.   Persistent intraventricular radioactivity
      c.   Lingering of radioactivity in the spinal canal
      d.   None of the above

A258: a. Although the cisternogram is somewhat helpful in distinguishing between Alzheimer's disease and normal pressure hydrocephalus, it should not be considered able to make a definite diagnosis.

Q259: In which illnesses are CSF measles antibodies found?
      a.   Alzheimer's disease
      b.   Creutzfeldt-Jakob disease
      c.   SSPE
      d.   Multiple sclerosis

A259: c, d

Q260: Which are characteristic features of the sleep patterns following sleep deprivation?
      a.   Early terminal awakening
      b.   Relatively normal REM distribution
      c.   Decreased REM latency
      d.   Increased sleep latency
      e.   Increased total sleep

A260: b, c, e

Q261: Which physiologic processes are found in sleeping people when the EEG shows great quantities of high-voltage, 1–3-Hz activity?
      a.   Some limb EMG activity
      b.   Relatively low blood pressure and pulse
      c.   Penile erections
      d.   Rapid eye movement

A261: a, b. (Such EEG activity is "slow wave" or deep NREM sleep.)

Q262: Which of the following conditions might cause rigidity and akinesia but no tremor in adolescents?

      a.   Huntington's chorea   e.   Tourette's syndrome
      b.   Wilson's disease   f.   Sydenham's chorea
      c.   Parkinson's disease   g.   Cerebral palsy
      d.   Medications   h.   Serotonin excess

A262: a, b, c, d, g

Q263: Which sleep changes are *not* associated with old age?
      a.   Multiple brief awakenings
      b.   Shift to earlier time of sleep and awakening
      c.   Increased amount of stage 4 NREM sleep
      d.   Shortening of total sleep time

A263: c

Q264–266: Match the illness that can cause mental changes with its physical manifestations:
      264. Porphyria   a.   Dermatitis, diarrhea
      265. Hypothyroidism   b.   Abdominal pain
      266. Pellegra   c.   Ataxia, coma

A264: b

265: c

266: a. Pellegra causes the "3D's:" dermatitis, diarrhea, and dementia.

Q267: Which conditions cause headache and ipsilateral ptosis?

<table>
<tr><td>a.</td><td>Trigeminal neuralgia</td><td>d.</td><td>Cluster headaches</td></tr>
<tr><td>b.</td><td>Temporal arteritis</td><td>e.</td><td>Ophthalmoplegic migraine</td></tr>
<tr><td>c.</td><td>Rupture of a posterior communicating artery aneurysm</td><td>f.</td><td>Diabetic oculomotor nerve infarction</td></tr>
</table>

A267: c, d, e, f

Q268: Which of the conditions listed above also produce pupil dilatation?

A268: c, sometimes e, very rarely f

Q269: A 30-year-old woman has the sudden onset of "the worst headache of her life." She has nuchal rigidity, but otherwise her neurologic examination is normal. A CT scan shows blood density material in the right sylvian fissure. What is the best diagnostic procedure to perform?

      a.   Lumbar puncture

      b.   EEG

      c.   Isotopic brain scan

      d.   Cerebral arteriography

A269: d. The patient probably has had a subarachnoid hemorrhage from a ruptured "berry"aneurysm. Cerebral arteriography would document the aneurysm, reveal its location and anatomy, and exclude the possibility of other sources of bleeding, such as a mycotic aneurysm or small arteriovenous malformation (AVM). A lumbar puncture would probably be superfluous and possibly dangerous because it could lead to a rerupture of the aneurysm or, if a large hematoma were present, transtentorial herniation.

Q270: In which brain region do patients with Alzheimer's disease have a pronounced neuron loss that results in an acetylcholine deficit?

      a.   Frontal lobe

      b.   Frontal and temporal lobe

      c.   Hippocampus

      d.   Nucleus basalis Meynert

A270:   d. The most important area is the nucleus basalis Meynert. Although patients also have neuron loss in the hippocampus, that loss is not associated with an acetylcholine deficiency.

Q271: Which processes are found in a sleeping person when the EEG shows asynchronous low-voltage fast activity?

<table>
<tr><td>a.</td><td>Increased intracranial pressure</td><td>d.</td><td>Pronounced ocular movement</td></tr>
<tr><td>b.</td><td>Absent limb EMG activity</td><td>e.</td><td>Polyspike EEG activity</td></tr>
<tr><td>c.</td><td>Increased pulse and blood pressure</td><td>f.</td><td>Erections</td></tr>
</table>

A271:   a, b, c, d, f. People in REM sleep have an EEG that is similar to an awake state EEG and so much autonomic nervous system activity that they are said to have "activated" sleep.

Q272: After a fall, an 80-year-old man who is known to have Alzheimer's disease begins to have the rapid loss of remaining cognitive function and then becomes lethargic. A CT scan shows swelling of the right cerebral hemisphere and shift of midline structures. Which structural lesions are most likely to have developed?

      a.   A CVA

      b.   A glioblastoma

      c.   A subdural hematoma

      d.   A pseudotumor cerebri

A272:   c. An *isodense* subdural hematoma appears as brain swelling, but infarctions and tumors are discrete lesions. People with cerebral atrophy, especially the elderly, are prone to develop subdural hematomas, which are usually radiodense (white) when acute and radiolucent (black) when chronic. At some time in their course, subdural hematomas are often isodense to the brain. They are probably more common than primary brain tumors and they are a correctable cause of dementia.

Q273: In which conditions is the choline acetyltransferase (CAT) concentration of the cerebral cortex markedly reduced?

    a.   Alzheimer's disease
    b.   Trisomy 21
    c.   Parkinson's disease without dementia
    d.   Huntington's chorea
    e.   Parkinson's disease with dementia

A273: a, b, e

Q274: In Alzheimer's disease, the concentrations of which substances are markedly reduced in the cerebral cortex?

    a.   CAT
    b.   Gamma-aminobutyric acid (GABA)
    c.   Somatostatin
    d.   Dopamine

A274: a

Q275: A 29-year-old homosexual man has weight loss, lymphadenopathy, change in affect, and two seizures of his left arm. CT scan shows a large circular lesion in the right frontal lobe. Which of the following tests should be performed and what results can be expected?

    a.   Mononucleosis spot test
    b.   Serum human T-lymphotropic virus type III (HTLV-III) antibody determination
    c   CSF examination for cryptococcus
    d.   Serum toxoplasmosis titer
    e.   Blood tests for syphilis

A275: b, d, e. This patient probably has acquired immune deficiency syndrome (AIDS). Since serum HTLV-III antibodies are present in 90 percent of AIDS patients, he will probably have a high antibody titer. When AIDS patients have signs of a cerebral lesion, such as focal seizures, CT scans are necessary to look for cerebral toxoplasmosis, lymphoma, or other mass lesions. Until such lesions are excluded, a lumbar puncture should not be performed. Cerebral toxoplasmosis, which typically causes hemiparesis and seizures, is a common neurologic complication of AIDS. With cerebral toxoplasmosis, serum toxoplasmosis titers are usually elevated. Also, since syphilis often develops in male homosexuals, blood tests may indicate that the neurologic problem is partly or entirely neurosyphilis.

Index